A·N·N·U·A·L E·D

MW01700898

Women's Health 99/00

Second Edition

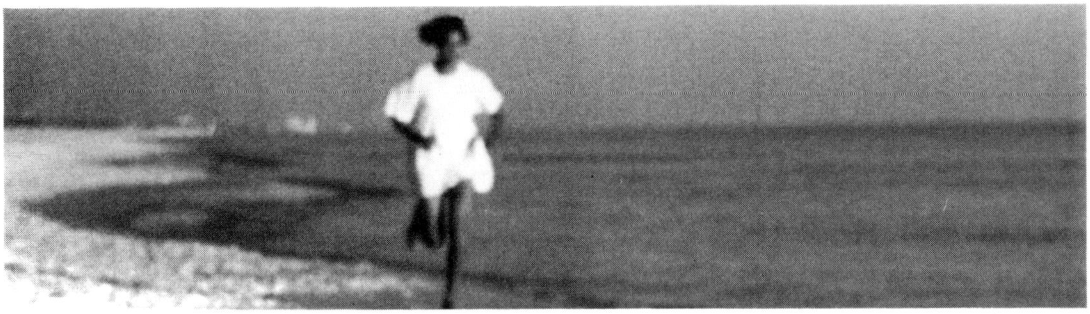

Editors

Maureen Edwards
Montgomery College

Dr. Maureen Edwards is coordinator of the Health Education Program at Montgomery College in Rockville, Maryland, and a faculty research assistant in the Department of Health Education at the University of Maryland, College Park. A private consultant in health behavior, her areas of specialization are stress management and gerontology. During her tenure at the University of Maryland Health Center, Dr. Edwards served as coordinator of the Stress Management Education Program. In addition, Dr. Edwards has served as a stress management consultant to a number of government and private agencies. Dr. Edwards holds a doctorate in health education from the University of Maryland.

Nora L. Howley
Montgomery College

Nora Howley is an adjunct faculty member in the Health Education Program at Montgomery College in Rockville, Maryland, where she teaches women's health, among other courses. In addition, she is a private consultant in health education. Ms. Howley is the former Health Educator for the Association of Occupational and Environmental Clinics, where she developed health education programs. Presently, she is a consultant to the American Federation of Teachers' Breast and Cervical Cancer Education Project. Ms. Howley has a master's degree in health education from the University of Maryland.

Dushkin/McGraw-Hill
Sluice Dock, Guilford, Connecticut 06437

Visit us on the Internet
http://www.dushkin.com/annualeditions/

Credits

1. Women and Health
Facing overview—© 1999 by PhotoDisc, Inc.
2. Nutrition and Fitness
Facing overview—© 1999 by Cleo Photography.
3. Gynecological and Reproductive Health
Facing overview—Dushkin/McGraw-Hill illustration by Mike Eagle. 68—photos by Richard Pierce.
4. Psychological Health
Facing overview—© 1999 by PhotoDisc, Inc.
5. Chronic Diseases
Facing overview—© 1999 by PhotoDisc, Inc.
6. Substance Abuse: New Trends for Women
Facing overview—EPA Documerica photo.
7. Violence in Women's Lives
Facing overview—© 1999 by PhotoDisc, Inc.
8. Special Issues for Older Women
Facing overview—© 1999 by PhotoDisc, Inc.

Copyright

Cataloging in Publication Data
Main entry under title: Annual Editions: Women's health, 1999/2000.
1. Women—Health and hygiene. I. Edwards, Maureen, *comp.* II. Howley, Nora L., *comp.*
III. Title: Women's health.
ISBN 0-07-035009-4 613.042'44'05 ISSN 1096-9713

Second Edition

Printed in the United States of America 1234567890BAHBAH54321098 Printed on Recycled Paper

Editors/Advisory Board

Members of the Advisory Board are instrumental in the final selection of articles for each edition of ANNUAL EDITIONS. Their review of articles for content, level, currentness, and appropriateness provides critical direction to the editor and staff. We think that you will find their careful consideration well reflected in this volume.

To the Reader

In publishing ANNUAL EDITIONS we recognize the enormous role played by the magazines, newspapers, and journals of the public press in providing current, first-rate educational information in a broad spectrum of interest areas. Many of these articles are appropriate for students, researchers, and professionals seeking accurate, current material to help bridge the gap between principles and theories and the real world. These articles, however, become more useful for study when those of lasting value are carefully collected, organized, indexed, and reproduced in a low-cost format, which provides easy and permanent access when the material is needed. That is the role played by ANNUAL EDITIONS.

New to ANNUAL EDITIONS is the inclusion of related World Wide Web sites. These sites have been selected by our editorial staff to represent some of the best resources found on the World Wide Web today. Through our carefully developed topic guide, we have linked these Web resources to the articles covered in this ANNUAL EDITIONS reader. We think that you will find this volume useful, and we hope that you will take a moment to visit us on the Web at ***http://www.dushkin.com*** to tell us what you think.

Dedication:

To our mothers Rita and Louise and the other women in our lives who have served as friends, mentors, and a constant source of inspiration.

In particular, special love and thanks to big sister Pat Brophy and to Ginny Keene (M.E.), and in memory of Barbara, Rachel, Molly, and Sally, the women who paved the way (N.L.H.).

In this, the second edition of *Annual Editions: Women's Health,* we continue to address the most current issues in women's health. With the help of suggestions by our readers and reviewers, we have attempted to broaden our perspective and have gathered information of interest to a more diverse group of women. We have included articles on health issues for women of color and have also tried to target some age-specific topics. What became immediately apparent to us in preparing this second edition is the tremendous growth of information about women's health that appears in the popular press. We have sifted through an incredible range and number of publications. One comment we received about the first edition was that we relied too heavily on popular rather than research publications for our selections. This was, however, done purposefully. We believe that it is very useful and instructive to note how the research is perceived and reported in the lay press. In addition, it is also interesting to note how the areas of interest change over time. In preparing this edition we noted that there was much more information available on chronic disease but not quite as much as in the past on addiction. We also found information on alternative medicine that we hope to include in the next edition. We will continue to sample and report on what is in the public consciousness at the time.

Not every issue is clear cut. Consensus does not always exist and we have continued to represent multiple and sometimes controversial viewpoints. You may not agree with or like every article we have selected. In fact, we hope that you don't. As educators we take great delight in encouraging students to think critically and independently. Our goal is not just to purvey information but to generate discussion. Out of such discussion, argumentation, and controversy we hope to generate a genuine and passionate interest in the field of women's health.

Women's health encompasses much more than reproductive health. Women's health includes nutrition, mental health, fitness, chronic disease and so on. We have tried to touch on as many of those areas as possible, without neglecting the reproductive arena. Women are not monocultural. We have tried to address some of the issues from the perspective of nonwhite women. We also hope that women from many different age groups will pick up this book; we have tried to find something for everyone from the young woman exploring contraception options to the older woman dealing with the cost of growing old.

The book is divided into eight units that correspond to major areas of health, such as nutrition and fitness and psychological health, or that address key topics, such as violence, chronic diseases, and reproductive health. The first unit, Women and Health, is designed to explore issues of how women participate in the health care system, including managed care. This unit is intended to provide an overview of the status of women's health and the leading issues in the field.

To facilitate the use of this volume by teachers and students of women's health, we have included a number of features. Because so many health issues cut across section headings, the *topic guide* provides a cross-reference for finding information on a topic in all the locations where it is addressed. In addition, *World Wide Web* sites, which are cross-referenced by number in the topic guide, can be used to further explore the topics. The *table of contents* also includes abstracts, in which we have tried to summarize the key points of each article. Instructors may find this useful in choosing readings to assign. Each unit begins with an overview, providing background information on the area as well as more detailed information on how articles were chosen. We have also included key points to consider to help students focus their reading.

We will be updating *Annual Editions: Women's Health* annually. It is our goal that this collection be useful and effective for those teaching and learning. We welcome your advice, suggestions, and comments. Please fill out the *article rating form* on the last page of the book. Thank you.

Maureen Edwards

Nora L. Howley
Editors

Contents

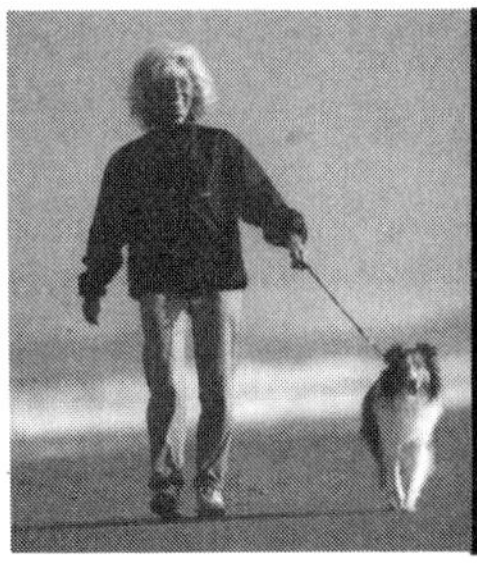

UNIT 1

Women and Health

The seven articles in this section consider the way women are treated in today's health care system.

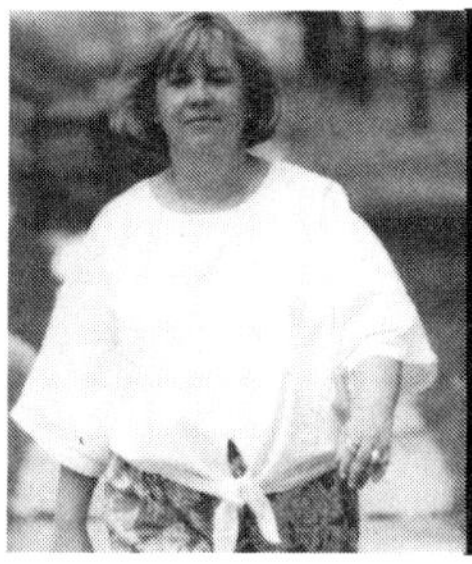

UNIT 2

Nutrition and Fitness

Seven selections in this unit look at the current popularity of dieting and the need for a healthful fitness program.

The concepts in bold italics are developed in the article. For further expansion please refer to the Topic Guide and the Index.

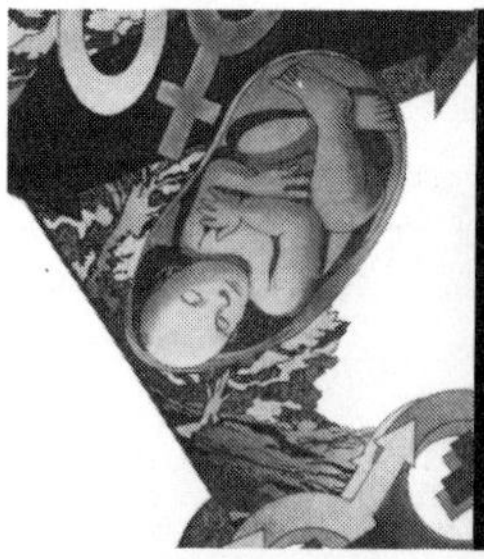

UNIT 3

Gynecological and Reproductive Health

In this section, seven articles consider the importance of periodic physical examinations, the latest data on birth control, and the abortion debate.

The concepts in bold italics are developed in the article. For further expansion please refer to the Topic Guide and the Index.

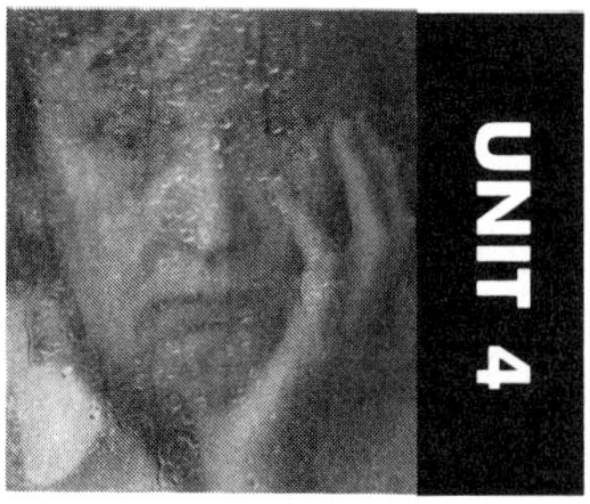

Psychological Health

Ten selections in this section look at how stress, depression, eating disorders, and children impact on a woman's psychological health.

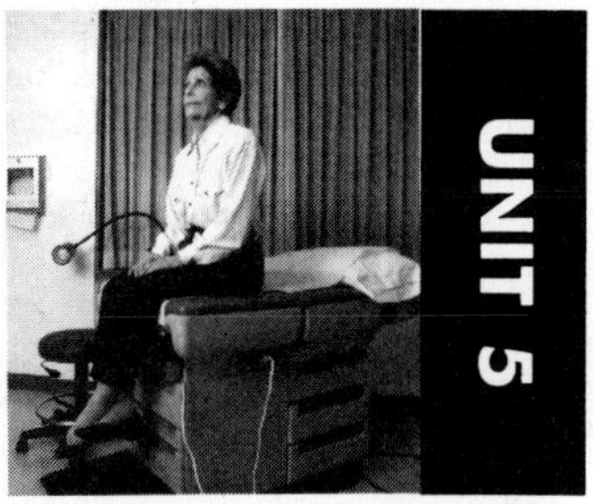

Chronic Diseases

How heart disease, cancer, and other chronic diseases affect women are addressed in the eight articles in this section.

The concepts in bold italics are developed in the article. For further expansion please refer to the Topic Guide and the Index.

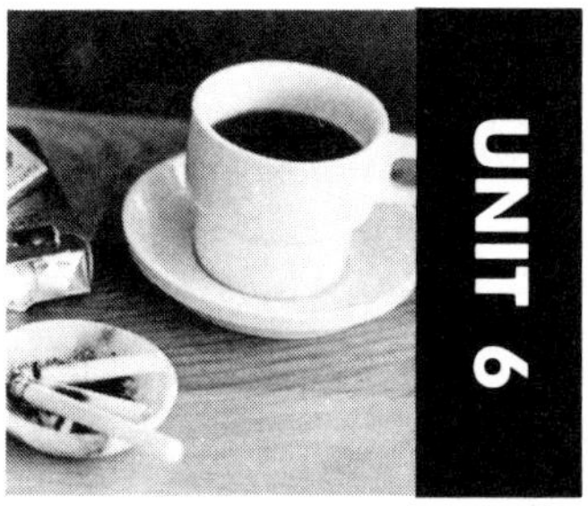

Substance Abuse: New Trends for Women

In this unit, nine articles look at the latest on women's abuse of tobacco, alcohol, and drugs.

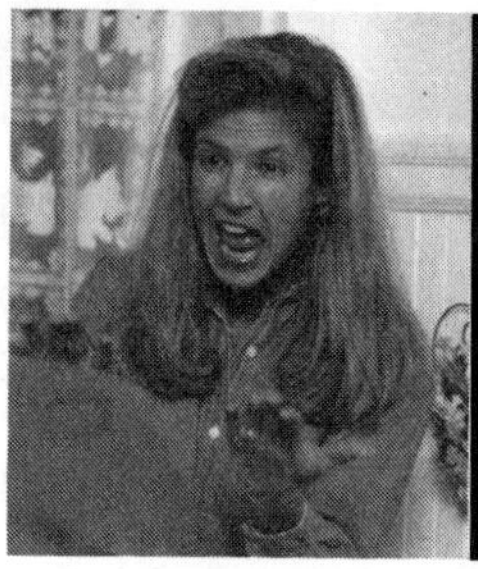

UNIT 7

Violence in Women's Lives

Five selections in this section discuss violence and women, particularly domestic violence and rape.

The concepts in bold italics are developed in the article. For further expansion please refer to the Topic Guide and the Index.

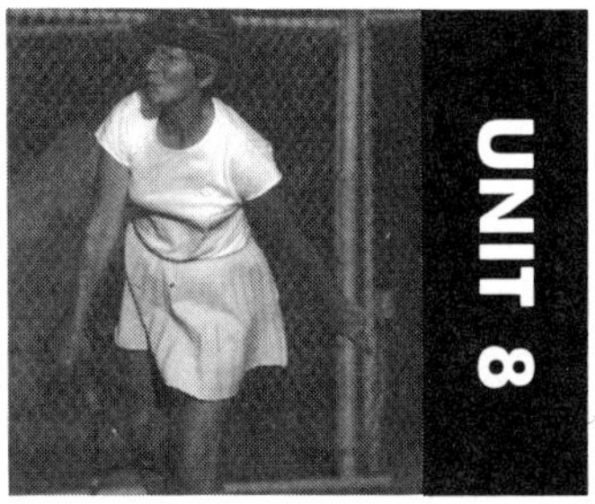

Special Issues for Older Women

The six selections in this section consider health challenges that older women face.

The concepts in bold italics are developed in the article. For further expansion please refer to the Topic Guide and the Index.

Topic Guide

This topic guide suggests how the selections and World Wide Web sites found in the next section of this book relate to topics of traditional concern to professionals and students of a course in women's health. It is useful for locating interrelated articles and Web sites for reading and research. The guide is arranged alphabetically according to topic.

The relevant Web sites, which are numbered and annotated on pages 4 and 5, are easily identified by the Web icon (◎) under the topic articles. By linking the articles and the Web sites by topic, this ANNUAL EDITIONS reader becomes a powerful learning and research tool.

TOPIC AREA	TREATED IN
Abortion	21. Truth about Abortion ◎ ***1, 2, 3, 4, 6, 8, 14, 15, 22***
Addiction/ Alcohol Drugs	40. What Does Being Female Have to Do with It? 41. Why Women Drink 42. Alcoholic in the Family 43. Prescription for Addiction 44. Stop Smoking 45. Kickin' Butt 46. Way Out West 47. Lethal Drugs' Lethal Side Effects 48. Prescription for Disaster ◎ ***22, 23***
Aging	54. Midlife Motherhood 55. Women & Estrogen 56. Estrogen to Prevent Alzheimer's? 57. Can You Afford to Get Old? 58. Harder Better Death 59. Taking Care of Mom ◎ ***8, 10, 14, 18, 19, 20, 21, 27, 28, 29***
Alternative Approaches	1. Women's Health Studies 30. Give Your Body Time to Heal 31. Female Brain 39. Healing Power ◎ ***11, 12, 13***
Cancer	4. Dangerous Legacies 9. Rebel against a Sedentary Life 20. Consensus: No Long-Term Link 21. Truth about Abortion 36. Stopping the Deadliest Cancer 38. Closing In on Cancer 44. Stop Smoking 45. Kickin' Butt 55. Women & Estrogen ◎ ***1, 2, 3, 4, 6, 7, 8, 9, 10, 20, 27, 28, 29***
Childless	1. Women's Health Studies 3. Forgotten Women 19. For Infertility Treatments 27. I Chose to Be Sterilized at 29 ◎ ***6, 14, 15***
Children	17. Other Epidemic 22. Forever Frazzled? 25. War Inside Your Head 42. Alcoholic in the Family 54. Midlife Motherhood 59. Taking Care of Mom ◎ ***14, 15, 16, 17, 19, 27, 28***
Contraception	15. Women and Sex 16. What Women Need to Know 17. Other Epidemic 18. Rethinking Birth Control 20. Consensus: No Long-Term Link 27. I Chose to Be Sterilized at 29 ◎ ***14, 15***
Depression	9. Rebel against a Sedentary Life 21. Truth about Abortion 28. Treat Depression 51. "I Was Raped" ◎ ***16, 17, 24, 25, 26, 27***
Diabetes	9. Rebel against a Sedentary Life ◎ ***19, 21***
Diet	8. Say Good-bye to Dieting 9. Rebel against a Sedentary Life 10. Who *Isn't* on a Diet? 12. Fat Chances 24. Dieter's Paradox 55. Women & Estrogen ◎ ***11, 12, 13***
Drugs	35. Heart Disease in Women 40. What Does Being Female Have to Do with It? 41. Why Women Drink 42. Alcoholic in the Family 43. Prescription for Addiction 44. Stop Smoking 45. Kickin' Butt 46. Way Out West 47. Legal Drugs' Lethal Side Effects 48. Prescription for Disaster ◎ ***22, 23***
Eating Disorders	10. Who *Isn't* on a Diet? 13. Dying to Be Thin 24. Dieter's Paradox 26. You're Not Fat ◎ ***11, 12, 13, 16, 17***
Estrogen	35. Heart Disease in Women 55. Women & Estrogen 56. Estrogen to Prevent Alzheimer's? ◎ ***14, 15, 18, 20, 27, 28, 29***
Ethics	4. Dangerous Legacies 5. Managed Care 21. Truth about Abortion 49. Female Genital Mutilation 51. "I Was Raped"
Exercise	8. Say Good-Bye to Dieting 9. Rebel against a Sedentary Life 11. How Far Should You Go? 12. Fat Chances 26. You're Not Fat 39. Healing Power 55. Women & Estrogen ◎ ***11***

DUSHKIN ONLINE

AE: Women's Health

The following World Wide Web sites have been carefully researched and selected to support the articles found in this reader. If you are interested in learning more about specific topics found in this book, these Web sites are a good place to start. The sites are cross-referenced by number and appear in the topic guide on the previous two pages. Also, you can link to these Web sites through our DUSHKIN ONLINE support site at *http://www.dushkin.com/online/*.

The following sites were available at the time of publication. Visit our Web site—we update DUSHKIN ONLINE regularly to reflect any changes.

General Health Sites

1. Healthfinder: Gateway Consumer Health and Human Services Information Web Site

http://www.healthfinder.gov

Healthfinder can lead you to selected online publications, clearinghouses, databases, Web sites, and support and self-help groups, as well as to the government agencies and not-for-profit organizations that produce reliable information for the public. This site is so popular that Healthfinder asks you to use *http://www.healthfinder.org* when you find it inaccessible due to heavy traffic.

2. National Institutes of Health: Health Information Index

http://www.nih.gov/health/

This index will help you identify the NIH's role and responsibility in all areas of medical research. It also links to a collection of NIH publications and a list of information clearinghouses with their phone numbers. From here you can also access Internet Grateful Med v2.3 for free access to the Medline and PubMed data bases.

3. NIH: Consumer Health Information

http://www.nih.gov/health/consumer/conicd.htm

The publications of the agencies of the National Institutes of Health are listed at this site and can be accessed online.

4. Starting Point: Health

http://www.stpt.com/health/health.html

Search engine to excellent resources on health and fitness. Click on Women's Health for complete menu of links to relevant sites.

Women and Health

5. American Medical Women's Association

http://www.amwa-doc.org

The home page of the AMWA, an organization of over 13,000 female physicians and medical students dedicated to the care of the woman patient, serves as a unique voice for women's health. Changing articles on a host of health topics can be found here and links to other sites.

6. Guide To Women's Health Issues

http://www.coil.com/~tsegal/womens_health.html

This guide is an effective launching site for gender issues in health care, and includes a Table of Contents and Emotional, Physical, and Sexual Health Issues, which can be accessed by topic. Abstracts help you decide whether or not to read further. Includes bibliographical material and links to the Argus Clearinghouse.

7. National Women's Health Information Center

http://www.4woman.org

This extensive new site contains the resources of the U.S. Public Health Service's Office on Women's Health and the Defense Women's Health Information Center. Add *nwhic/minority.htm* to the URL and reach an extensive list of links to health resources for women of color.

8. National Women's Health Resource Center

http://www.healthywomen.org

The NWHRC is a complete woman's health resource that includes Web resources and links as well as questions and answers about every woman's health issue from adolescence to the aging process.

9. Program on Women's Health

http://www.cmwf.org/programs/women/index.asp

This is the Commonwealth Fund's site for its program on women's health. The Table of Contents leads to Overview of Program, Work in Progress, and Completed Initiatives.

10. Women's Health Initiative

http://www.nhlbi.nih.gov/nhlbi/whi1/

The WHI is one of the largest preventive studies of its kind in the United States. It focuses on the major causes of death, disability, and frailty in postmenopausal women, with a goal of reducing coronary heart disease, breast and colorectal cancer, and osteoporotic fractures among this study group.

Nutrition and Fitness

11. FitnessLink: The Health and Fitness Source

http://www.fitnesslink.com

An excellent resource for fitness information, FitnessLink includes the following indexes: Nutritional Information and Mind/Body Connection, each of which is useful to a discussion of women's health.

12. Food and Nutrition Information Center

http://www.nal.usda.gov/fnic/

Run by the Agriculture Network Information Center, this Web site contains a Search Engine plus Publications and Databases, and also links to information produced by other USDA agencies, as well as an Index of Food and Nutrition Internet Resources.

13. Mayo Clinic Diet & Nutrition Resurce Center

http://www.mayo.ivi.com/mayo/common/htm/dietpage.htm

At this site find many new diet and nutrition articles, plus a Virtual Cookbook: Send your recipes and have them altered for health; also Ask the Mayo Dietician; Quizzes that test nutrition knowledge; Reference Articles; and Links to Other Organizations.

Gynecological and Reproductive Health

14. A Forum for Women's Health

http://www.womenshealth.org

This Internet resource for women's health information hosts a collection of information, advice, and suggestions to help women deal with their health concerns. Organized under Ask a Woman Doctor; Subjects (such as Reproductive, Social/Psychological, and Wellness); Lifecycle (containing Girls' Reproduction, Midlife, Mature); What's New; Search the Forum; and Links. Helpful place to deal with birth control and pregnancy issues.

15. Women's Health Interactive

http://www.womens-health.com

This interactive learning environment facilitates the exchange of information among participants and motivates individual proactive responses. Featured are The Infertility Center, The Gynecological Health Center, and comprehensive health resources. Special services include Bleeding Assessment Diary and Infertility Insurance Advisor. Interactive sites are Assessment of Pregnancy Factors, Assessment of Gynecological Factors, Symptoms, and Cardiovascular Health Assessment.

Psychological Health

16. Mental Health Net: QuickFind Results

http://www.cmhc.com/search.htm

Link to many articles on women and stress by using the search engine at this site. Then explore this comprehensive guide to mental health online, which contains information on depression, substance abuse, eating disorders, and much more. You can also take a Self-Help Quiz.

17. Women's Mental Health Resources

http://mentalhealth.miningco.com/msub15.htm

From this site, the special issues of women and mental health can be researched. Examples of resources include the Division of Society, Women, and Health at the Clarke Institute of Psychiatry, women's self-help articles on women's mental health issues, and a site on seasonal affective disorder, a syndrome that affects women differently than men.

Chronic Diseases

18. Heartinformation Network: Women's Health

http://www.heartinfo.org/reviews/wmhd.htm

This site links interesting articles about heart disease and other chronic diseases of women to other sites that discuss women's health.

19. Mayo Clinic's Women's Health Resource Center

http://www.mayo.ivi.com/mayo/common/htm/womenpg.htm

In addition to Ask the Mayo Physician and a comprehensive collection of articles covering women's health issues, as well as articles for the Mayo Clinic's own Women's Health Resource Newsletter, click on Cancer Center, Heart Center, Pregnancy and Child Health Center, and Diet and Nutrition Center for additional information and links.

20. NCI's CancerNet Cancer Information for Patients

http://wwwicic.nci.nih.gov/patient.htm

A wide range of accurate, credible cancer information is at this site, from peer-review statements from PDQ (Physicians Data Inquiry) covering latest cases, to cancer fact sheets and other publications. All have been reviewed by oncology experts and are based on results of current research. Some examples: Prototype Breast Cancer Resource and Information for Ethnic/Racial Groups. The site includes a glossary and global resources.

21. Search Federal Health and Human Services

http://www.hhs.gov/search/

At SEARCH enter "articles-about-cancer-in-women" and a list of 50 articles will appear at this site of the Department of Health and Human Services. Go to *http:www.hhs.gov* also and explore What's New. Use the Search feature to initiate your own quest.

Substance Abuse: New Trends for Women

22. National Clearinghouse for Alcohol and Drug Information

http://www.health.org/women.htm

Material from many sources about alcohol, tobacco, and other drugs can be accessed at this clearinghouse. Bibliographies are also available. Click on Making the Link: Alcohol, Tobacco, and Other Drugs & Women's Health for Women's Health, Sex under the Influence, Pregnancy and Parenthood, and Alcohol, Tobacco, and Other Drugs.

23. National Institute on Drug Abuse (NIDA)

http://www.nida.nih.gov/WHGD/WHGDHome.html

The mission at this site is to promote the conduct and dissemination of research on women's health and gender differences concerning substance abuse and other health problems. There are also links to other Web sites of interest.

Violence in Women's Lives

24. Crisis Resources

http://www.access.digex.net/~nova/resource.htm

This page of crisis resources contains toll-free and toll numbers for information and referrals on victim's rights, services, and criminal justice issues; Web resources that offer help; and links to victims, survivors, and grassroots organizations related to issues of violence.

25. Domestic Violence

http://www.s-t.com/projects/DomVio/domviohome.HTML

The main page of this site leads to 60 articles that explore domestic violence—its causes, victims, and some solutions. There is also a special help file and a guide to resources on the Internet.

26. Sexual Assault Information Page

http://www.cs.utk.edu/~bartley/saInfoPage.html

This page covers every issue connected with sexual violence toward women from acquaintance rape to domestic violence, to incest, to post-traumatic stress disorder, and to sexual assault.

Special Issues for Older Women

27. Lifecycle: Mature

http://www.womenshealth.org/lifecycle/mature.htm

This page addresses some of the issues that concern older, postmenopausal women. Issues covered include the reproductive system, pertinent medical issues, social and psychological issues, wellness questions, and finding appropriate health providers.

28. National Institute on Aging

http://www.nih.gov/nia/

The main page of the NIA leads to What's New, NIA Research, Health Information, and Related Sites, many of which concern the health problems of older women.

29. National Survey of Women's Health

http://www.cmwf.org/programs/women/whhilite.asp

Survey results of major health problems that affect older women are included in this study.

We highly recommend that you review our Web site for expanded information and our other product lines. We are continually updating and adding links to our Web site in order to offer you the most usable and useful information that will support and expand the value of your Annual Editions. You can reach us at: *http://www.dushkin.com/annualeditions/*.

Unit 1

Unit Selections

1. **Women's Health Studies,** *Harvard Women's Health Watch*
2. **Work with Me, Doctor: How to Get Better Care,** *Women's Health Advocate Newsletter*
3. **Forgotten Women: How Minorities Are Underserved by Our Health Care System,** Lisa Collier Cool
4. **Dangerous Legacies,** Dana Hawkins
5. **Managed Care: How to Protect Yourself,** *Women's Health Advocate Newsletter*
6. **More Research, More Profits, More Conflict,** Laura Mansnerus
7. **There Is No Women's Health Crisis,** Sally L. Satel

Key Points to Consider

- What are some of the reasons why minority women may receive substandard care? How can this be changed?
- Genetic testing raises many questions regarding privacy, ethics, and effectiveness. What are some of the pros and cons of genetic testing for diseases like breast cancer?
- Have women been neglected in medical research? Is there a women's health crisis? Defend your answer.

DUSHKIN ONLINE Links

www.dushkin.com/online/

5. **American Medical Women's Association**
   http://www.amwa-doc.org
6. **Guide To Women's Health Issues**
   http://www.coil.com/~tsegal/womens_health.html
7. **National Women's Health Information Center**
   http://www.4woman.org
8. **National Women's Health Resource Center**
   http://www.healthywomen.org
9. **Program on Women's Health**
   http://www.cmwf.org/programs/women/index.asp
10. **Women's Health Initiative**
    http://www.nhlbi.nih.gov/nhlbi/whi1/

These sites are annotated on pages 4 and 5.

Women and Health

The purpose of this first chapter is to provide an introduction to some of the issues facing women in the changing health care environment. The existence of women's health as a discipline of study is the result of a long history of advice and activism that has pushed the particular issues of women out of the background and into the light.

After many years of neglect by the medical establishment, women's health has been discovered. The studies described in the article "Women's Health Studies" are a response both to the realization that "one size does not fit all" in health care and to years of advocacy and pressure from women. The process of investigating what is unique about women's health will provide the basis for women's health courses for years to come. In keeping with the commitment to provide diverse views, we offer a selection by Sally Satel that argues that there is no women's health crisis.

While women as a group have been neglected by the health system, minority women have received a double dose. Lisa Collier Cool, in "Forgotten Women: How Minorities Are Underserved by Our Health Care System," demonstrates that minority women, whatever their insurance status, do not get as many screenings, may receive less aggressive care, or may not be told of new treatment options. Historically, they have been neglected by the research trials both as women and as minorities. The implications of this for women's health are also discussed.

Several new areas of challenge face all women in the health care system. Managed care has become more of an issues for many Americans. Two articles discuss the challenges of managed care, "Work With Me, Doctor: How to Get Better Care" and "Managed Care: How to Protect Yourself." As health care becomes every more complicated and perceived by many to be highly impersonal, more and more high-tech tests, such as genetic testing, are becoming increasingly available. However they can cause more confusion than certainty. "Dangerous Legacies," by Dana Hawkins, offers a look at the issues that must be faced when research is used for screening.

In reading this section, we hope that you will see the common thread that unites these articles. As health care in the United States changes and evolves, women are faced with a myriad of questions and challenges. The primary challenge is how to receive appropriate care in a system that is just beginning to learn what works for women.

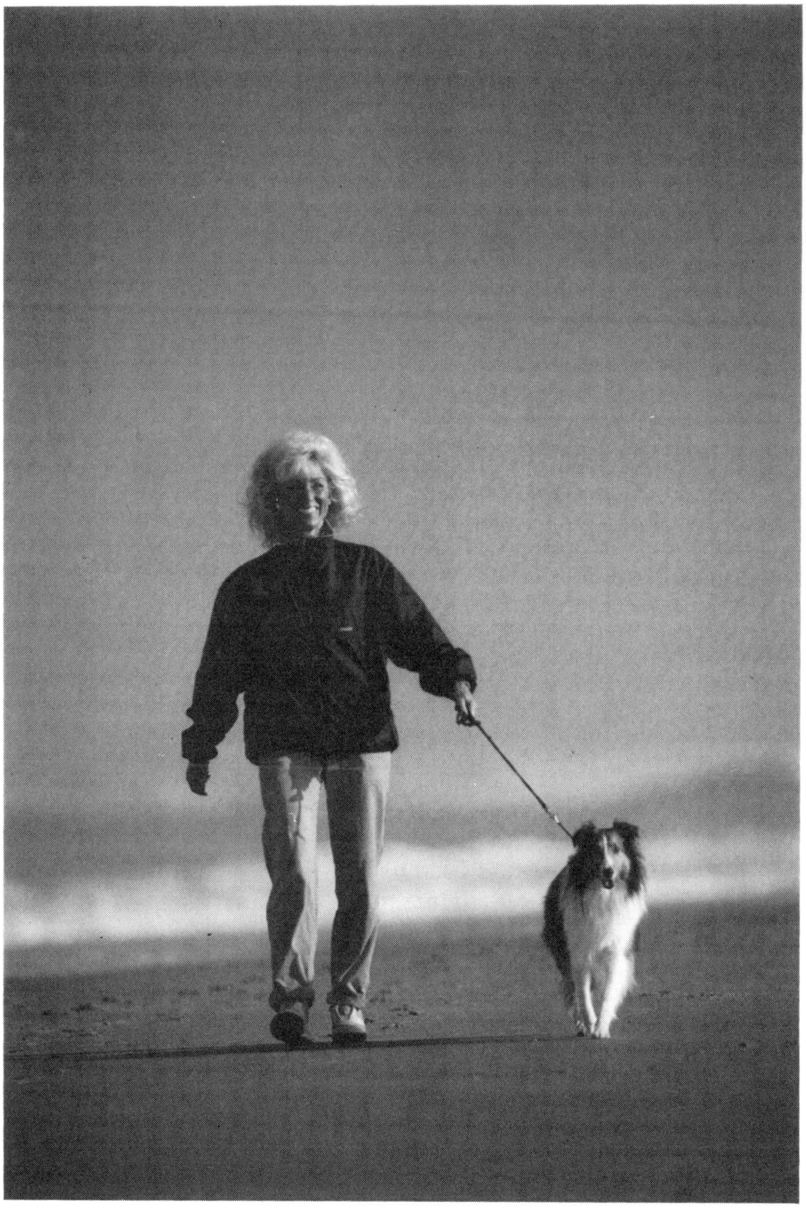

Women's Health Studies

The gender gap in medical research is closing. It has been since 1990, when the Office of Research on Women's Health was established at the National Institutes of Health to address the underrepresentation of women in medical studies. Since then, women in such investigations have increased not only in number, but also in diversity. Postmenopausal women, once all but ignored in scientific investigations, have become the focus of several new projects, and efforts to include African-American, Asian, and Hispanic women have expanded. These studies should provide information to guide us in reducing our risks of heart disease, cancer, osteoporosis, and other degenerative diseases. They generally take one of two forms — observational or interventional investigations.

Observational studies are designed to reveal possible associations between physical characteristics or health habits and disease. They usually include large numbers of people who are followed for several years. The participants may answer periodic questionnaires and may also be tracked through hospital records, tumor registries or death records.

Interventional studies are designed to determine the effects of specific treatments, diets, or health practices. Controlled trials are considered the gold standard of interventional studies. In these investigations, participants are randomly assigned to groups and each group follows a certain treatment, with at least one of the groups receiving a placebo or no treatment at all. At the end of the study, the results in each of the groups are compared.

The following studies are the first major investigations to deal exclusively with health issues of women at mid-life and beyond.

• *The Women's Health Initiative.* The largest study of women to date, the WHI includes both observational and interventional components. Researchers at 40 centers around the country are studying 160,000 healthy, postmenopausal women who were between the ages of 50 and 79 when they enrolled.

In the Observational Study, 100,000 women will undergo a physical examination upon entry and again after 3 years. Every year, the participants will complete questionnaires on their health habits.

The remaining 60,000 women are being enrolled in one or more of three controlled trials — the Dietary Modification (DM) Study, the Hormone Replacement Therapy (HRT) Study, or the Calcium and Vitamin D Supplementation (CaD) Study. The DM is designed to determine whether a low-fat diet reduces the risk of breast and colorectal cancer. The CaD study will test the effects of taking calcium and vitamin D supplements on osteoporosis risk.

The HRT Study should help to determine whether postmenopausal hormone supplementation actually lowers the risk of heart disease and osteoporosis and increases the risk of breast cancer, as some observational studies have indicated. It may also help to resolve the question of estrogen's effect on mental acuity and on the risk of developing Alzheimer's disease: women over age 65 will take annual examinations to test memory and reasoning. To enroll in this study, call 1-800-54-WOMEN.

• *The Nurses' Health Study.* This ongoing observational study, conducted by researchers at Brigham and Women's Hospital, Harvard Medical School, and Harvard School of Public Health, was inaugurated in 1976, when 120,000 women between the ages of 30 and 55 were enrolled. They are asked to fill out extensive questionnaires about their health and lifestyles every two years. By changing the questions asked, the researchers are able to examine the relationship between different lifestyle factors and medical outcomes. The more than 100 reports emanating from this study have provided the foundation for additional research into women's health risks. These reports have, among other things, indicated that there are health benefits in regular exercise, diets high in fruits and vegetables, and maintaining a lean body mass. They have suggested that oral contraceptive use does not increase the risk of cardiovascular disease, that postmenopausal replacement therapy with estrogen alone is linked with an increased risk of endometrial cancer, that drinking alcohol increases the risk of breast cancer, that the risk of gallstones rises with obesity, that suntanning increases the likelihood of melanoma, and that aspirin, estrogen, and exercise may reduce the risk of colon cancer.

The participants in the Nurses' Study are now between 50 and 75. Not only have their answers changed with age — more have suffered heart attacks, osteoporosis or cancer — but the questions have, too. The next round of inquiry is designed to obtain information on the psychosocial factors, such as stress, anxiety, social isolation and mood changes, that may influence health and longevity.

• *Study of Women's Health Across the Nation* (SWAN). This observational investigation, sponsored by the National Institute on Aging, is underway at seven medical centers in the United States. Researchers are selecting 3,200 women between the ages of 42 and 52, whom they will track for about five years. The project will focus on the physical and psychological differences among African-American, Hispanic, Asian-American, and Caucasian women during menopause.

The researchers will look at body composition, bone density, hormone levels, cardiovascular function, and menstrual bleeding. They will also consider psychosocial influences, such as sexuality, interpersonal relationships, commitment toward work, social values, and attitudes toward aging. Lifestyle factors — diet, exercise, smoking, and alcohol consumption — will also be included.

This is the first of a two-part story on how to get better care, whether you're covered under traditional insurance or are in a managed care plan.*

Work with Me, Doctor: How to Get Better Care

It's the best of times and the worst of times to be a patient. The advances of the last 50 years have been breathtaking, and never has so much medical information been available directly to health care consumers.

What's more, the doctor-patient relationship has undergone a subtle shift in the last 10 to 15 years. Paternalism is out; partnerships are in. Many doctors today are more attuned to patient advocacy issues, and patient satisfaction is a topic that appears more and more often in physician publications, says Mike Donio, director of projects at the People's Medical Society.

However, this shift in power is occurring simultaneously with a profound shift in the way medicine is practiced. Increasingly, managed care—HMOs, PPOs, and other corporate-influenced arrangements—is the name of the game.

As a result, the doctor-patient relationship often includes a third party—and many third parties carry a big stick. In some HMOs, doctors who would like to spend more time listening to their patients and providing them with more information simply can't. Thus, any advice on how to form a "health care partnership" with your doctor is, by necessity, general and subject to adaptation to individual circumstances.

Ten Steps to Better Care

In the best of all worlds—and under the ideal insurance plan—here are some steps you can take to help forge a satisfying doctor-patient relationship. (Most of these approaches will work well under any type of provider relationship, although next month's issue of *WHA* will carry tips on navigating the world of managed care.)

1 Schedule an interview. If you have a choice in physicians, get recommendations. Find out from the office staff whether the doctor is accepting new patients. If so, ask for other basic information, such as the doctor's specialization, training, fees, and office hours.

Then arrange for a get-acquainted interview. (If the doctor refuses, go on to the next physician on your list.) Be aware that some physicians charge for a get-acquainted visit; others don't.

This first-time interview may take about 10 to 15 minutes. Ideally, it should be conducted in person, although it can be done over the phone. Either way, this is the time to ask about things that are important to you, such as wellness and screening strategies and attitudes toward vitamins or alternative treatments.

Evaluate your "gut level" response—did the doctor seem harried? distracted? irritated or offended by your questions? Or did he or she make good eye contact, listen, and take your concerns seriously? Were things explained in terms you could understand? Will you feel comfortable in revealing important information to him or her? Most importantly, do you feel that this is someone you can work with?

2 Come prepared. Before your first medical visit to any new doctor, gather all relevant information about all major illnesses and treatments. List current medications and any problems you've had with particular drugs. Bring copies of relevant test results—mammograms or other x-rays, for example. Include your family medical history—first- or second-degree relatives who've had heart disease, cancer, diabetes, or other chronic diseases.

3 Jot it down. Before an appointment, make a list of any questions or concerns. A written list is more time-efficient, and it can keep you from forgetting to ask something important. Keep a notebook handy for taking notes.

If you're facing a complex medical procedure, consider taking along a family member or friend to help you remember important details.

You might also ask the doctor if you can tape record a lengthy or complicated discussion. If your doctor's initial reaction to this request is a negative one, point out that you don't want to miss or forget something.

4 Be observant. You are the only person who can describe how you feel. When you have a problem, keep track of your symptoms and write down anything that might be helpful.

For instance, if you're experiencing pain, when does it occur? How long does it last? What does it feel like—jabbing, squeezing, or a dull ache? The more specific you can be, the better.

5 Tell the truth. Be honest about eating, exercise, smoking, drinking, and other habits. Holding back information because you're embarrassed—or you're trying to avoid conflict—could jeopardize your health.

The same is true when a treatment is prescribed. For instance, if you aren't taking your medication or you haven't consistently altered your eating habits, let your doctor know. It isn't easy to admit to noncompliance, but being evasive can lead to diagnostic confusion and perhaps to a more complicated or invasive treatment than you actually need.

And if a doctor wants you to do something you suspect might be a problem—such as waking up in the middle of the night to take a pill—be honest about your concerns. There may be an alternative.

6 Do your homework. Find out all you can about your particular medical condition or the drug you're taking. The purpose isn't to diagnose your own illness but to learn what questions to ask and help you negotiate with your doctor.

7 Don't be afraid to ask. If you don't understand a medical phrase, or something is unclear, say so. Above all, don't leave your doctor's office until you're clear about your diagnosis and any treatment or follow-up plan.

8 Speak up. If you run into a problem—if, for instance, you don't feel as if your doctor is spending enough time with you or taking your problem seriously—you need to speak up and make your feelings known.

An assertive, straightforward expression of your feelings usually can bring an end to the bothersome behavior. For example, if the doctor regularly conducts post-examination discussions while you're still on the table in a paper gown, you might say, "I feel uncomfortable when our discussions take place in the examining room; I'd like to get dressed first."

If you find it hard to express yourself during an office visit, Donio suggests writing the physician a letter or calling later and asking for a brief appointment to discuss your concerns. If your physician responds negatively or continually ignores your wishes, it's time to find a new doctor.

9 Don't be intimidated. Even the most involved patients have been known to fall into the trap of letting themselves be intimidated by a doctor's perceived prestige or expertise.

It's important to remember two things: First, behind the starched white persona is a human being. Secondly, you're paying for his or her services.

10 Consider a second opinion. If you're facing an invasive procedure, are told you have a life-threatening illness, or are uncomfortable with—or uncertain about—the diagnosis or recommended treatment, tell your doctor that you'd like to get a second opinion.

If your doctor balks at the request, find another physician. For one thing, such consultations are common. More importantly, it's your right—and your duty to yourself—to ask for and receive the kind of medical care you need.

Resources:
Related stories published previously in *WHA* include: How to find medical information (July 1995); how to keep your own medical history (December 1995); and older women's health care rights (October 1996).

People's Medical Society. Write 462 Walnut St., Allentown, Pa. 18102, or call (800) 624-8773.

*See "Managed Care: How to Protect Yourself," from *Women's Health Advocate,* May 1997 on page 17 of this volume.

Assertiveness Helps Your Health

What's an ounce of assertiveness worth? Your health, perhaps. Consider the following:

Tufts University researchers conducted four separate trials in which patients with a chronic illness—hypertension, ulcers, diabetes, or breast cancer—were assigned to one of two groups.

In each trial, patients in the first group were given general information about their particular disease and the importance of self-monitoring and self-care.

Those in the second were given this basic information plus training in assertiveness and communication techniques. These patients also were shown their own medical records and given information on treatment strategies; their training session took place immediately before a scheduled office visit.

Six to eight weeks later, researchers assessed each patient's health status, measuring it subjectively (via the patient's own assessment) and objectively (through medical tests).

The findings: In all four trials, patients who had had the assertiveness training were in better health.

Similar research has supported these findings. What's the underlying connection between good health and assertiveness? It may be feelings of self-confidence or a sense of control. Over the years, numerous studies have suggested that a sense of control over one's situation—be it a job or a health condition—lowers stress and boosts mental and physical well-being.

Forgotten Women: How Minorities Are Underserved by Our Health Care System

LISA COLLIER COOL

Imagine living in a place where going to a doctor involves a difficult or even dangerous trek to a distant, overcrowded clinic where you wait hours for a few minutes of questionable medical care—a place where preventive treatment is so lacking that breast tumors sometimes protrude through the skin before they are diagnosed.

You might expect these conditions in a third world country, but actually they're faced every day by minority women in some parts of the U.S. Statistics show that "an African-American woman born in Harlem today has less chance of surviving to age 65 than a woman from Bangladesh, one of the poorest nations on earth," says Colin McCord, M.D., associate director of surgery at Harlem Hospital in New York City.

Although you may think that poverty is to blame, the truth is that even affluent minority women—whether black, Hispanic, Asian-American or Native American—fare poorly in our medical system. "An African-American woman who earns triple what a Euro-American female earns still has a greater chance of mortality from disease like breast cancer," says Faye Gary, Ed.D., distinguished service professor at the College of Nursing of the University of Florida in Gainesville.

What makes this all the more shocking is that even as progress has been made in women's health as a whole, the health disparities between black and white women have remained. Mortality from heart disease and cancer has fallen among white women, yet is unchanged in blacks. At every age, "African-American, Native American, Hispanic and Asian-American women suffer from poorer health and greater risk of premature death," says Dr. Gary.

Deadly Discrimination Socioeconomic factors explain only some of these inequities. While it's true that black women have triple the rate of poverty of white women and are slightly less likely to be insured, research reveals that they're also the victims of subtle but potentially fatal

YOUR HERITAGE, YOUR HEALTH

Here's how your background may affect your disease risk. (Except where noted, individual groups are compared to U.S. women as a whole.)

Native American women:

- are 10 times likelier to suffer from diabetes.
- have 12 times the odds of dying from alcohol-related causes before age 34.
- are much likelier to live more than half an hour away from the nearest health facility.

Hispanic women:

- are 60% likelier to say their health is fair or poor.
- have a greater risk of obesity.
- have the greatest rate of severe depression.

Black women:

- have quadruple the high blood pressure risk of whites in young adulthood and a higher rate of serious complications, including stroke, later in life.
- have the highest death rate from colon cancer.

Asian-American/Pacific Island women:

- are least likely to be satisfied with their health care.
- have the highest rate of stomach cancer.
- are at greater risk for the genetic disorders alpha- and beta-thalassemia, which cause retardation, as well as for hepatitis B.

From *American Health for Women*, May 1997, pp. 37-38, 40.

medical bias. A recent study at Boston University found that at every income level, black women over age 64 are only half as likely as whites to have a mammogram ordered for them by a doctor, even if they see a primary-care physician just as often. Mammography rates are even lower for Native American women. The result is that black and Native American women have a 30% higher risk of dying of breast cancer, despite the fact that the disease is much less common in these groups than in whites.

The same pattern of prejudice prevails in hospital care: A study at Beth Israel Hospital in Boston found that doctors order 1½ times as much surgery and other high-tech treatment for whites as for equally ill blacks. It's not just costly procedures these patients are shortchanged on, either: 20% of Latinas and 65% of Korean Americans have never had a Pap smear, yet lab costs start at $16.

Even in the emergency room, your race or ethnicity can have more impact on your care than your condition, says Jane Delgado, Ph.D., president and CEO of the National Coalition of Hispanic Health and Human Services Organizations in Washington. "A study of people treated for a broken leg showed that the single greatest predictor of who got painkillers was whether they were Hispanic," she says. "The doctors often withheld painkillers from Hispanic patients even though Hispanic and non-Hispanic patients rated their pain as equally severe." This reminds Dr. Gary of the segregated care she received growing up in the South in the '50s. "My parents had to drive 100 miles to take me to the only white dentist who would see black people," she recalls. "I remember feeling grateful when he yanked out my teeth at his kitchen table, because I wasn't allowed into his office."

Deep-Rooted Stereotypes Not only are minorities' medical needs dangerously neglected, but doctor prejudice can also result in substandard care for those who get treated, says Claudia R. Baquet, M.D., associate dean for policy and planning at University of Maryland School of Medicine in Baltimore. "In focus groups," she says, "minority women say that doctors assume they have multiple partners or start having sex at an early age. Racial and ethnic stereotyping is still rampant and a barrier to quality care."

Minority women are doubly disadvantaged because they may be subjected to sexism in addition to racial bias, notes Aida Giachello, Ph.D., director of the Midwest Latino Health Research, Training and Policy Center at the University of Illinois in Chicago. Many Latinas report that doctors dismiss their complaints. "The stereotype is that Latinas overuse the health system," says Dr. Giachello. "But when we did a focus group with these women, the reality was that they had to go to their doctors over and over with the same symptoms, because the physicians would say it was stress while the real problem went undiagnosed, sometimes causing serious complications."

Equally damaging are the assumptions physicians may make if they judge a patient's ethnicity based on her skin color or surname. "If a Native American woman from the Southwest has a Latino last name, a doctor may misclassify her and not test for gallbladder disease, which is epidemic in that population," says Dr. Baquet. Others question the medical value of determining ethnicity at all. "Asking someone what race she considers herself to be doesn't tell you what her genetics are," points out Olivia Carter-Pokras, Ph.D., an epidemiologist and public health analyst at the Office of Minority Health in Washington. "Even sickle-cell anemia, thought of as a 'black' disorder, also appears in white people of Mediterranean origin."

Research Bias More serious still is the situation in clinical trials, where scientists develop the medicine of the future by testing new drugs, diagnostic techniques and other treatments. Despite laws mandating the inclusion of women and minorities in trials sponsored by the National Institutes of Health, many doctors don't seem to have gotten the message, reports Dr. Carter-Pokras, who says she constantly sees unconscious or even overt prejudice on the part of researchers. "A doctor may decide to recruit from her own clinic, never stopping to think that since her patients are 80% white, she needs to be aggressive about finding minority cases," she says. Investigators often try to recruit Spanish speakers with no

Equal Opportunity Health Resources

To lobby for better care for minority women, or to get more information about minority women's health risks, contact the following:

- **Minority Health Consortium,** in Richmond, VA (804-355-4502), offers free women's health pamphlets and referrals to other resources.
- **National Black Women's Health Project** in Washington (202-835-0117) provides free information on subjects of special interest to black women.
- **National Coalition of Hispanic Health and Human Services Organization** in Washington (202-387-5000; http://www.cossmho.org) offers a free catalog listing bilingual literature, videos and hot lines.
- **Office of Minority Health Resource Center** (800-444-6472; http://www.omhrc.gov) provides customized database searches and referrals.

translators or bilingual materials. Not only do such attitudes reduce minority women's access to state-of-the-art care, but also underrepresentation in studies ensures that the second-class medical care will continue for decades to come.

Increasing the number of women of color participating in medical studies is important, but Dr. Gary feels it doesn't go far enough. "There also needs to be better representation of ethnic groups among the people who do the studies," she says. Despite doctors' best intentions, subtle biases and cultural differences can still interfere with good research.

Constructive Changes The outrage from women of color is finally starting to be heard on Capitol Hill. To determine how to end these inequities, 740 experts convened in Washington last January for the nation's first minority women's health conference, sponsored by the U.S. Public Health Service's Office on Women's Health. The agency is developing a culturally sensitive women's health curriculum for medical and nursing schools, and it has started programs to recruit more minority women into health careers and as participants in clinical trials.

Other federal agencies are creating their own initiatives. The Centers for Disease Control and Prevention is funding studies of chronic disease that affect women of color disproportionately (see "Your Heritage, Your Health"). But it's still up to women to help alert doctors to the potential for bias in diagnosis and treatment and to become more attuned to how our racial or ethnic background may affect our health. Each of these efforts shares the same crucial goal: to create a healthier tomorrow for *all* women.

Award-winning journalist Lisa Collier Cool lives in Pelham, NY.

Dangerous legacies

New gene tests provide fresh grounds for discrimination

BY DANA HAWKINS

The quartet of smiling women in the gold-leaf-framed portrait share the same high cheekbones and hazel eyes. The youngest balances a chubby baby boy on her hip. Susan McGuire, 46, arranged for the photograph of herself with her grandmother, mother, daughter, and grandson shortly after her mother was diagnosed with ovarian cancer two years ago. Since then, her mother's luxuriant white hair has been lost to chemotherapy.

McGuire would like to take new tests that would probe her genetic blueprint, or DNA, and reveal whether she carries mutations that increase her chances of developing ovarian or breast cancer. They are known as the BRCA tests (after *br*east *ca*ncer, though they test for ovarian cancer, as well). She can trace this destructive legacy back two generations. In that span, five members of her family have battled ovarian cancer; three have died. If she tested negative, she and her husband could breathe easier. If the results were positive, she says, she would have her ovaries removed to reduce her risk of getting the disease.

Like countless other women with family histories of cancer, however, she is afraid to take the BRCA tests—and for good reason. She is not the only one who might obtain the results. Potential employers and insurers could at least theoretically get hold of the information, perhaps making it difficult for her to find work or be insured. In the year since the BRCA tests became commercially available, Congress has passed no bills to prevent discrimination against people on the basis of genetic information. Some two dozen states have enacted protective statutes, but they vary widely. In Illinois, for instance, the results of genetic tests may be released only to the person tested; in New Jersey, neither employers nor insurers may use the results of tests to discriminate. Two years ago, the federal Equal Employment Opportunity Commission issued an interpretation of the 1990 Americans with Disabilities Act stating that workers should be protected from genetic bias, but the issue hasn't been tested in court.

Pandering? Some people contend that any woman who can pay the fee, which ranges from $300 for a basic test to $2,700 for a comprehensive screening, and wants the test should take it. Dr. Harvey Stern, director of the BRCA testing program at Genetics and IVF Institute (GIVF) in Fairfax, Va., has screened patients with no family history of breast or ovarian cancer. "Am I pandering to their neurotic fear of cancer? I don't think so," he says. "If this gives them inner peace—fine."

Yet many women's health experts, including Dr. Susan Love, author of the best-seller *Dr. Susan Love's Breast Book*, believe women should not have themselves tested until a federal antidiscrimination law is in place—and until a lot more is known about the medical significance of a positive result. As Love points out, many women have heard that 1 in 8 of them will develop breast cancer at some point in their lives, but few realize that the gene mutations identified by BRCA tests account for only 5 to 10 percent of breast and ovarian cancers. The rest of the cancers may be caused by various other risk factors, including mutations in other genes and lifetime exposure to estrogen and other hormones.

A negative result on the gene test doesn't mean that a woman won't get cancer—nor does a positive result mean that she will. Until last spring, health experts believed that a woman with a BRCA mutation probably would develop breast cancer at some point in her life. Estimates said the risk was from 50 to 90 percent. But the results of a newer, broader study suggest that the risk could be lower.

WAITING ON CONGRESS

Susan McGuire wants to take the BRCA tests to learn if she's at greater risk for ovarian cancer. But only if Congress passes an antidiscrimination law.

Questionable value. Some experts argue that even a positive result is not useful clinically because there's nothing anyone can do to avoid developing the disease. Last spring, the *Journal of the American Medical Association* published the first set of guidelines for doctors with patients who have mutations identified by the BRCA tests. The report said it isn't yet clear whether pre-emptive removal of breasts or ovaries helps avoid cancer because, even after surgery, tumors may develop in nearby tissues. Other experts disagree, relying on the work of researchers at the Mayo Clinic who found that preventive mastectomies appear to reduce an at-risk woman's chances of getting breast cancer by about 90 percent.

More and more Americans are facing similar dilemmas about testing as scientists identify a growing roster of genetic mutations linked to common diseases. This fall, for instance, a gene test for hemochromatosis, which causes the body to store excess iron in the organs and is the most common genetic disease in the United States, reached the market. A new test for colon cancer is moving rapidly from the lab to doctors' offices. As the list grows, so do concerns about discrimination based on them. Civil rights attorneys are concerned that employers who insure their own workers (about 10 percent of employers) as opposed to signing on with a group plan may turn down job applicants with a genetic predisposition to various types of cancer because of the high cost of treatment.

While there have been no population-wide surveys of genetic bias, many people have reportedly suffered discrimination after being identified as having, or being at risk for, an inherited disease. Even before DNA gene tests, doctors could get clues about a person's future by studying family medical histories or by analyzing blood and urine samples for biochemical indicators of disease. In 1992, in one of the first papers published on genetic discrimination, Dr. Paul Billings, chief medical officer of the Heart of Texas veterans hospitals, described a pregnant woman in Louisiana whose fetus tested positive for cystic fibrosis. After the woman's managed-care health plan got the news, it said it would limit coverage of her pregnancy and child. (The plan said it would cover the cost of an abortion, however.) A Harvard Medical School study published last year documented 200 cases of genetic discrimination. One woman was fired from her job as a social worker after her bosses learned she was at risk of developing Huntington's disease, a fatal disorder that causes uncontrollable movements and dementia.

So far, no one has taken an employer or insurer to court for discrimination on the basis of BRCA test results. But such discrimination and lawsuits are likely to happen soon, according to Wendy McGoodwin, the executive director of the Council for Responsible Genetics in Cambridge, Mass., a nonprofit bioethics group. "We now have a huge new pool of people who are vulnerable to genetic discrimination," she says.

Congress is considering a number of bills that would limit discrimination against people with faulty genes, an idea backed by President Clinton. The proposals vary. Some would prevent medical, life, or disability insurers from dropping individuals with positive results or raising their premiums. Others would forbid employers from discriminating in hiring and promoting workers.

Insurance companies say they have a right to see their clients' test results. Life insurers argue, for instance, that people who test positive for mutations linked to life-threatening diseases might load up on insurance because they expect to die at a relatively young age, raising rates for others in the pool. Similarly, the Health Insurance Association of America is worried that previously uninsured people who learn they have a genetic predisposition to a disease will purchase insurance, incur high medical costs, and drive up premiums. The group is also lobbying against the bills on grounds that companies that insure individuals or small groups need to know genetic information so they can exclude high-risk people or charge them more for coverage.

Susan McGuire, whose family has a history of ovarian cancer, knows federal antidiscrimination legislation is not expected to pass this year, but that doesn't stop her from checking the newspaper each morning—just in case. McGuire says she'll get tested the moment such a bill is signed. Now she has an added sense of urgency. This week her sister, 47, expects to learn whether the growth she recently had removed from her uterus was cancerous.

How to get better care, part 2: Navigating the world of managed care.

Managed Care: How to Protect Yourself

In the golden days of health insurance coverage, if you were dissatisfied with your doctor, you simply "voted with your feet" and went elsewhere.

Things have changed. Today, some 150 million Americans are in managed-care plans. In all fairness, it must be noted that many of them are satisfied with their coverage. However, we rarely hear testimonials from contented patients. Instead, we hear the horror stories—"drive-by" deliveries and mastectomies, "gag rules" limiting patient-physician communication, and denials of emergency care, among other disasters.

Fighting Back

As with finding a physician under a traditional insurance plan, the best way to prevent problems is to make the right match at the outset (see "Buyer Beware").

But if you find yourself with a mismatch, what are your options? Ideally, your primary care physician (your "gatekeeper" in the plan) will go to bat for you. However, as Mike Donio, director of projects for the People's Medical Society, points out, patients in an HMO really are negotiating with an insurance company, not an individual doctor.

Thus, advice about how to communicate with your physician goes only so far. If you're denied access to a specialist or to appropriate diagnostic tests and treatments, you may have to resort to other tactics to get the treatment you need. Here are a few approaches that may help:

1 **Ask for an explanation.** Ask why you're being denied access, and write the reasons down.

2 **Provide justification.** Look for medical articles that support your belief that you need specialized or additional care. Overviews of "current practice" or "review" articles often provide good summaries of state-of-the-art diagnosis and treatment. (For information on finding medical information, see the July 1995 issue of *WHA*.) Keep copies of all documentation in case you need to file written complaints later.

3 **Try negotiating.** Try proposing a time frame for reevaluating your condition—for instance, "If this pain hasn't gone away by next Monday, I would like to come back in for further tests."

4 **Call their bluff.** Tell the doctor that you plan to file an appeal. Ask, "Do you really want me to take this step?" or "Do you think this is the best way for me to proceed?" If you like, you can raise the issue of financial incentives—"I understand that some organizations offer incentives for limiting care. Is that what's going on here?"—but don't expect a cordial response.

5 **Be stubborn.** Demand, in no uncertain terms, to be given access to the doctor or care that you need. If you're still rebuffed, get the person to put the denial in writing.

6 **File a complaint.** By law, HMOs must have an appeals process, and they must tell you how to proceed with a formal appeal. The plan may have a hot line you can call; if not, check with the member services department.

When you begin, be aware that you're likely to run up against the very person who denied you coverage in the first place.

If the dispute can't be resolved over the phone, prepare a written appeal. Be sure to follow the plan's rules exactly.

If you have a good working relationship with your HMO doctor—and the doctor isn't bound by rules barring this step—ask him or her to support you in your appeal. The physician should write a letter stating that he or she deems the treatment medically necessary.

As you prepare your appeal, provide full documentation—names, dates, stated reasons for refusal, details about your condition, and copies of relevant professional articles to support your position.

7 **Do an end run.** If you can afford to, go outside of your plan for a second opinion. Ask this doctor to write a letter stating the details and medical necessity of the care. Send copies to your doctor within the HMO, to the HMO's medical director, and to the plan's president.

8 **Tell the state.** File a complaint with the state insurance department (see "Resources"). Remember, HMOs are insurance companies that provide health care. As a result, they

are governed by the state insurance department. (In some states, a special division of the state health department is the governing body.) Provide all the documentation noted above plus a record of how you have tried to resolve the problem.

9 Tell your employer. If you're covered through work, inform your company's benefits manager. Even if this person can't step in, complaints can serve notice that the company needs to find another HMO, especially if a number of employees are involved.

10 Tell your legislator. Oversight of managed care is a hot topic at both the state and federal level, so take advantage of this momentum.

Above all, remember these basics:

- **Keep track.** Be meticulous about documenting everything—who, what, and when. Keep copies of all letters and any supporting documentation. Use registered mail.

- **Keep your cool.** Your rage may be completely justified, but don't unleash it on a harried physician or hapless clerk. You want these people to be absolutely clear about what you need in terms of information or behavior—and you want them to cooperate with you.

- **Keep the pressure on.** Don't accept indefinite promises to "look into things." Pin the person down—"When will you get back to me?"—and follow up, both on the phone and in writing.

Resources:
How to Find the Best Doctors, Hospitals, and HMOs for You and Your Family (New York: Castle Connolly Medical Ltd., 1995). This comprehensive guide includes extensive appendices with addresses and phone numbers of state insurance departments, medical specialty boards, and more.

Buyer Beware

If you have a choice in plans, here are some questions to consider:

- Are the physicians board-certified? As a general rule, a higher proportion of board-certified doctors means better-quality care.

- How does the plan rate in such areas as consumer satisfaction and physician turnover? How many complaints have been filed against the plan? (See "Resources.")

- How are the doctors paid? Some are paid a discounted fee for services rendered. Others are *capitated*—that is, paid a flat fee per plan member per month (also known as "PMPM" in HMO lingo). Under this system, the doctor is paid whether or not you walk through the door.

Employers and the government love capitation because it makes health care costs predictable. However, critics charge that capitation provides an incentive for the physician to skimp on treatment or tests. That's especially true if the physician is both *capitated* and *at risk*—in this instance, the doctor must pay for any costs of treatment that exceed the capitation fee out of his or her own pocket. (Some doctors have "stop-loss" insurance, which covers part of these costs.)

- Is the list of participating physicians up to date? It's up to you to confirm that any physician you're interested in is still with the plan and accepting new patients.

- What's the policy on referrals and preauthorizations? For instance, what kind of approval is needed before you can be hospitalized? How easy is it to be referred to a specialist, especially if you have a chronic condition? What about referrals to gynecologists? Are there any other restrictions placed on access to specialists? For instance, in some plans, a specialist may be able to treat you only if you live in the county in which he or she practices.

- How easy is it to change doctors within the plan?

- Do you have the option of going outside of the network to see a physician? (Such arrangements are known as "point-of-service" plans and usually require you to pay a greater portion of the cost.)

- What hospital is the plan affiliated with? A community hospital is fine, but you'll also want access to a university or teaching hospital.

- What is and isn't covered? For instance, what's covered under preventive health? What about emergency care, after-hours care, and coverage while you're traveling? If you take a particular drug, is it covered? And what about other options that are important to you, such as infertility treatments, mental health benefits, home health care, physical therapy, or alternative treatments such as acupuncture?

Some consumer advocates advise thinking of "worst-case" scenarios. For instance, do you have a family history of a particular illness? If you developed that illness, what would be covered?

- What treatments aren't covered because they're deemed experimental? "Experimental" can mean different things to different health plans.

- What kind of appeals process does the HMO have? By law, you have the right to file an appeal. Thus, if a plan can't give you a clear explanation of its appeals process, be suspicious.

More Research, More Profits, More Conflict

By LAURA MANSNERUS

NEVER before have women meant so much to so many. Recognized as the health care system's biggest customers, they are being treated as such: researched and marketed to, tracked and talked about.

Consider: Premarin, an estrogen replacement, is the most widely used prescription drug in the United States. From 1991 to 1992, the number of hospitals with a women's health center rose 19 percent, according to a survey by the American Hospital Association. In many cities, Atlanta and Dallas among them, hospitals are competing for pregnant Medicaid patients; among the lures are free Disney movies for the older children, infant car seats, baby showers, insulated beverage flasks and monogrammed blankets.

Even the women who coalesced 30 years ago into something loosely called the women's health movement are struck by the mix of responsive medicine and commercial grasping that the 1990's have delivered. It is both more and less than these mothers of intervention bargained for.

"As a lasting legacy of the women's movement, health care is one of our shining moments," said Dr. Susan Reverby, a professor of women's studies at Wellesley College, who recently served on an obstetrics and gynecology advisory panel for the Federal Food and Drug Administration.

While acknowledging that "the health care system is relentless in its ability to figure out where the next buck is coming from," Ms. Reverby said the medical profession had become more aware of women's concerns, especially those beyond the gynecologic. "There's much more consciousness about what women's issues are," she said. "We can now talk about heart disease and about AIDS."

But not all women applaud the results of that new consciousness.

Rachel Fruchter, an associate professor of obstetrics and gynecology at the State University of New York Health Science Center in Brooklyn, said she was appalled that women were pursued so avidly as consumers, particularly by pharmaceutical companies whose advertisements picture radiant middle-aged women and counsel, "Ask your doctor."

"The pretense that that's what the women's health movement wanted is a bad joke," Ms. Fruchter said.

In the beginning, the women's health movement talked mostly about abortion and contraceptives. But as its baby boomer leaders have reached the age of influence—and the age of menopause—the health concerns of older generations have taken on new urgency. That urgency is also fueled by the fact that women are living longer—on average, more than seven years longer than men—

WHAT WOMEN SAY: FROM A NEW YORK TIMES / CBS NEWS POLL

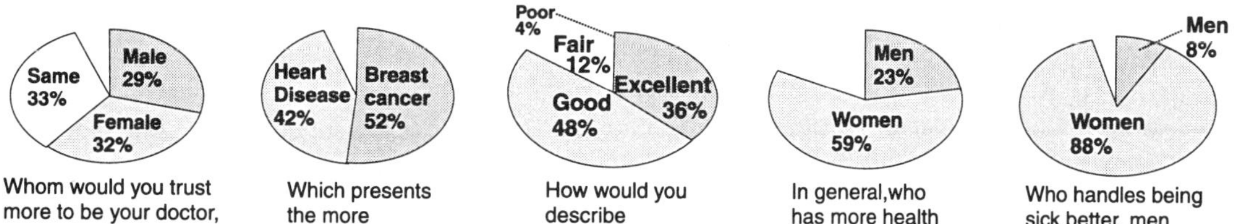

Whom would you trust more to be your doctor, a man or a woman? | Which presents the more serious risk? | How would you describe your health? | In general, who has more health problems? | Who handles being sick better, men or women?

and are thus suffering from the crippling diseases of old age, like arthritis and osteoporosis.

At the same time, women have not just been complaining about doctors but have been becoming doctors. The influx has made female patients happier and helped bring new emphasis to the doctor's role as interviewer, said Dr. Charlea Massion, a family doctor at the Santa Cruz Medical Center in California and a clinical faculty member at Stanford University.

"Women physicians do have, and linguistic studies show this, a different way of communicating," Dr. Massion said, adding: "I don't think women physicians are necessarily interested in women's health just by being women, and I don't think women physicians are more open-minded or have a more comprehensive approach just because they are women. But most of the innovative thinking that's being done in health care is being done by women."

That does not mean that women believe they are being well served.

Like many of the other early participants in the women's health movement, Ms. Fruchter views the issue as a matter of social justice. She noted that many women cannot afford the health care that is being urged upon them.

She said that she addressed Brooklyn community groups and churches on cancer screening but that many of the women she saw could not pay for it: they are the working poor, not insured by employers and not old enough to qualify for Medicare. And they have an array of health problems.

"They say breast cancer is important," Ms. Fruchter said, "but there are other things. What about their blood pressure, their diabetes, their disabled child?"

Much of the attention to women is undeniably genuine, even if it feeds advertising campaigns. Federal funds for breast cancer exceeded $600 billion in the current fiscal year, up from $90 billion in 1990. The National Institutes of Health, the source and overseer of money for most of the nation's biomedical research, established an Office of Research on Women's Health in 1990 and has undertaken two huge studies of heart disease and cancer among women.

A half-dozen new medical journals on women's health have sprung up in the same period. But even these cannot contain the academic attention: while a survey of Medline, a data base of medical journal articles, turned up 159 entries under the heading "women's health" from 1986 through 1991, it found 1,426 entries from 1992 through 1996.

Some scholars argue that men are now being slighted by researchers.

Still, women's health remains a fractious business. Even some of the most commonplace decisions women make—yearly mammograms for 40-somethings? hormones for 50-somethings?—are subject to wild disagreement.

Many women say that focusing on disease and treatment misses the point. "It's easier to prescribe a pill than to address the precarious economic status of women," said Dr. Judith G. Gonyea, a professor of social work at Boston University who specializes in women and aging. "People's health is about their housing, their nutrition, about feeling socially connected, which all may have a much greater bearing on their physical health status than their level of estrogen does."

In research, especially, the line between science and politics has been tested in the debate over whether women have been shortchanged.

"There's a perception that women and their diseases have been studied less than men," said Dr. Curtis L. Meinert, an epidemiology professor at the Johns Hopkins University who specializes in clinical trials. "That's so totally dead wrong it's painful."

When they surveyed research published from 1980 to 1993, Dr. Meinert and two colleagues, both of them women, found that the number of projects studying just men and the number studying just women were virtually equal.

In public research dollars spent, it does not seem that women have been slighted. In 1996, the last year for which figures are available, 16 percent of National Institutes of Health funds went to study diseases exclusive to women, 5.7 percent to diseases exclusive to men and 78.3 percent to diseases afflicting both. A decade ago, when the first breakdown by sex was calculated, the figures were 13.5 percent, 6.5 percent and 80 percent. And on a per-fatality basis, the National Cancer Institute spends much more on cancers that afflict only women than it does on prostate cancer.

Some researchers say age is more important than sex in determining where the money goes. Compare, for example, the hundreds of millions of dollars spent on breast cancer, which strikes many women in the prime of life, with the much smaller sum spent on prostate cancer, a disease of elderly men.

But Dr. Vivian Pinn, the director of the N.I.H. Office Research on Women's Health, said: "Budget figures can fool you. You have to figure out where you have gaps in knowledge, and we know there are great gaps of knowledge in women's health."

The sharpest contention centers on introducing a form of affirmative action in clinical trials of new drugs and treatments for both men and women. Though the N.I.H. prodded researchers to include women in more clinical trials in the 1980's, the General Accounting Office reported in 1990 that the policy was often ignored. Then in 1993, Congress mandated the inclusion of women in most trials in numbers sufficient to analyze sex differences in the way a disease and its treatment play themselves out.

Many researchers resented the intrusion—the phrases "research by quota" and "politically correct trials" were invoked—and argued that in many trials, including enough women to yield reliable comparisons would be prohibitively expensive.

Cardiovascular disease raises especially perplexing questions. Because its incidence during middle age is so much higher in men, any clinical trial requires many more female than male subjects to assess risk factors and treatments for women—and more still to analyze the differences between men and women.

That is why, researchers say, they have focused on men. But when women reach their 70's, their risk of cardiovascular disease rises sharply. Yet a lack of data makes it unclear whether they respond to preventive measures and treatments in the same way that men do.

Some epidemiologists, like Dr. Meinert, maintain that in terms of most diseases and treatments, women do not differ significantly from men, so including women in most clinical trials is unlikely to produce useful information. Others respond that this issue is, at the least, woefully underinvestigated.

Some women contend that sex differences are important and complicated enough to warrant a new specialty—women's medicine—analogous to pediatrics or geriatrics. "We're not talking about lady doctors delivering medical care to lady patients," said Dr. Eileen Hoffman, a co-director of the women's health program at Mount Sinai Medical Center in New York. "We're talking about an art and science that's focused on the female."

"Female," in Dr. Hoffman's view, is a distinction that applies at every physiological level, down to the cellular, and should not be the province of obstetrics and gynecology alone. Besides, she added, "medicine only takes something seriously when it occupies an official space in the academic hierarchy."

Dr. Hoffman and other doctors and researchers have formed the American College of Women's Health Physicians, which is working toward recognition as a new specialty. But not without opposition. Many women argue that anything labeled "women's medicine" is unnecessary and, worse, bound to be marginalized.

"My response," Dr. Hoffman said, "is that women's health has already been marginalized by ob-gyn. Many women in this country only see a gynecologist for care. But lung cancer is the leading cause of cancer death in women, and heart disease kills 10 times more women than breast cancer."

To some, the notion that women have been underserved by American medicine is amazing. In a 1995 article in The Atlantic Monthly, Dr. Andrew G. Kadar, an anesthesiologist on the clinical faculty of the University of California at Los Angeles, wrote that if either sex needs better health care, it is the men.

"There is no question that women seek out medical attention more," Dr. Kadar said in an interview. "Whether they are less healthy is another issue and much more difficult to sort out, especially since there are diseases that keep you from feeling your best but don't shorten your life expectancy."

A better measure of health, he said, is mortality rates, reflected in the 7.5-year gap between men's and women's life spans. "You can't get any sicker than dead," he said.

But the trends in women's health care are likely to be determined more by market imperatives than by medicine or politics. "We made people aware of how health care works," Ms. Reverby said. "We couldn't control the economics of it." Neither, to their dismay, could doctors.

The march of managed care, most public health experts say, is good news and bad news for women.

"Women want respect; they want choices; they want preventive care," said Sally Rynne, a health care consultant in Evanston, Ill. "That's what women have clamored for." And the intent today, Ms. Rynne said, is to get people to take care of themselves because it is cost-effective.

"The other side of that," she said, "is, Are women going to be denied certain procedures or treatments that they feel they really need? That's the dance we're in right now."

Managed care also means that patients spend less time with doctors, though surveys consistently show that women prize such time. Health care providers have tried to address the problem by offering women's centers, which join specialists under one roof and use nurses and physicians' assistants to help coordinate medical care.

"Right now, it's a big marketing attempt," Dr. Hoffman said. "Let's be clear about that."

But the centers are hugely popular. "Women love them" said Dr. Carol Weisman, a professor and health services researcher in the Johns Hopkins University School of Public Health who has surveyed women's health centers nationwide.

Whether the clinics provide better care, Dr. Weisman said, is a separate question, and an all-but-unexamined one. It is not clear that any attempts to make medicine more responsive to women have brought measurable results. Regard[less] of whether the big push in research will lead to big advances in treatment, no answers are expected in this century.

Plenty of people are working on it, though. So far this year, Medline lists more than 80 articles under "women's health." There is no heading for "men's health."

There is no women's health crisis

SALLY L. SATEL

IN 1993, First Lady Hillary Clinton rather dramatically remarked upon "the appalling degree to which women were routinely excluded from major clinical trials of most illnesses." Or as Secretary of Health and Human Services Donna Shalala sweepingly put it: "Women have good reason to be cynical about whether this country cares about women's health." These sentiments are shared by an army of special interest groups that lobby Congress on behalf of what has become known as women's health. Active participants in this campaign include the Society for Advancement of Women's Health Research, which has collaborated extensively with the Congressional Women's Caucus, the Center for Women's Policy Studies, the National Women's Health Network, Jacobs Institute of Women's Health, the American College of Women's Health Physicians, and even Hadassah, the old and venerable Jewish women's organization.

The understanding that biomedical research focuses more on the health problems of men is one reason the Department of Health and Human Services (HHS), the Centers for Disease Control (CDC), the Food and Drug Administration (FDA), and the National Institutes of Health (NIH) have created special offices for women's health; five state governments now have their own offices, as well. In addition, both the NIH and the FDA have been criticized for inattention to women's health. Federal law now mandates that all NIH-funded clinical research include women, and the FDA is currently considering a rule to do so.

It was against this backdrop that the heated mammogram debate took place in Congress last February. In the crossfire was an independent panel convened by the NIH that advised women in their forties to decide for themselves, with advice of their doctors, whether to get breast X-rays. Given the high rates of false-positive mammogram results, leading some women to undergo needless surgery, and the negligible reduction in

Reprinted with permission of the author from *The Public Interest,* No. 130, Winter 1998, pp. 21-33.

mortality associated with screening of women in their forties, the panel concluded that a universal recommendation for annual or biannual mammography was unwarranted. Senator Olympia Snowe nevertheless introduced a non-binding resolution in favor of mammography for women in their forties. With a vote of 98 to 0, Congress brazenly called on the National Cancer Institute of the NIH to issue its own recommendation in favor of regular mammography for women in their forties. One month later, it did.

Predating the mammogram debate by a few months was the passage of the Newborns' and Mothers' Health Protection Act requiring health plans to provide a minimum hospital stay of 48 hours following a non-surgical delivery. This popular initiative was followed by the introduction of the Women's Health and Cancer Rights Act, which would make "drive-by" mastectomies illegal. And, in July of 1997, Senator Barbara Boxer introduced the Women's Cardiovascular Diseases Research and Prevention Act. Representative Maxine Waters submitted a companion bill in the House. The bill authorizes $140 million to the National Heart, Lung, and Blood Institute (NHLBI) of the NIH to "draw resources to cardiovascular disease which strikes so many of our grandmothers, mothers, aunts and daughters," the Senator's press office said.

The problem with all this activity is that it was partly driven by a false assumption about the status of women's health. The fact is that it is far from appalling. Not only are women well represented as subjects in clinical research but their diseases are now getting more attention than men's. Furthermore, historical claims that researchers discounted women's health and routinely excluded them from study are overstated. The evidence, which follows, indicates that women have long been regularly represented in medical research. Sometimes, they have been overrepresented.

Perceiving underrepresentation

The current focus on women's representation in biomedical research began in the 1980s. A 1981 paper in the *Annals of Internal Medicine*, titled "Underrepresentation of Women in New Drug Trials," called attention to the FDA policy of barring pregnant women and those of childbearing potential from participating in drug-safety tests (an exception was granted if the woman had a life-threatening illness). Then, in 1985, the U.S. Public Health Service produced the much publicized *Task Force Report on Women's Health Issues*. To redress "gender bias in research," the report called for "expansion of research to ensure emphasis on conditions and diseases unique to, or more prevalent in, women in all age groups." It highlighted many areas requiring further clinical knowledge, including cancers of the breast and reproductive system, sexually transmitted diseases, osteoporosis, arthritic conditions, and certain mental disorders, including depression, late onset schizophrenia, and alcoholism. Hormonal therapy for pre- and post-menopausal symptoms and the afflictions of older women were also emphasized. In response to the report, the NIH devised a policy in 1986 urging all researchers to include women in clinical research and to evaluate any sex differences in response to treatment. However, it did not publish guidance for its implementation until 1989.

In the spring of 1990, the General Accounting Office (GAO) released its report, "Problems in Implementing Policy on Women in Study Populations." Requested by Representative Henry Waxman, the GAO report concluded, "NIH made little progress in implementing its (1986) policy to encourage the inclusion of women in research study populations." The report also pointed out that the NIH continued to receive grant applications for all-male studies, as well as applications that failed to mention how many men and women would be included in the study, and others that provided no information on the sex of the study population. As a result, the GAO said, "It is impossible to determine the impact of the [inclusion] policy."

In the fall of 1990, due largely to the inconclusive findings of the GAO report, the NIH created the Office of Research on Women's Health (ORWH), whose mandate was to track compliance with agency guidelines that required female access to trials and to ensure that the NIH "adequately addresses issues regarding women's health." Early on, ORWH commissioned the National Academy of Sciences' Institute of Medicine to study, among other things, the ethical implications of including pregnant and fertile women in clinical trials. Although the Institute of Medicine (IOM) was not specifically asked to explore the more general topic of women's inclusion in clinical trials, a large portion of its 1994 report, *Women and Health Research*, examined that subject in depth: It found no evidence of systematic exclusion of women from treatment trials. As Ruth Faden, co-chair of the IOM report committee, said, "The one thing the [IOM report] committee failed to nail down was the truth of the perception that women have been underrepresented."

By 1993, women's health became an unprecedented subject of legislation—still, despite the fact that there was little evidence of gender bias. Public Law 103-43, the NIH Revitalization Act of 1993, mandated that government-funded clinical researchers include women in their clinical research. The law specifically required that "women [be] included as subjects in each project of research" and that trials be "designed and carried out in a manner sufficient to provide for a valid analysis of whether the variables being studied ... affect women ... differently than other [male] subjects."

When women were excluded

The three issues that have sparked criticism of the research establishment are: (1) that pregnant and fertile women were excluded by the FDA from determinations of drug safety; (2)

that women were omitted from early key studies on cardiac disease and AIDS; and (3) that, even when women were included, researchers failed to determine whether their responses to drugs differed from men's.

Consider the first issue—that the FDA unwisely and unfairly excluded pregnant and fertile women from participating in the toxicity testing of pharmaceuticals. This refers to a 1977 policy (since withdrawn) that evolved in the wake of birth-defect tragedies associated with thalidomide and diethylstilbestrol (DES). Women were excluded from the so-called Phase I and II clinical trials, the small-scale safety-testing phases of pharmaceutical trials, to protect the fetus and, to some extent, to avoid liability. But critics argued that, unless fertile and pregnant women were studied, there was no way to detect potentially harmful fetal effects. After all, an all-male study on a drug with fetal toxicity certainly would not shield the manufacturer from liability; it would merely delay legal repercussions until women who took the drug began having deformed babies. Furthermore, FDA critics argued that such a policy smacked of paternalism: A woman well-informed about the risks of participating in research, they said, should be allowed to make her own decision. These are reasonable objections, but to charge that the FDA's exclusion policy was rooted in lack of interest in women is unfounded.

The second observation involved women's inclusion in clinical trials that test the effectiveness of various drugs—the step following safety testing. These are also called late Phase II and Phase III trials. Here, a number of omissions did occur, documented most thoroughly by the 1994 IOM study. Looking mainly at large-scale government-funded studies, the IOM identified the 1958 Baltimore Longitudinal Study of Aging (BLSA) as the earliest example of women's exclusion. Although the NIH-funded BLSA was not a clinical trial—it was an observational study of diseases of aging—its failure to include women was striking, especially in light of women's disproportionate representation among the elderly. In 1978, women were added to the study. They have been there ever since.

Regarding female omission from other NIH-funded clinical trials, the IOM identified two areas: studies of intervention for heart disease and AIDS. Several specific studies of heart disease were singled out for excluding women, including: the Multiple Risk Factor Intervention Trial (MFRIT), Lipid Research Clinics Coronary Primary Prevention Trial (CPPT), and the Coronary Drug Project. Initiated 20 to 30 years ago, these studies evaluated the roles of diet, salt restriction, blood-pressure medication, weight reduction, smoking cessation, and cholesterol-lowering drugs on the development and course of heart disease in men. In 1981, the Physician's Health Study examined whether daily aspirin and beta carotene (a precursor of Vitamin A) influenced the development of heart disease and cancer also exclusively in men.

Another concern was whether the findings of clinical research can be generalized. Thus, when the Physician's Health Study mentioned above found that aspirin did indeed cut men's risk of heart disease, women's health advocates noted that this information was not useful to them because it was derived from a study based on male physiology. But even when women had been included in trials, their numbers were sometimes too small to detect whether they responded to medications differently from men. While technically true, these observations have been misconstrued as evidence of callous disregard for women's health.

Just the facts, ma'am

The reality is that women as a group are not discriminated against in medical research. According to the Office of Research on Women's Health at the NIH, women represented 52 percent of the more than one-million participants in NIH-funded research in 1994 (the most recent statistics). And women were six times more likely than men to be the subjects of single-gender studies. The NHLBI, which is largely devoted to the study of heart disease, reports that every one of its 60 trials active in 1996 included women. Eleven were women only; none were male only. As early as 1979, according to NIH, 268 of the 293 active clinical trials involved males and females; of the remainder, 13 were all-female, 12 all-male.

Today, one could safely make the claim that women are actually favored in the allocation of research dollars. Breast-cancer research, for example, has received more money than any other type of cancer research each year since 1985, when the National Cancer Institute began keeping track of disease-specific funding. (Notably, it is lung, not breast, cancer that is the biggest cancer killer in women.) And breast cancer has always received many times the funding of prostate cancer, about 5 times more in 1997. This is the case even though more men get prostate cancer than women get breast cancer (however, slightly more women die of their disease than men of theirs, and some of these women die at a young age).

The Women's Health Initiative, begun in 1991, is another instance of the government's and the medical community's interest in women's health. It examines preventive effects of hormone-replacement therapy, calcium and vitamin D supplements, and diet modification on osteoporosis, cancer, and cardiovascular disease in post-menopausal women. At $625 million over 14 years, it is the most expensive and ambitious NIH trial ever funded. Lastly, exclusive women's diseases (e.g., reproductive cancer, menopause-related problems) receive fully 14 percent of the clinical-research budget.

Despite these expenditures, the Society for the Advancement of Women's Health Research (SAWHR) decries the fact that "only 52% of the population receives barely 14% of federal health research funding." Apparently, SAWHR counts as benefiting females only the portion of the NIH's research budget earmarked for diseases of women—not the great mass of research on human health generally. Indeed, less than 10 percent goes to clinical research on all-male diseases like male reproductive cancers (and even some of the research on hormonal treatment for prostate cancer may be applicable to breast cancer and visa versa). That means that at least 75 percent goes to diseases that affect both sexes. Thus, more accurately, 52 percent of the population benefits from 90 percent of the research budget.

Women in the journals

The representation of women in medical publications and studies also appears robust. Johns Hopkins University researchers Adele Gilpin and Curtis Meinert conducted an exhaustive analysis of all published clinical trials (over 15,000 of them between 1983 and 1993) reported in English-language medical journals and listed in the Abbreviated Index Medicus. They found that women were included in 60 percent to 70 percent of all studies over that decade. (About 20 percent of the journal articles failed to identify the sex of the subjects.)

For such diseases as depression, osteoporosis, and arthritis, women have been studied more than men. This should come as no surprise, since physicians tend to study the group most at risk. Arthritis, for example, is at least twice as prevalent in women. And women thus represented 69 percent of all subjects in FDA-required tests of newly approved anti-inflammatory drugs (intended for arthritis) in 1988.

Similarly, osteoporosis mainly afflicts women. A review of the three leading medical journals, the *New England Journal of Medicine, Journal of the American Medical Association*, and *Annals of Internal Medicine,* reveals that 116 articles on characterization and treatment of osteoporosis in women had appeared between 1978 and 1988. The 20 percent of osteoporosis cases that are male must draw upon these female-only studies. FDA surveys from 1983 and 1988 found that "women represented a majority of patients ... in data bases of drugs used to treat conditions more common in women (or more commonly treated) such as arthritis." And, even when women were less likely to suffer a condition, they still comprised a sizable minority of subjects, about 30 percent or more, in clinical trials testing medications for those conditions.

Chloe E. Bird of the Harvard School of Public Health surveyed all clinical trials published in the *Journal of the American Medical Association* in 1990 and 1992 and found that 17 percent of studies had no women and 32 percent had one-third or fewer women. The male-only studies tended to be the ones conducted where mostly men were found—in Veterans Affairs Hospitals, the armed services, and prisons. Or they were the studies concerned with male-specific diseases. Trials with fewer than one-third women were mostly concerned with conditions predominantly found in men.

How research works

When women are omitted from clinical trials, it is generally for two reasons: Either they were not known to be at risk for a particular illness at the time the research was conducted, or they possessed clinical characteristics that made them difficult and expensive to study.

Early clinical trials involving patients with HIV and AIDS fall into the first category. In the early 1980s, homosexual men were the only group identified by the CDC as being at risk. But, as it became clear that women were also at risk for HIV/AIDS, they were recruited into clinical trials. In 1986, for example, only 2 percent of subjects in clinical trials were women; by 1992, over 18 percent were women; today, they make up a little over 30 percent of NIH-funded AIDS clinical trials, twice their 15 percent representation among all AIDS cases. According to Wanda Jones of the Office of Women's Health at the CDC, "women-friendly" trial sites that offer child care and transportation are able to recruit participants without much trouble.

Failure to recognize that women were at risk for cardiac disease, especially heart attack, also explains their absence from the large NIH-funded trials mentioned earlier. Ironically, researchers gained this impression from early analyses of the first major federally funded cardiac study, the Framingham study. Begun in 1948 (and still active), fully 55 percent of its subjects were women. While we now know that women are stricken with heart attack—though about 20 years later than men—the women in the Framingham study were all under 68 years old. As a cohort, they had barely entered the phase of risk that begins around that age. Had the early Framingham women been followed for a longer period of time, however, their vulnerability to heart attack would have become obvious. (By contrast, risk for high blood pressure was long recognized as afflicting both men and women of middle age, and thus women were routinely included in NIH-funded trials on treatment for high blood pressure, most notably the large 1973 Hypertension Detection and Follow-up Study, funded by NHLBI, which enrolled more women than men.)

Based on the early Framingham results, initial spin-off studies on heart disease did not include women. The Coronary Drug Project (CDP), designed in the early 1960s, looked at the benefit of cholesterol-lowering drugs in people under 65 with a prior history of heart attack. By the early 1970s, when a number of large-scale cardiac studies were launched, researchers and physicians were beginning to recognize that women were indeed at risk for heart attack. Yet, women were still excluded from the large Multiple Risk Factor Intervention Trial (MRFIT) and the Lipid Research Clinics-CPPT. These analyzed subjects between the ages of 37 and 57, and 37 and 59, respectively, periods of the life cycle when women rarely develop heart disease. Why didn't these studies include older subjects?

One reason is that older subjects are harder to study. Since women tend to be older when they manifest heart disease, they are more likely to suffer additional age-related illnesses, for which they take other medications. These variables—concomitant illness plus medications—make it difficult to assess the impact of the medication being studied. Also, the elderly subjects are sometimes too frail to tolerate the study procedure itself; this was the case with treatment trials of angina (cardiac-related chest pain), which usually require vigorous treadmill exercise tests. A 1992 article in the *Journal of the American Medical Association* by J. H. Gurwitz and co-workers, "The Exclusion of the Elderly and Women from Clinical Trials in Acute Myocardial Infarction," captured the phenomenon nicely. In reviewing trials from 1960 to 1991, the authors found that over 60 percent of the trials excluded people over age 75. They concluded that age, not sex, determined who was enrolled.

Other reasons for excluding women are convenience and expense. In the 1981 Physicians Health Study (PHS), which included subjects up to age 84, a pragmatic decision was made to include only male physicians. Physicians were selected as the study population because of their likely high rate of compliance with the self-administered protocol. Male physicians in particular were selected because very few female doctors (about one for every 10 males) were old enough to be at risk for heart disease when the trial began. To study only young female doctors would have meant either enrolling many more subjects (to enhance the chances of "catching" the few at risk) or observing them for a longer period of time than male enrollees. Consider this fact too: about 260,000 male physicians were screened for inclusion in the PHS study in order to recruit the 22,000 who actually entered. Had the study been performed on women, according to the NHLBI, the number of subjects screened, and then randomized to the placebo and active arms of the trial, would have had to be three times as large—and the study at least three times as expensive—in order to obtain the same magnitude of results found in the men. The same was true of the MRFIT and Lipid Research Clinics-CPPT.

Advocates took these omissions as evidence of the devaluation of women's health. More accurately, they simply reflect the way research legitimately proceeds: Researchers first study the group most at risk or the group least medically complicated. This allows for control of as many variables as possible. The findings gleaned will determine whether future testing, in women (as well as older men), is warranted. After all, as Curtis Meinert of Johns Hopkins wrote in the journal *Science*, "There is no point in worrying about whether a treatment works the same or differently in men and women until it has been shown to work in someone." And once shown to work in men, treatments are studied for their effectiveness in older women. Indeed, a 1983 FDA survey revealed that cardiac trials with patients over 70 years old contained as many women as men.

Inclusion for inclusion's sake

As of 1993, the FDA strongly recommended, and the NIH required, that adequate numbers of women be used in trials in order to conduct what is called a "subgroup gender analysis"; that is, to assess how well a drug works in women compared to men. The problem with subgroup analysis, a kind of statistical test, is that it requires a bigger total sample—and a more costly study—than simply assessing the degree of a drug's effectiveness, relative to a placebo, in male and female subjects. More important, the expense of an inclusion-for-inclusion's-sake approach may not always be justified since men and women tend to respond similarly to most medications.

Indeed, doctors have been successfully extrapolating from women to men in the treatment of a number of conditions, such as osteoporosis, rheumatoid arthritis, breast cancer, and eating disorders. Consider the recent report in the journal *Circulation* that warned about the cardiac risks of second-hand smoke. The data were based on an all-female sample, the Nurses Health Study. On careful reading, the study's conclusions don't stand up—the design was too weak to discern a correlation. But the key point here is that neither the Harvard researchers who conducted the study nor anyone else shied away from applying the study's findings of the risk of second-hand-smoke exposure beyond women to men.

This is not to say that meaningful sex differences don't exist. Hormonal fluctuations of the menstrual cycle and menopause, as well as the use of oral contraceptives, may interfere with the effectiveness of medications. Often such interactions can be determined biochemically in the laboratory using a blood sample, though sometimes clinical studies may be needed. The question, of course, is the clinical relevance of these interactions. Epidemiologist Janet Holbrook of Johns Hopkins University, intrigued by the increasing emphasis on finding gender differences in treatment response, examined published reports of multi-center clinical trials between the years 1990 and 1994. All trials were large enough to include both men and women in adequate numbers to detect a difference if it existed. Interestingly, 78 percent of trials in her sample were both gender, 18 percent of trials were female only, and 4 percent male only. Among the two-gender studies that showed a treatment effect, Holbrook found no subgroup differences based on sex.

Perhaps this is because the physiological differences between men and women don't always translate into meaningful clinical effects. Leslie Z. Benet, chairman of the Department of Pharmacy at the University of California, San Francisco, writes, "'Will differences in drug response due to gender be clinically significant?' My answer is, 'Rarely if ever.'" Furthermore, physicians tailor the medication dose to the patient; sometimes this is a function of body mass and kidney function; other times—as when medicating for mania or psychosis—dosage is based on intensity of symptoms and then lowered if side effects are too uncomfortable. Either way, patients generally end up on individualized, empirical dosing schedules that don't rely on a set formula derived from gender-comparison research. In the case of drugs that are therapeutic at one dose, but toxic at a slightly higher dose (narrow therapeutic index), meticulous personalized dosing can be lifesaving. According to Benet, in situations where there is a large discrepancy between positive effect and toxicity (broad index), "the variability in the male population most likely already encompasses the difference between the male and female population."

Assuredly, there is more to know about the treatment of diseases in women. We need to know more about the way natural hormones, contraceptives, and replacement hormones affect other medications women may take. Increasingly, there is evidence that pre- and post-menopausal women may metabolize drugs differently. And we need to know more about the symptoms of heart disease in women and better ways to interpret diagnostic tests for chest pain. But it is wrongheaded to confuse the need to know more—an imperative that will always be with us—with the notion that women are second-class subjects of medical research. Such confusion leads to an agenda of inclusion for inclusion's sake and, in the end, will divert precious dollars from medical research that could benefit us all.

Unit 2

Unit Selections

Key Points to Consider

- What are the factors that influence women's view of their bodies? What role does culture play in these factors?

- Many people seek out quick fixes for health problems. What impact does this view have on long-term weight and health status?

- Nutritional information can be very confusing. Summarize the current recommendations in a form that can be easily understood and implemented.

- Exercise (or activity) has a number of physical and psychological benefits. What are these and how can they be integrated into your lifestyle?

- The image of the "ideal" woman has changed over time. Describe some of the past views of the ideal woman and how they compare with the present view. Are any of them more realistic?

DUSHKINONLINE Links

www.dushkin.com/online/

11. **FitnessLink: The Health and Fitness Source**
    http://www.fitnesslink.com
12. **Food and Nutrition Information Center**
    http://www.nal.usda.gov/fnic/
13. **Mayo Clinic Diet & Nutrition Resurce Center**
    http://www.mayo.ivi.com/mayo/common/htm/dietpage.htm

These sites are annotated on pages 4 and 5.

Nutrition and Fitness

The United States has a national obsession with thinness, which is particularly focused on women. Until very recently, the hot look for female fashion models was an emaciated thinness, achievable only by those on drugs or with severe eating disorders. At the same time, as a country we are heavier than ever. We also suffer from a variety of chronic diseases (which will be discussed in more detail in a later unit) that are caused by or influence by our nutritional and fitness behavior.

Our decision to pair these issues is based on the belief that, as we look at the role of each in women's health, they cannot be separated. We also note that the new generation of diet pills provides yet another "quick fix," which may have unintended consequences.

As Laura Fraser points out in "Say Good-bye to Dieting," the thinness many women strive for can, in fact, cause ill health. The focus on "dieting" as opposed to healthy eating leads many women to choose behaviors that are both physically and psychologically dangerous. Exercise can help to provide the balance between a need to feel good and to eat a well-balanced diet.

In "Who *Isn't* on a Diet?" Michelle Stacy discusses the historical changes that have lead us to a point where "normal" for American women means to be concerned about food and weight. In fact, it could be argued that most American women demonstrate some level of disordered thinking about food.

Several articles address the balance between diet and exercise. These include "How Far Should You Go to Stay Fit?" and "Fat Chances." In "Dying to Be Thin," the author examines the deadly consequences of eating disorders.

Finally, the highly medicalized state of our culture and the desire for quick fixes has led many women to seek a pill that will provide a quick-fix weight loss. "Diet Drugs: As Fen-Phen Alternatives Emerge, Safety Questions Go Unanswered" examines the newest generation of pills designed to promote weight loss. While many people see these drugs as a panacea, the article points out that they can have serious consequences and that all the side effects are not yet known.

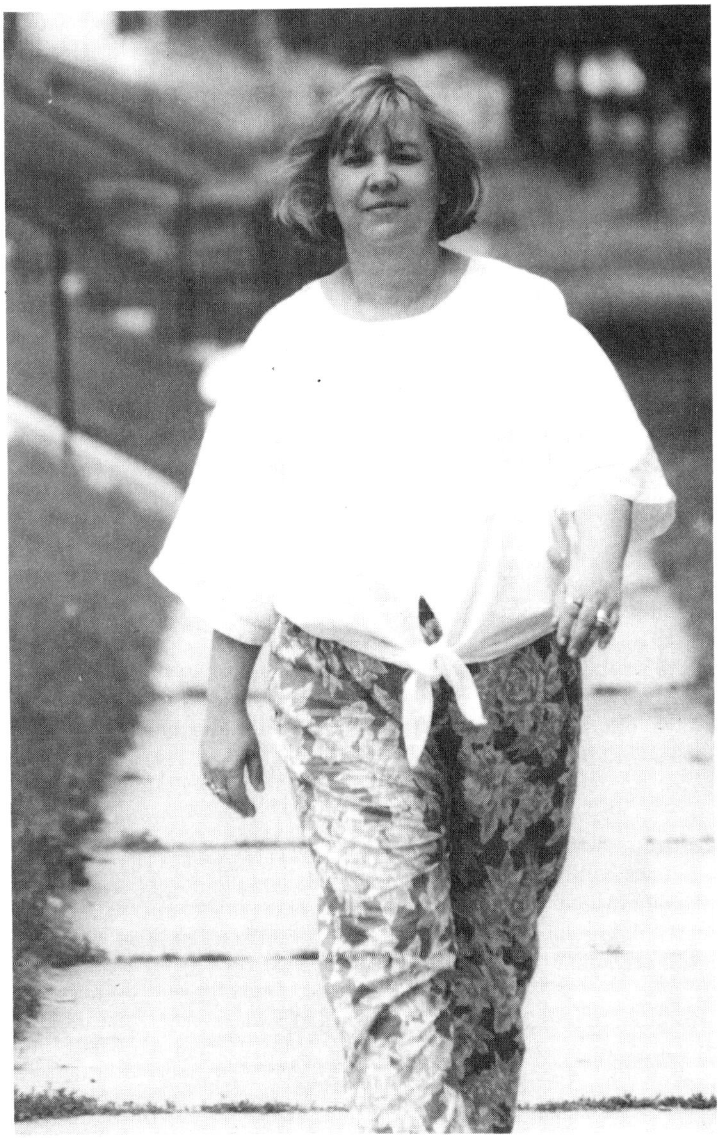

For years women have been driven by their desire to be thin. Now research shows you don't need to lose weight to be healthy. And you sure don't need to be skinny to look great.

SAY GOOD-BYE TO DIETING

By Laura Fraser

LAST SUMMER I went to the beach with a friend who, at age 42, looks lean and carefree in a bikini. Lying in the sand beside her, I wondered: What would it be like not to have to think about sucking in your stomach? Not to have to wrap a towel around your waist to hide your chubby thighs? Not to feel embarrassed during that awful moment when you drop the cloth and head for the water? I envied her, and like so many other women who have avoided two-piece swimsuits all of their lives, I wished for the zillionth time that I was thin.

Later that day my friend, who is an art teacher, commented that when I merged from the ocean after my swim, waves lapping at my ankles, I looked like a figure from a 16th century painting. "A venus," she said. With my smallish waist, slightly rounded tummy, ample hips, and fleshy thighs, I do have some traits in common with Titan's famous *Lying Venus.* But I don't have her lusciously confident gaze, and frankly, I don't even like being compared to her.

"Great," I told my friend. "But we're living at the end of the 20th century." And with this body, that's not always easy.

A blanket of fat was once a sign of prosperity and sexuality, but over the past century or two our culture has turned its back on the plump female physique. Chubbiness stopped being a badge of status as soon as everyone had plenty to eat. And when women started to demand roles other than mother and housekeeper, they shunned the maternal shape that symbolized former constraints. Thinness came to represent everything modern, disciplined, and healthy. If Titian were painting the ideal female today, he would hardly need to color in between the lines.

Most of us realize that the ideal put forward in ads and magazines is unattainable. But that doesn't stop us from wanting to be runway thin ourselves. And too often losing weight becomes so important we lose our marbles instead.

Like many otherwise sensible women, I'm astonished at the stupid things I tried over the years to shed a few pounds: 500-calorie-a-day diets, fat-free junk food binges, fruit juice fasts, even bulimia. Fortunately, I'm older now, and the years have brought not only some reason to my chaotic eating habits and a weariness with the whole topic of weight, but also an acknowledgment that women in their mid-thirties aren't meant to have prepubescent-looking bodies.

So I stopped dieting. But even so, I often felt the sting of shame about my size.

Famous Dieters

Who Lost—and Who Won

YOU AND ME, WE PUT ON A FEW POUNDS and sigh as we struggle to fasten our pants. Celebrities gain weight and there's a national lynching. When actress Alicia Silverstone (*Batman and Robin*) appeared at the 1996 Oscars a bit chunkier than her *Clueless* size, the tabloids proclaimed: FATGIRL. Alicia took her personal trainer and slunk away, not to be seen again until she lost those extra pounds.

But if we delight in guffawing at overweight celebrities, we've also been eager to snap up their diet books to learn how they went from whale to wisp in 30 short days. For years this was our mistake; stars were wedded to the strict calorie counting we now know is a prescription for disaster. But some notables are learning. Here we grade the decade's celebrity diet books by the quality of the advice. Just as researchers have discovered that the only smart way to "diet" is to eat sensibly, exercise, and learn to accept your body as it is, thankfully, so have Oprah and a few others. —*Danelle Morton is a writer at People.*

Elizabeth Taylor
Grade: D+

BOOK: *Elizabeth Takes Off, 1987*
PRE-DIET WEIGHT: 180 +
DESIRED WEIGHT: 122
PLAN: 1,000 calories a day for 14 days, with some swimming or walking

A good way to drop pounds quickly but an impossible way to live. Liz soon regained most of what she'd lost and returned to covering up all of the mirrors in her house except the hand mirror—her standard denial strategy when she thinks she's overweight.

Victoria Principal
Grade: D

BOOK: *The Diet Principal*, 1987
PRE-DIET WEIGHT: 140
DESIRED WEIGHT: 105
PLAN: As little as 800 calories a day for 30 days

Having just lost a coveted part because she wasn't rail thin, Principal cut her calories to this unhealthy level—a bad idea for anyone, even a work-starved Hollywood actress. Also troublesome is her ban on fatty or sugary foods you love; allow yourself a nibble, she says, and you'll lose control.

Oprah Winfrey
PART I
Grade: F

"The Oprah Winfrey Show," 1988
PRE-DIET WEIGHT: 211
DESIRED WEIGHT: 140
PLAN: Four months on Optifast liquid protein with minimal exercise

It seemed like a triumph. But in retrospect, hauling a little red wagon filled with 76 pounds of beef fat on stage to let people see exactly how much weight you lost makes you a caricature of a yo-yo dieter. Two years later she was back over 200.

Jane Fonda
Grade: C +

BOOK: *Jane Fonda's New Workout & Weight-Loss Program,* 1986
PRE-DIET WEIGHT: 125
DESIRED WEIGHT: 125
PLAN: 1,200 calories a day on a high-protein, high-carbo diet with an hour of aerobic and floor exercise

For years Jane's big problem was eating too *little*. Why? As a plump child she saw her older sister had written: "June is busting out all over." She misread it as: "Jane is busting out all over." This plan is still too strict with calories, but it helped her drop the illusion that she was overweight.

Susan Powter
Grade: B

BOOK: *Stop the Insanity!* 1993
PRE-DIET WEIGHT: 260
DESIRED WEIGHT: 127
PLAN: About 2,300 calories a day (mainly carbohydrate and vegetables) along with abundant exercise

The buzz-cut infomercial queen lets you eat all you want of some healthy foods, and it's a delight to come across a dozen pages of her and an overweight woman demonstrating exercises. But her ban on sweets is insupportable; in her nutritional worldview, one cookie equals *20 cups* of rice.

Angela Lansbury
Grade: B-

BOOK: *Angela Lansbury's Positive Moves,* 1990
PRE-DIET WEIGHT: 165
DESIRED WEIGHT: 150
PLAN: Low-fat, high-fiber eating plus walks and gardening

She was prompted to eat better when she discovered that the "Murder, She Wrote" wardrobe guy bought her clothes at the plus-size shop. Egad! "Don't count calories" is good advice. But she advocates a lifetime of tiny portions—which you halve during an initial period of weight loss.

Oprah Winfrey
PART II
Grade: A

BOOK: *Make The Connection* (with Bob Greene), 1996
HEALTHY WEIGHT: 150
PLAN: Eat a balanced, low-fat diet full of fruits and vegetables; commit to exercising five times a week; and let your body settle at its ideal weight.

Oprah's unrestricted-portion, whole-food recommendations deserve applause, as do the daily 45-minute walks or bike rides. Not bad for someone who once broke a diet by eating defrosted, two-year-old hot dog buns slathered with pancake syrup.

And year after year, experts' proclamations reminded me anew that, at 5 foot 6 and about 155, if I didn't lose 20 pounds, I was endangering my health.

But recently that view changed. First, researchers revisited long-ignored findings that dieters are vulnerable to depression and rarely keep off lost weight. Then, last year, studies found that being overweight is not as risky as we once thought. For many women, in fact, it isn't risky *at all*.

These are two heady notions: Diets are bad for us. We don't need to lose weight to be healthy. From them has sprung an alternative to dieting that every woman should consider.

WHY DOES DIETING seldom work? University of Toronto psychologists Janet Polivy and Peter Herman were the first to show that people on diets binge more often than normal eaters. In one study the researchers gave dieters and nondieters milk shakes before a snack. The nondieters did what makes sense: They ate less after the drink. But the dieters did the opposite, eating much more. The reason, Polivy and Herman decided, is that people on diets don't eat according to whether they feel hungry or full but according to their sense of whether they're being "good" or "bad." When they're bad (the milk shake), they figure they've blown their diets and, like a coil wound too tight, tend to spring apart—losing control and binging. Such episodes intensify dieters' anxieties about their weight and spawn new vows to do "better." This cycle is familiar to anyone who has ever tried to lose weight, but researchers now say we should give ourselves a break: It's the diet, not the dieter, that's to blame.

The problem with limiting food is that the body reacts as if it's being starved. Neurotransmitters in the brain start clamoring for food, producing cravings. Metabolic rate slows so the body can survive the apparent famine. And then the mind starts a rebellion. "It's the deprivation effect," says Polivy. "If you're told you can't have something, then that's what you want. You want it so much, in fact, that you become preoccupied with food at the expense of emotional stability." Many obesity researchers now agree. "Clearly the psychological consequences of dieting are horrible," says John Foreyt, a psychologist at Baylor University.

Nevertheless, few medical experts have challenged the practice of treating overweight people with diets. Drastic measures were necessary, doctors said, for patients with this serious health problem. The so-called healthy weight tables developed years ago by the life insurance industry told physicians which patients should lose pounds. And the message that weight kills kept getting confirmed by new, similar studies.

Then, in 1986, gerontologist Reubin Andres looked at the data behind the tables and wasn't impressed. The studies making connections between obesity and death made no allowance for whether the subjects smoked or were ill. They also ignored many elderly people's need for extra pounds to fend off osteoporosis. Other researchers went further, showing that a person's weight alone—without regard to body shape, blood pressure, cholesterol levels, and fitness—was essentially useless as a predictor of health.

Last year, when Cornell University nutrition professor David Levitsky and his colleagues analyzed 19 studies of weight and mortality, they found that only people at the extremes of weight died younger than the general population. Levitsky's conclusion: If they don't have other health problems, even the most overweight people have no additional risk of dying early. "Nobody ever dies of obesity itself," he says.

Then Steven Blair, an epidemiologist at the Cooper Institute for Aerobics Research, reviewed the health of 25,000 men and found that once he accounted for how much exercise they got, their weight had no bearing on their life span. Blair and Levitsky are quick to say that all people—fat or not—must exercise and eat well to cut their risk. But they also point out that it does no good to tell anyone except those who are excessively fat—50 to 100 pounds heavier than average—to lose weight.

Make no mistake, there's still heated debate over whether they're right. But more and more experts agree with Andres. "Extreme obesity is dangerous," he says, "but I don't think we're doing a service to the rest of the American public to create massive anxieties about weight."

THAT IS comforting news, but how many of us are neurotic about our weight because we want to live longer? If Satan offered us slenderness in exchange for five years off our lives, many of us would take the deal.

In this culture it's easy to get stuck disliking our bodies and believing we should deprive or punish ourselves to look better. Sometimes, when I stand in front of the mirror and acknowledge that I will never pass for svelte (not even dressed all in black), I still get depressed. But with researchers now debunking diets, things are clearer to me. I realize that my obsession with weight made me lose touch with myself. It may be easier to face a weight-loss program than to tackle the vague project of learning to listen to, and respect, your body. Over many years I have learned to eat when I feel hungry rather than when a diet plan says I can.

Think of this approach, which experts call internal regulation, as nature's feeding plan. Left to themselves, children will choose a variety of foods and stop eating when they've had enough, according to research by Penn State psychologist Leann Birch. By adulthood physical signals have often been drowned out, usually by judgments from a parent or a diet identifying "good" and "bad" foods. The way back to normal eating, psychologists say, is to stop listening to anyone's advice about weight or food. What it meant for me was to quit tracking how many calories I'd eaten in a day or burned at the

> One day when I was feeling depressed, I asked an old friend the question men dread most: "Do you think I'm fatter?"

QUIZ

ARE YOU HUNG UP ABOUT YOUR WEIGHT?

EAT WHEN YOU'RE hungry, stop when you're full, and choose foods that are good for you. Oh, and while you're at it, learn to love your body, whatever its shape or size. If only it were so simple. But experts say that until we learn to respect our natural hunger signals and to accept the way we look, we'll never be able to kick the dieting habit. To find out how close you are to that healthy goal, pick up a pencil and circle true or false for each of the following statements.

My life would be better if only I could lose some weight.

TRUE or FALSE

I often eat when I am upset, depressed, anxious, or angry as a way of feeling better.

TRUE or FALSE

I tend to overeat in social situations.

TRUE or FALSE

I avoid mirrors.

TRUE or FALSE

I keep eating even when I'm full.

TRUE or FALSE

If I ate whenever I wanted to, I would get very fat.

TRUE or FALSE

I choose clothes that hide the size of my body.

TRUE or FALSE

I often feel guilty after I eat.

TRUE or FALSE

I'm afraid to have even a taste of dessert because I might lose control and eat too much.

TRUE or FALSE

I have tried many diets.

TRUE or FALSE

I prefer to make love in the dark because I'm embarrassed about my body.

TRUE or FALSE

I eat even when I don't feel hungry.

TRUE or FALSE

I compare my body unfavorably with those of others.

TRUE or FALSE

I eat normally when I'm with friends; when I'm by myself I tend to pig out.

TRUE or FALSE

I think about food nearly all the time.

TRUE or FALSE

I'm embarrassed about the fact that I like to eat.

TRUE or FALSE

.... **Total number of trues**

FIVE OR FEWER TRUE

Congratulations. You're in tune with your hunger, and you've resisted the pressures—cultural or otherwise—that make so many women dissatisfied with their bodies.

SIX OR MORE TRUE

You probably realize that your relationship with food and your view of your body are somewhat troubled. Try to ease up on yourself and take steps to relearn a more natural way of eating.

Making Peace With Your Body

Make mealtimes sacred. Rather than reading or working while you eat, focus on the food; chew slowly and savor each mouthful. Also, pause periodically to see if you're still hungry. It takes roughly 20 minutes from the time you start eating before your stomach lets your mind know you've had enough.

Don't deprive yourself. It's better to eat one or two cookies than to swear off sweets entirely, say experts. Deprivation only makes people unhappy, which in turn makes them much more likely to overindulge.

Get moving. The evidence is overwhelming. Not only does exercise help you stay healthy and live longer, it also makes your body look better. A combination of aerobic exercise and weight training will tone you up—and help you go down a size or two in clothes—even if you don't lose any weight.

Accentuate the positive. Play up the parts of your body you *do* like. Get a great haircut, wear a low-cut dress, find a sweater in a color that flatters your complexion. And console yourself with the fact that almost all women, thin or not, are unhappy with some parts of their bodies.

Know thyself. Figure out whether your concerns about weight could be substituting for other unmet needs. Too many women try to eat their way out of anxiety, boredom, or loneliness, and their bodies—and minds—are paying the price. If that sounds like you, reach out to your friends, rethink your job, figure out what's missing in your life and how you can work on getting it. If necessary, seek professional help.

FOR MORE INFORMATION

***Overcoming Overeating* (Fawcett Columbine Trade Paperbacks, 1989, $11) and *When Women Stop Hating Their Bodies* (Fawcett Columbine, 1996, $23), by Carol Munter and Jane Hirschmann, are both invaluable resources for women dealing with weight and body-image issues.**

gym, give up weighing myself, and start trusting myself to make what are actually pleasurable choices about what to eat and when to exercise.

The irony about my to-hell-with-diets attitude is that I've developed habits obesity doctors would love all their patients to have. For exercise I choose only activities I enjoy, and I've reached the point where I feel restless if I don't have a chance to get sweaty every day. With bingeing no longer a part of my life, I've discovered I'm not that fond of junk food. I gravitate toward fruits, vegetables, and pasta; occasionally I eat a few cookies but never the whole bag. I check in with myself: Do I really want the rest of this angel hair, or should I ask the waiter to pack it up for lunch tomorrow?

Through it all, my weight has stayed more or less the same (without a scale all I can say is my size 12 jeans still fit). That weight is about 20 pounds lighter than it was when I was bingeing and 20 pounds heavier than what some doctors might say it should be, but it seems to be the weight my body likes. And I feel good.

One day a few years ago when I was feeling depressed, I asked an old college friend the question men dread most: "Do you think I'm fatter?"

Brave and foolish man, he answered me honestly. "You're definitely heavier," he said. "But you're much sexier because you look like you live in your body." And I suppose that's true. I feel like I carry myself with a confidence that makes fewer concessions to my weight.

I've discovered nothing magical, of course. I've just had to learn the hard way what some women know intuitively from the start. Your body is all you've got. Accept it. Yet even if you can start to live more cheerfully and rebelliously with a less-than-ideal figure, you may not feel fabulous in a bikini. I don't.

But does anyone in this culture feel completely comfortable in her body? I take perverse pleasure in knowing that even those people who are genetically slender would probably change something about their bodies if they could. Maybe they wish they didn't have knobby knees and scrawny arms. Maybe, just maybe, they wish they were blessed with a few more curves, like me.

Contributing editor Laura Fraser is the author of Losing It: America's Obsession With Weight and the Industry That Feeds on It.

Cars. Desk jobs. Escalators. It's hard to be active these days. Yet researchers now know that when it comes to health, the single most important thing you can do is live your life on the go.

REBEL AGAINST A SEDENTARY LIFE

By Katherine Griffin

A DECADE AGO MOST of my ideas about exercise came from my housemate John, a former cross-country runner. For exercise to do you any good, he told me, you have to get your heart pounding and keep it that way for at least 20 minutes, or even better, an hour. John's endless energy made him a persuasive advertisement for long runs and killer bike rides. I was sufficiently impressed that I allowed him to haul me out of bed at 6:30 several times a week to go running, a feat I haven't repeated since.

These days John lives nearby, and I still see him bounding off for two-hour runs. But I'm now paying more attention to a neighbor who embodies a strikingly different approach. Her name is Emma, and she's 92 years old. Every morning as I'm drowsily returning to consciousness, the *skritch-skritch* of a rake outside lets me know that Emma has started her workout. She spends a couple of hours each day raking everybody's leaves, up and down our block and around the corners. Her back is bent and her hair a white, wispy puff, but from a distance, watching her stab the rake at the leaves, stuff the leaves into bags, and haul the bags away, you'd swear she wasn't a day over 50.

Emma is modest about her labors. "Don't have anything else I have to do," she says, with a slightly embarrassed shrug. But in my eyes, she's doing more than defying expectations about how someone her age behaves. She's living proof, in my front yard, of the most important health finding of the decade: Just working movement into everyday life can be a veritable fountain of youth.

The irony is, we've discovered this just as we've created a society that compels us *not* to move. Today the average person going about her everyday life burns a whopping 800 fewer calories a day than she would have 20 years ago. That's the equivalent of three hours of daily walking that have simply vanished. Take even a cursory look at how most of us live and it's not hard to see why we move less. Most jobs require nothing more physically taxing than pecking at a computer. Growing numbers of us live in suburbs laid out so it's practically impossible to

HOW "Go for the Burn" BECAME "Easy Does It"

AFTER SOME FALSE STARTS, in 1978 the high priests of fitness declared the road to health was paved with three to five hard workouts a week. The then-20-something boomers dashed out to do right. But just as that dictum became a burden for a generation facing 50, the experts gave everyone a new goal to chase: exercise lite.

1951 Fifteen years after opening the nation's first health club, Jack LaLanne airs "The Jack LaLanne Show." "I'm going to build a new and lovelier you!" he tells his 6 million viewers before putting them through his workout. "We're going to reduce"—pause to touch his rump—"the old back porch!"

1963 Alarmed that baby boom children are weaker than European kids, the new President's Council on Physical Fitness instructs schools to get us exercising. Setting an example, the Kennedys turn family touch football games into a national pastime.

1968 In his best-selling *Aerobics,* Kenneth Cooper of the Cooper Institute argues that four workouts a week prevent heart disease. "I've been called a zealot, yes. But this is an idea that could reshape the lives of millions." Not until 1984 will a study finally tie exercise to longevity.

1977 Once-chubby ex-smoker Jim Fixx brings Cooper's message to the masses with his evangelical *Complete Book of Running.* Everyone perceives an irony when he later dies of a heart attack while running, but he had inherited heart disease.

1982 Jane Fonda's Workout video kicks off the aerobics craze. "Namby-pamby little routines that don't speed up your heartbeat and make you sweat aren't really worth your while."

1987 By touting beauty benefits, the *Buns of Steel* videos trigger another hard-core fitness wave and go on to sell 13 million copies. But when a study finds people who just walk or garden regularly earn exercise's health dividends, experts rethink their advice.

1991 Despite more than a decade of pleas from fitness experts, two in three women get no regular exercise—more than in 1985.

1993 A study at Tufts University finds that lifting weights reverses muscle and bone loss, and may be as important to good health as walking, jogging, swimming, or other aerobic exercise.

1993 Taking the just-get-moving cue, 14 million Americans now go walking at least twice a week, up almost 40 percent in six years. Leading the way is girl-next-door walking enthusiast Kathy Smith.

1996 The surgeon general's report on exercise makes it official: Doing any moderate exercise for 30 minutes a day can help unclog arteries, lower diabetes risk, delay osteoporosis, and lengthen life.

go anywhere without getting into a car. There are drive-through restaurants, banks, even liquor stores. In a thousand ways both big and small, our landscape shouts, "All right, nobody move!"

Some 15 percent of us, including my friend John, have compensated for this immobilization by making time for hard workouts. But for the great majority of us who have failed at that, the only answer is to become more active without formal exercise. And that calls for no less than an outright rebellion against the conveniences that cushion our lives.

Emma, for her part, refuses to pay for a gardener—or to let her neighbors hire one. How will the rest of us revolt? I don't know, but we'd better start plotting. Because either we move, or we die.

RESEARCHERS AREN'T JUST playing cheerleader when they say that movement is a genuine magic pill. They've piled up a mountain of proof that activity can stave off the killer diseases that steal vitality and life from millions every year. In 1996 the first surgeon general's report on physical activity exhaustively detailed that evidence. Think of an illness that someone you love has died from—cancer, heart disease—or an ailment that has hobbled someone you're close to—high blood pressure, osteoporosis, diabetes, depression—and chances are that moving around helps prevent it.

Meanwhile, the dangers of a sedentary life have become alarmingly clear. We're used to thinking of cigarettes as the number one health threat, but overused recliners are just as treacherous. Last July Steven Blair, an epidemiologist at the Cooper Institute for Aerobics Research in Dallas, published the first comprehensive study to compare the effects of a lack of exercise with other health dangers. Following 32,000 people for eight years, he found that those whose only risk was inactivity were more likely to die prematurely than those who had high cholesterol, high blood pressure, *and* a smoking habit but who got some exercise each day.

And forget "no pain, no gain" and all those eighties-style exercise mantras. In 1984 University of Pittsburgh epidemiologist Ronald LaPorte found that mail carriers who merely *walked* seven miles a day were as healthy as distance runners. "Workouts" like Emma's are where the vast majority of benefits lie. This means at least 30 minutes per day of activity that's as demanding as a brisk walk. Being about that active, Blair has found, cuts your odds of an untimely death by more than half. The risk for those who follow a hard-core regimen declines further but not by much more. In addition, the experts say, you can pile up activity in short bursts throughout the day.

It sounds simple: Get back to moving

QUIZ

ARE YOU ACTIVE ENOUGH?

DON'T WORRY IF you can't find the time to get to the gym, experts now say. Accumulating 30 minutes of vigorous movement—taking the stairs, mowing the lawn, pedaling your bike around the block—can offer the same benefits as a full-fledged workout. The trouble is, our lives have become so convenient that even getting bits and pieces of exercise takes a concerted effort. To find out how well you're doing, circle true or false for each of the statements below.

I always take the stairs instead of the escalator.

TRUE or FALSE

I usually walk or ride my bike to do errands.

TRUE or FALSE

I do my own housecleaning and laundry.

TRUE or FALSE

My job involves a lot of walking or lifting.

TRUE or FALSE

I do my own yard work.

TRUE or FALSE

I play active games with children a lot.

TRUE or FALSE

I resist the impulse to find the closest parking space.

TRUE or FALSE

I have stairs in my house.

TRUE or FALSE

I often do exercises while watching TV—at least during commercials.

TRUE or FALSE

My hobbies involve a lot of activity.

TRUE or FALSE

I take a 30-minute walk or go to the gym five times a week.

TRUE or FALSE

.... **Total number of trues**

SIX OR MORE TRUE
You're probably managing to work in at least 30 minutes of activity a day.

FIVE OR FEWER TRUE
You need to get moving. Make some small changes to rally yourself.

Walking Away From Convenience

Get out of the car. Whenever possible, go partway to your destination by car, park, then walk the rest. Or even if you simply trade time in the car for time on a bus or train, the walk to and from the station will add valuable active minutes to your day.

Go on three-minute walks. Piling up short periods of activity appears to be as good as exercising all at once, so take "moving" coffee breaks or lunchtime walks.

Swear off E-mail. Communicating by computer is sure to keep you in your chair all day. Walk over and talk to your coworkers face-to-face.

Make chores your workout. Scrub the floor. Weed the garden. Bike to the store. Everyday activities count as exercise as long as they're strenuous enough to leave you slightly winded.

Shun escalators. Elevators may be hard to forswear if your office is on the eighteenth floor. But escalators are usually only a flight or two long—and they're often right next to the stairs.

around, a little bit here, a little bit there. But don't fool yourself. The promise of the 20th century was that technology would transform our lives, freeing us from the drudgery of manual labor. For most Americans that promise has been fulfilled, and we aren't begging to chop wood and haul water again. "All through the course of evolution, people had to be active to survive," says Philip James, an obesity researcher at Rowett Research Institute in Aberdeen, Scotland. "Now, for the first time, we have constructed a world in which you have to go out and make a conscious decision to be active."

It was James who calculated that the average person now burns 800 fewer calories each day than she did in 1975. The main culprits? Cars, freeways, offices, and suburbs spreading willy-nilly across the land (the typical American spends 45 minutes each day sitting behind the wheel of a car); televisions glowing in every home (three hours per day); and computers humming in every workplace.

The evils of automobiles and desk jobs are frighteningly familiar to 46-year-old Susan Donahue of Davis, California. Until three years ago her job as a veterinary technician at the local university kept her hopping. "I was always chasing sheep around or carting stuff to the lab," she says. But since becoming the editor of the university's veterinary newsletter, she spends her days behind a terminal, chasing deadlines instead of sheep.

Once movement was gone from her job, she was appalled to realize that she'd turned into the stereotypical sedentary American. "I'd drive to work, drive home, and that was it," she says. Years earlier she had gardened during the week and hiked or skied on weekends. But as she got busier and added a computer to her home, those hobbies slipped out of Donahue's schedule. "When life speeded up," she says, "exercise was the first to go."

Having too much to do, of course, is the epidemic of our era. And Americans pinched for time can find mechanized ways to make any chore far less time-consuming. Can't spare an hour for the lawn? Invest in a sit-down mower and a leaf blower. No time to scrub the car? Drive it through the car wash. Even conveniences that seem innocuous contribute to the decline in activity: Just adding a second phone in your house means you may walk 70 fewer miles a year.

"Everything we do—cleaning, cooking, yard work—burns fewer calories than it used to," says Blair. "It's the accumulation of tiny little increments, but they add up to a lot."

Eventually Susan Donahue got fed up. After casting a critical, almost subversive eye on her surroundings, she seized one big opportunity for movement: She gave up the sticker that allowed her to park on campus and started cycling the flat, four-mile round-trip to work. "Instead of mindlessly driving along with all the other driver-drones, I just told myself that I was going to make this happen," she says. "Everything else would have to adapt to it." No more excuses about being too busy, no more oversleeping and flying out the door late.

Three years later she still bikes every day, rain or shine. Sometimes it's a hassle. She has to allow more time to get to work. Her skirt gets stuck in the spokes. Rainy days find her wearing plastic bags over her shoes and looking, she admits, like a fashion outcast. But she won't give up her daily ride. "It's a wonderful thing to work into my day," she says. "Now when I get home I feel energized." So much so that she also takes evening walks with her husband, keeps up with the yard work, and goes on weekend rides with a local bicycle club.

How did Donahue manage to buck the system? Researchers who study why people get moving would ascribe it to some combination of her self-confidence, enjoyment of the activity she chose, and support from others. As a student years before, Donahue had bicycled everywhere, so there was a part of her deep down that knew she could switch from car to bike. And once she was back to cycling, the joy of being outdoors, seeing things she'd otherwise miss, motivated her to stick with it even on cold, windy mornings when the car tempted her. Finally, Donahue's husband was a longtime cycling enthusiast who was thrilled when she started to ride and got her involved with the bike club.

Donahue's path was further smoothed by the fact that she lives in Davis, a town where visionary planners had created a network of bike lanes and greenbelts. Today one in four commuters in Davis cycles to work, compared with 3 percent nationwide.

When Donahue bicycles in other cities, though, she can see why everyone drives. Exhaust fumes and traffic too often make human-powered transport unpleasant and even dangerous. And when she has to hunt around the back of a building before she can find its dirty and poorly lit stairwell, she understands why everyone takes the elevator. Such barriers help explain why people don't make the effort to move and why many experts think that the only sure way out of our bind will be to change our environment.

"Ideas have been floated that range from feasible to ridiculous," says Blair, who mentions levying a tax on recliners, funneling highway money into bike and walking paths, requiring office buildings to have centrally located and attractive stairs, and restricting driving in downtown areas to get people out walking.

This kind of social engineering may sound preposterous, but think back 20 years. Who would have imagined no-smoking restaurants and bars, or forlorn smokers huddled outside office buildings? Now that we know sitting around is as perilous as smoking, shouldn't we, as a society, create opportunities to bustle about, so it's not just the determined few who make movement routine?

> Now that we know sitting around is as perilous as smoking, why don't we create more opportunities to bustle about?

In the meantime, those of us who want to thrive at Emma's ripe age will have to change our lives on our own, each finding her own carpet of leaves to attack on sunny—as well as chilly—mornings.

"Don't like to sit around all day," Emma says.

Such a simple idea. Why does it have to be so complicated?

Katherine Griffin has been a staff writer at the magazine since 1989.

Who *Isn't* on a Diet?

In search of sensible eating. BY MICHELLE STACEY

Show me a woman who spreads real butter heedlessly on a baguette and I'll show you a woman of uncommon independence (or uncommon genes). She is also a member of an ever-diminishing minority: women who don't diet. We have reached, in the last decade or so, a remarkable turning point in the annals of dieting, a point of redefinition that threatens to turn the universe of eating on its head. In short, restricting one's intake in some fashion has become so common that "normal eating" is no longer, well, normal eating.

"Normal" eating used to be a fairly simple affair. You got hungry, you ate; you got full, you stopped. American culture devised patterns that most people followed: breakfast started the day, lunch kept it going, dinner (once called supper) finished it off. Sometimes, of course, in the face of tradition (Thanksgiving) or great temptation (chocolate cake) one overindulged and kept eating past satiety. Normal, after all, essentially means "the norm," or what most people have decided is sensible, and once upon a time the norm was not to skip meals or to skim fats but to eat in a manner that might be called natural—that is, being attuned to one's internal signals of hunger and fullness, rather than attuned to external expectations of slenderness or self-denial.

Those impossible expectations, and the feast-or-famine behaviors they give rise to, have slowly been severing our ties with our previous, well-fed notions. Consider this: a friend of mine confessed to a "big lunch" that necessitated skipping dinner entirely. The big lunch consisted of a roll with butter, three-quarters of a plate of gnocchi, two diet sodas and a *gelato* shared among four women. Our mothers would consider that normal (albeit not exactly nutritionally balanced), maybe even on the skimpy side—after all, she didn't clean her plate. Or consider this: an advertisement touts "Now you can have a sliver this big"—showing a piece of cheesecake that fills a magazine page—because the cake is made from nonfat cheese. Is that normal?

Eating-disorder researchers Janet Polivy and C. Peter Herman of the University of Toronto put it this way in an article in the *Journal of Consulting and Clinical Psychology:* "It is now 'normal' for individuals in our society to express concern about their weight and to engage in fitful attempts to change it.... Normal eating now requires periodic dieting." Polivy and Herman simply established what those of us sitting at the table have long known in our hearts about women and eating: it is becoming more and more difficult to eat without neurosis. Years, even decades, of power struggle with food—denying our hunger, trading off a dressingless salad for lunch with a chocolate mousse dessert at dinner, fretting and stewing over whether we had one smidgen of toast too much—have forced a sea change not only in the language of food but in its very reality.

From *Town & Country,* June 1996, pp. 144-146.

Here are some of the voices of the new normality, or abnormality, about food. Not surprisingly, they are anonymous. Who would want to admit to these utterances?

- "I love the kind of vacation where you work out a lot, because then you don't have to worry about what you eat."
- "I weigh myself every day, because otherwise I'd be at the mercy of my subjective feelings about whether I'm heavier today: I would drive myself crazy."
- "I eat a Wasa cracker with lunch because if I eat bread it tastes so good I just can't stop."

Writer Barbara Grizzuti Harrison believes dieting has become one of the defining rituals of our lives. "We live in a time largely devoid of ritual: dieting is the ritual of the secular cult of fitness," writes Harrison, a self-described fat person. The ritual brings a sense of control; it sometimes feels oddly cleansing and comforting. Underlying that clarity, however, are confusion and some free-floating anxiety: what on earth are we supposed to eat? Any coherent answer to that question can be worth literally millions: *In the Kitchen With Rosie: Oprah's Favorite Recipes,* which describes the food that helped engineer Oprah Winfrey's seventy-two-pound weight loss, became the fastest-selling hardcover in history two years ago, selling 1.4 million copies even before its official publication date.

There are several ironies in all of this. Americans are, on average, fatter now than they were even ten years ago; one-third qualify as obese, up from one-quarter, according to the National Institutes of Health. Yet we have never before been as well informed (or as confused) about nutrition and weight loss. Yo-yo dieting is indicted, then cleared. Low-fat, high-carbohydrate diets are universally touted as the only key to weight loss, then we start hearing about something called insulin resistance and the dangers of eating too many carbohydrates. We are barraged with facts: fat contents, calories per ounce, sodium, transfatty acids. Perhaps the greatest irony of all in this orgy of obsessing and restricting is that the word "diet" has completely fallen out of favor. Diets don't work, proclaim an increasing number of obesity experts (and headlines). What you need is an "eating plan," a "lifestyle change," not a temporary restriction in calories. So why are most of us dieting, secretly or shamelessly?

To understand that conundrum, it may be comforting (or not) to know that although diet mania is hitting a new high, it is not something born of recent neuroses. Historians have traced a trail of "reducing" (America's first term for dieting) back to the 19th century. An early hint of body consciousness occurred at the end of the 18th century, when the fashion was simple Empire-style dresses that draped straight from the bustline to the ankle (though the bodies beneath these often revealing dresses were still rounded).

The first wholesale move toward an ideal of slenderness, in the 1830s, came at the prompting of a fashion magazine, *Godey's Lady's Book,* according to Roberta Pollack Seid in *Never Too Thin: Why Women Are at War With Their Bodies.* The newly fashionable slim body carried a moral message as well: all bodily appetites were coarse and impure, and good women were expected to be above the desires of the flesh. These ideas gained force during the Victorian era, when it was considered indelicate for women to consume hearty foods like meat. Salads, breads and cakes were appropriate feminine foods, and among young girls the pallor and languor caused by iron-deficiency anemia (then called chlorosis) were considered signs of beauty.

The first diet book, William Banting's *Letter on Corpulence,* appeared in 1864; anorexia nervosa was first diagnosed, as a mysterious, psychologically induced loss of appetite that usually appeared among upper-class adolescent girls, in 1873. Although the ideal female form swelled to larger proportions at the turn of the century, the Edwardian woman—wearing a bustle to exaggerate her hindquarters—proved to be the last stand for the rounded figure. Fashions became more revealing, and the infrastructure of undergarments—corsets, hoop skirts, crinolines, bustles—that had helped shape the out-of-shape disappeared (only to make a fanciful reappearance in the 1990s via such designers as Karl Lagerfeld, Vivienne Westwood, Valentino and Dolce & Gabbana, but not in any manner meant to be of help to the hefty). The culture of dieting had begun. By 1914, a writer for *Living Age* magazine was describing a "cult of slimness," and after World War I, flapper styles brought in the first truly androgynous look. The first best-selling weight-loss book, *Diet and Health,* with "Key to the Calories," was published in 1917; by 1959, ninety-two diet books were in print.

The '50s marked the beginning of the modern diet age, according to Seid. The decade also ushered in fad diets (the Revolutionary Rockefeller Diet, the dextrose diet), diet foods (low-cal sodas, Metrecal), a perfectly formed Barbie doll that came with her own scale (set at 110 pounds) and a televised Miss America contest (in 1954). In the '60s we got Dr. Taller's *Calories Don't Count* (1961), the Stillman diet (1968), Tab, Diet-Rite, Overeaters Anonymous (1960), Weight Watchers (1963) and Twiggy (5 feet 7½, 91 pounds). The '70s brought Dr. Atkins' *Diet Revolution* (1972, one million copies sold in seven months) and *Fasting as a Way of Life* (1977), the exercise imperative and cellulite.

You know the rest: a steady slide into Lycra dresses, nonfat cookies and Stairmaster addiction. We seem at least to have acquired some skepticism about the craziest of fad diets (Oprah's Optifast may have been the final loss of innocence), and membership in organized diet programs has dropped significantly in the last few years (Nutri/System has half the number of centers it had five years ago; the number of new participants in Jenny Craig dropped by one-third between 1993 and

1994; Weight Watchers saw a 15 percent decline in membership in 1992 and 1993).

Yet this seeming modification of the dieting impulse is up against a powerful force in shaping women's collective self-image; depictions of ideal female forms that are, for most women, unrealistic or even unattainable. A study of Brandeis University a few years ago found that female models are 9 percent taller and 16 percent thinner than the average woman. "Models fall at the extreme of the distribution of body types in the population," explains Joseph Cunningham, a professor of psychology at Brandeis, who helped conduct the study.

Can we blame media images for our permanently restrained, or at least self-conscious, eating patterns? Certainly there's a connection, but nothing is quite that simple. "I think it's pretty clear that the Twiggy and post-Twiggy models through the '70s and into the '80s did create a lot of pressure on the average woman to diet," says Richard Gordon, a professor of psychology at Bard College and author of *Anorexia & Bulimia: Anatomy of a Social Epidemic.* "This kind of look is a very dangerous thing, a very negative kind of image to be beaming, and I think it's been a contributing factor in what appears to be an increase in disorders over that period. But you can't totally blame the fashion industry, because while fashion leads and creates imagery, it also reflects."

What exactly is this ambient thinness reflecting? Perhaps, some social critics suggest, there is a strain of misogyny, a horror of female fleshiness, in our glorification of slim-hipped, boyish figures. Look at how models and actresses rebound from pregnancies. And, just as in Victorian days, the act of eating is saturated with moral meaning: chocolates are "sinfully delicious"; we are naughty when we eat meat or butter; we are pure and "doing the right thing" when we consume oatmeal or some other fibrous, low-fat food. The very act of self-restraint brings with it a sense of mastery and status. ("It makes me feel powerful to be hungry," a thin Ivana Trump announced bluntly in 1986.) Only the well-to-do, after all, can afford not to eat, and only an exceptionally self-controlled woman can turn down what every cell in her body is screaming for. Eating well—high-veggie, low-fat, slenderizing—has become a stylish must, a politically correct choice.

But the control that goes into making such choices has a way of backfiring. Perhaps this is why we are, in this age of food obsession, gaining weight. Diet experts say binging is not a naturally occurring phenomenon: it happens only after previous starvation and is the expression of a powerful physiological drive to refeed. "The bottom line is that the research shows very clearly that very restrictive diets don't work," says John Foreyt, director of the Behavioral Medicine Research Clinic at Baylor College of Medicine and coauthor of *Living Without Dieting.* "What happens is that physiology overwhelms psychology—hunger and

Fear of Fat

If every decade or so has its diet mantra, the '90s dictum is clear: "Fat makes you fat." Or, conversely, if you drain the fat out of your diet you will—effortlessly, almost automatically—lose weight. The bible of this movement is Dr. Dean Ornish's 1993 bestseller *Eat More, Weigh Less,* in which he advocates a 10-percent-fat diet that excludes all meat, fowl, fish and dairy (allowing only nonfat yogurt). Ornish's message is echoed by the less-credentialed but even more high-profile diet-and-exercise maven Susan Powter, author of *Stop the Insanity!*: "It's not food that makes you fat. It's fat that makes you fat."

Fat mania has driven SnackWell's fat-free cookies to the top of the grocery-store hierarchy, along with the hundreds of other reduced-fat, low-fat or nonfat products that are introduced each year. Fat paranoia has also led to such absurdities as reduced-fat peanut butter (which still has six grams of fat per tablespoon) and reduced-fat cake (if you're going to eat it, why not go for the real thing?). Now, predictably, we are entering a backlash period, in which experts are worrying that those on super-low-fat diets may not get enough of certain fatty acids, and others are suggesting that such dieters may actually put on weight by eating too many simple carbohydrates.

The bottom line as usual, moderation. Eating less fat can help you lose weight because fat is more calorie-dense and also may be stored more easily as fat in your body. But you must replace the fat you cut out with complex carbohydrates—fruits, vegetables, whole grains—not simple carbs like those in sugary nonfat goodies. Many experts also agree that a 10-percent fat diet is so low that it's hard to maintain, and suggest that 20 percent is just as effective and a lot more tasty. Two other caveats: you must still keep portion size within reason (just because pasta and breads are low- or nonfat doesn't mean their calories don't count) and, for any weight-loss regimen to produce lasting results, you must add physical activity.

M.S.

feelings of deprivation will overwhelm will power." Indeed, the failure rate of old-fashioned low-calorie diets is about 95 percent. And worse, chronic dieting—the new "normal eating" that has self-restraint as its byword—makes it ever harder to get back in touch with the reality of food. "The dieter learns to ignore signals from her body about hunger," explains Janet Polivy, a professor of psychology at the University of Toronto and coauthor of the "normal eating" theory. "Hunger and eating no longer go together. When people lose track of their hunger through dieting, it makes them more prone to overeat and binge eat."

But if expert opinion seems to be coalescing nicely in opposition to restrictive dieting, the question of what to put in its place—of how, after all, we ought to be eating—seems foggier than ever. Is there an "obesity gene"? Will everyone lose weight on a low- or nonfat diet? Even the experts seem confused.

There is a central mystery here that defies solution, that seems to deepen the more we learn about eating and our bodies. It now looks as it our bodies may have an intrinsic wisdom of their own, a "normality" they force upon us despite the blatant abnormality of our eating.

Some of that wisdom may come from simple hunger, once seen as a threat but now often a secret friend to be courted, a sign that we are doing the right (abstemious) thing. A thin friend of mine, who says she only feels anxious when she is full and comfortable when she is hungry, once moaned to me, "If only I could eat when I'm hungry and not eat when I'm not hungry. I'd be fine." Dr. C. Peter Herman, coauthor with Janet Polivy of the "normal eating" theory, calls this system "the Garden of Eden version of eating": what eating was before our loss of innocence, before we began to distrust our bodies' innate wisdom.

Many eating experts speak now of rediscovering the rightness of hunger. Several new nondiet weight-management books speak of "intuitive eating" and of "mouth hunger" versus physical hunger. New programs tout customized eating plans and the reorganization of goals: recognizing that, despite what Susan Powter screams at us, not everyone will be a size 4. The next wave in eating may involve making peace with food, this beleaguered pleasure that we have transformed from a comfort to an adversary. Perhaps we can learn to create our own culinary Eden, where the greatest sin would be to *not* savor every bite, be it of carrots or creme brûlée.

How far should you go to stay fit?

The battle between tough and tame

BY LYNN ROSELLINI

Oh, the horror. OK, so it's not really the final reckoning, but for nine women on black Reebok stationary bikes, it might as well be. Grunting and grimacing, they pedal madly in a windowless, mirrored room at the Tenley Sport & Health Club in Washington, D.C. The smell of perspiration hangs in the air, and sweat drips off noses, making handlebars slippery. "Tough it out!" shouts aerobics instructor Jan Wright above the sound of whirring wheels and pounding jazz.

Upstairs, a less taxing routine is in progress. Listening to disco music through her earphones, her breathing rate barely elevated, Catalina Rizo strides briskly around the club's rubberized indoor track. "I've read that walking can be just as effective [as aerobics classes] if you do it at a certain pace," says Rizo, 58, whose pink T-shirt and sweats give her the air of a tourist out for a stroll around the Jefferson Memorial. "They say any exercise is good."

That may be the only point exercise experts agree on these days. The contrasting fitness routines on display at the Tenley club illustrate two warring philosophies about how much and what kind of exercise Americans should get.

Too good to be true? Wright's cycle class harks back to the dogma of the late 1970s, amplified by exercise gurus like Jane Fonda and Jim Fixx: A minimum of 20 minutes of continuous running, cycling, or other vigorous activity at least three times a week is essential to guard against heart disease, high blood pressure, and other diseases.

Rizo's workout reflects the revisionist message of a 1993 report from the federal Centers for Disease Control and Prevention and the American College of Sports Medicine. At the time, the new public-health message seemed impossible but delightful, at least to couch potatoes: Just 30 minutes of ordinary activities—like walking, playing with a child, or gardening—most days of the week could enhance cardiovascular health. That half-hour could be pieced together from several shorter bouts of activity, such as a morning walk to the bus stop and an evening stint of lawn mowing.

Now it turns out that the government's recommendations may have been too optimistic. A cadre of researchers contend that the panel let public-health advocacy get in the way of good science. "I think it was deliberate on the part of the CDC and ACSM to make their guidelines more palatable [to the public]," says Paul D. Thompson, director of preventive cardiology at Hartford Hospital in Connecticut and president-elect of the American College of Sports Medicine. The CDC/ACSM panel "really made those recommendations without solid scientific proof," he says.

Risky calculation. Exercise experts are not simply squabbling over details. How much Americans exercise has an enormous impact on public health. The CDC estimates that lack of regular exercise kills as many as 250,000 Americans each year—about 12 percent of the total who die. People who don't exercise have twice as great a risk of coronary heart disease as those who exercise regularly. Middle-aged women are more likely to die of heart disease than breast cancer by a factor of more than 2 to 1. Moderate to strenuous exercise also lowers chances of developing diabetes, osteoporosis, colon cancer, anxiety, and depression.

The most roundly criticized aspect of the government's report was the contention that short, intermittent bouts of exercise are as good for health as a solid half-hour workout. The dispute stems partly from the CDC/ACSM panel's interpretation of studies that measured health gains among men who had a variety of weekly exercise routines. The men reported the amount they exercised but did not specify whether the activity was continuous or intermittent. The panel assumed that the men's workouts were broken up into short segments, although two of the scientists who conducted the studies contend that the nature of some of the activities, such as swimming, indicates that subjects often exercised for sustained periods.

Critics also fault the panel's interpretation of the results of other studies, including one by the Cooper Institute for Aerobics Research in Dallas. That 1989 study assigned 13,000 men and women to one of five fitness categories, based on their performances on a treadmill. Over an eight-year period, researchers found that the least fit group had proportionally many more deaths than did those in the next, slightly fitter, group. The Cooper researchers didn't report on their subjects' exercise routines. But from studies showing that people have to exercise only moderately to become as fit as the slightly fitter group, the researchers concluded that moderate physical activity lowered death rates.

> **THE EASY-DOES-IT OPTION**
>
> **Some experts say that an adult who gets 30 minutes of ordinary activity most days of the week, like playing with a child, will enjoy better cardiovascular health**

The main problem with relying on those conclusions, critics say, is that the panel used measures of fitness, not actual physical exercise, to come up with its

From *U.S. News & World Report,* November 10, 1997, pp. 95-96.

workout guidelines. Fitness is determined by more than just exercise; another key factor is genetic predisposition, points out Paul Williams, an exercise researcher at Lawrence Berkeley National Laboratory in Berkeley, Calif. "This is the government policy that confused genes with walking shorts," he says.

Members of the panel counter that they assessed dozens of studies that, when taken as a whole, show that moderate amounts of exercise can help prevent disease and promote good health. Russell Pate, the lead author of the report and an exercise physiologist at the University of South Carolina, now concedes that panel members took their best guess when they asserted that intermittent activity confers the same health benefits as continuous activity, but he says, "I have great confidence in the fundamental conclusions [of the guidelines]."

The purpose of those conclusions, supporters of the guidelines say, is to get the public off its duff. Despite all the publicity about the health value of physical activity, some 60 percent of Americans engage in little or no exercise. "The public-health approach is, 'Get them started, something is better than nothing,'" says University of Minnesota epidemiologist Arthur Leon, one of the authors of the report.

But in the effort to get people started, critics say, the panel may have set the bar too low. By exaggerating the benefits of moderate exercise, according to Williams, the government may have discouraged some people from the kind of rigorous workouts that yield far greater health benefits.

To date, however, the guidelines appear to have done little to alter the way Americans exercise. "There's no data to say with any confidence that anything has changed," says Carl J. Caspersen, a physical activity epidemiologist for the CDC.

Despite the controversy over the benefits of low-sweat exercise, the experts have reached a consensus on a couple of basic rules: The more variety you have in an exercise program—mixing running, swimming, and cycling, for instance—the less likely you are to get injured. And, in most cases, the more exercise, the better.

Williams's studies of female runners, for instance, show that those who increase their mileage from 10 miles a week to 40 miles a week can expect to decrease their chances of coronary heart disease by 29 percent (while incurring a somewhat greater risk of injury as a result of the increased mileage). To him, and to other experts, those taunting mottoes from the '80s—"no pain, no gain," "go for the burn"—were right, after all. Oh, the horror . . .

Fat Chances

Given the limited success of dieting—and the risks—is it better just to stay plump?

by Carol Ezzell

I couldn't believe my eyes. But there it was, printed in an editorial entitled "Losing Weight—An Ill-Fated New Year's Resolution" in the January 1 *New England Journal of Medicine*: "Unfortunately, the data…showing the beneficial effects of weight loss are limited, fragmentary and often ambiguous."

For someone like me who has struggled with her weight for years, this dry pronouncement from the medical profession's equivalent of the Voice on High was nothing short of a revelation. As a chubby child, a "baby-fat" teenager and a Rubenesque woman, nearly all my visits to doctors have inevitably ended with some version of the statement, "If you could lose 10/20/30 pounds, you would sleep better/have more energy/have lower blood pressure/(fill in blank here)."

Lose weight? In theory, it's no problem. I'm an expert at counting calories, calculating fat grams and figuring out just how much time on the StairMaster absolves the sin of eating an Oreo. I'm a veteran of the Grapefruit Diet, Weight Watchers and Diet Center, and I even survived the deadly liquid-protein diets of the 1970s. I took my first diet drug—one of Mother's prescription tablets cut in half—at age 10. I calculate that since the age of 18, I've lost (and gained and lost again) a total of at least 120 pounds—and at 5′6″ I've never weighed more than 196.

The pitfall to losing weight, as every serious dieter knows, is that what comes off doesn't usually stay off. A group of experts convened in 1992 by the National Institutes of Health concluded that at least 90 percent of dieters put the pounds right back on within five years. And losing weight and keeping if off becomes harder and harder as we get older; even thin people tend to gain between 10 and 20 pounds between their 20s and 60s.

So I found myself cheering inwardly when I read the *New England Journal* editorial. Could this mean that it's okay—healthwise, if not socially—to be fat? Should people like me call a truce in their battles with their bodies and just get on with life? Or would we just be deluding ourselves?

A Widening Problem?

There are a lot of us. Indeed, a startling percentage of women in the U.S. fall into the category "obese," including some who might be startled because they probably consider themselves simply plump. The National Center for Health Statistics says that more than one third of all American women are overweight, including nearly half of those between the ages of 55 and 64. The market for women's plus sizes (sizes 16 and up) is a booming $22.7 billion a year.

African-American and Latin-American women are even more likely than Caucasian women to be obese: the Second National Health and Nutrition Examination Survey found that 44 percent of black women and 35 to 40 percent of Hispanic-American women are overweight, compared with 25 percent of white women.

Although socioeconomic factors and cultural differences in diet undoubtedly play a role in the racial breakdown of obesity, most obesity researchers believe genetics is also important. (That is, after all, why they study the genetics of mouse strains with names like Obese and Tubby.) In a telling study reported earlier this year, Claude Bouchard of the University of Laval in Quebec and his colleagues found that both members of 12 pairs of adult male twins who ate 1,000 extra calories a day for 100 days gained the same amount of weight. But the exact amount of weight the men gained varied up to sixfold between sets of twins. Such indications that human obesity has a genetic underpinning don't shock me: both my grandmothers and most of my great-aunts tipped the scales at 250 plus, even though the tallest was 5′5″. (Of course, it could have been the family recipe for that time-honored Southern dish, pecan pie.)

The Risks of Being Fat

Despite the fact that obesity is so prevalent, sound medical advice is hard to come by. It's tough to know whom to believe. When launching the nonprofit organization Shape Up America! in 1994, former Surgeon General C. Everett Koop said obesity causes 300,000 deaths in the U.S. every year, second only to smoking. But in their January editorial, the *New England Journal*'s top editors, Jerome P. Kassirer and Marcia Angell, called the 300,000 figure "by no means well established" and wrote that it is "derived from weak or incomplete data."

So what are healthy figures—both in terms of statistics and body weight? Prompting the editorial was a report published in the same issue of the journal by June Stevens of the University of North Carolina at Chapel Hill and her colleagues. Stevens and her co-workers reported the results of analyzing health data gathered from 262,019 female and 62,116 male non-smokers during the American Cancer Society's Cancer Prevention Study I, which was conducted between 1960 and 1972. The researchers found that excess body weight slightly increases the risk of death from any cause among people between 30 and 74 years of age.

The Stevens report was by no means an unusual finding: in 1995 the *New England Journal* published a study linking body weight and mortality in 115,195 women between 30 and 55 years old who were part of the massive, ongoing Nurses' Health Study. And last year the *Journal of the American Medical Association (JAMA)* weighed in with two reports on the health hazards of obesity in women. In a separate report in *JAMA* on data from the Nurses' Health Study, a group from Harvard Medical School found that women who put on weight as adults were more likely to develop breast cancer after menopause. And in yet another report, some of the same researchers found that overweight women have increased risk of stroke. Other studies have linked obesity with gallstones, noninsulin-dependent—or Type II—diabetes and joint degeneration.

But in most of these studies, the relative risk conferred by carrying some extra weight was less than 2.0, which means that fat women were not even twice as likely to die or suffer breast cancer or stroke than their thinner counterparts. In epidemiological terms, this just isn't much.

The Risks of Dieting

So if obesity confers only a modest increase in mortality, what about the risks of striving to be thin? Extreme diets are known to pose health risks by depleting the body of vitamins and nutrients. But what about the new wonder drugs?

They, too, can be dangerous. By now, most people have heard of the demise of the diet-drug combo fen-phen (fenfluramine/phentermine). Fen-phen crashed and burned last September when Wyeth-Ayerst Laboratories took half of the duo—fenfluramine—off the market at the behest of the Food and Drug Administration. The decision followed reports that some women who had taken fenfluramine developed abnormalities in their heart valves, apparently because the drug elevated blood levels of the neurotransmitter serotonin, the same neurochemical boosted in the brain by Prozac. Wyeth-Ayerst also pulled fenfluramine's chemical cousin, dexfenfluramine (Redux), from pharmacy shelves.

In the aftermath of fen-phen, Knoll Pharmaceuticals delayed marketing its new drug sibutramine (Reductil), which increases brain levels of serotonin and another neurotransmitter, noradrenaline. And on March 13, an FDA advisory committee deadlocked over recommending Hoffmann–La Roche's orlistat (also called Xenical), which blocks the enzymes that break down fat in the intestines, allowing fat to pass through the gut undigested. The panel said it was confounded by evidence that the drug might cause or exacerbate breast cancer.

Confusion Reigns

So I'm back to where I was when I first saw the *New England Journal* editorial. Given the current state of affairs, no wonder we're all confused. Depending on your state of mind, you can find enough scary medical evidence to get you back to eating rabbit food or sufficient uncertainty to justify an apologia for staying adipose.

The bottom line is that researchers still don't know why some of us are fatter than others. The interpersonal differences in body fatness can't be explained by food intake, physical activity, genetics or metabolism alone.

Some researchers argue that drugs such as fen-phen, sibutramine and orlistat will never eliminate obesity, because the system of body-weight maintenance is like a balloon: pinch it at one end, and it will compensate by swelling at the other. In the January issue of the *American Journal of Clinical Nutrition*, Jules Hirsch of the Rockefeller University wrote that the mechanisms that determine body weight are carefully balanced. Accordingly, taking a drug to reduce hunger might just cause a reduction in metabolism to save energy, and a drug that ramps up metabolism just might make someone eat more to keep up.

So, is it time to join the National Association to Advance Fat Acceptance? That's up to you. Myself, I draw comfort from a study published in *JAMA* last year by the Cooper Institute for Aerobics Research in Dallas that found that fat people who exercised on a regular basis were less likely to die prematurely than thin people with poor physical fitness. So I'm going to continue to Jazzercise, swing dance and scuba dive—and try to eat moderately and well. I'm not going to take any more diet drugs, but I'm also not going to give up the good fight to be healthy.

Are You Obese?
(You Might Be Surprised)

It's a loaded word that no one wants pinned to them. Think "obese," and an image like the circus Fat Lady pops into mind. That's right, of course: a consensus statement developed by the National Institutes of Health has defined "extreme obesity" as weighing twice the desirable weight for one's height or being 100 pounds over that desirable weight. But the NIH also indicated that being 20 percent heavier than the desirable weight for your height is considered obese.

Where do you fit? To find out, calculate your body mass index (BMI).

$$\text{Your BMI} = \frac{\text{Your weight in pounds} \times 700}{(\text{Your height in inches})^2}$$

Scientific studies have used a wide range of BMIs—from below 27 to over 30—to define obesity. But most researchers say if you're a woman and your BMI is greater than 27, you're obese. The optimal BMI is generally considered to be 21.

What does someone with a BMI of 27 look like? Emme, the plus-size supermodel and host of *Fashion Emergency* on E! Entertainment Television, wears a size 14 or 16 and weighs 190 pounds at 5'11". That makes her BMI 26.4. —*C.E.*

Dying to Be Thin

Eating disorders cripple—literally—millions of young women, in large part because treatments are not always effective or accessible

by Kristin Leutwyler,

I don't own a scale. I don't trust myself to have one in the house—maybe in the same way that recovered alcoholics rightfully clear their cabinets of cold medicines and mouthwash. At 5′7″, I know that I usually weigh 118 pounds, and I know that is considered normal for my frame. But 13 years ago, when I was 15 years old and the same height, I weighed 67 pounds, and I thought I was grossly, repulsively obese.

My own bout with anorexia nervosa—the eating disorder that made me starve myself into malnutrition—was severe but short-lived. I had a wonderful physician who worked hard to earn my trust and safeguard my health. And I had one great friend who slowly, over many months, proved to me that one ice cream cone wouldn't make me fat nor would being fat make me unlovable. A year later I was back up to 95 pounds. I was still scrawny, but at least I knew it.

I was—am—lucky. Eating disorders are often chronic and startlingly common. One percent of all teenage girls suffer from anorexia nervosa at some point. Two to 3 percent develop bulimia nervosa, a condition in which sufferers consume large amounts of food only to then "purge" away the excess calories by making themselves vomit, by abusing laxatives and diuretics, or by exercising obsessively. And binge eaters—who overeat until they are uncomfortably full—make up another 2 percent of the population.

In addition to the mental pain these illnesses cause sufferers and their families and friends, they also have devastating physical consequences. In the most serious cases, binge eating can rupture the stomach or esophagus. Purging can flush the body of vital minerals, causing cardiac arrest. Self-starvation can also lead to heart failure. Among anorexics, who undergo by far the worst complications, the mortality rate after 10 years is 7.7 percent, reports Katherine A. Halmi, a professor of psychiatry at Cornell University and director of the Eating Disorders Clinic at New York Hospital in Westchester. After 30 years of struggling with the condition, one fifth die.

Because studies clearly show that people who recover sooner are less likely to relapse, the push continues to discover better treatments. Eating disorders are exceedingly complex diseases, brought on by a mix of environmental, social and biological factors. But in recent years, scientists have made some small advances. Various forms of therapy are proving beneficial, and some medications—particularly a class of antidepressants known as selective serotonin reuptake inhibitors (SSRIs)—are helping certain patients. "SSRIs are not wonder drugs for eating disorders," says Robert I. Berkowitz of the University of Pennsylvania. "But treatments have become more successful, and so we're feeling hopeful, even though we have a long way to go to understand these diseases."

Weighing the Risks

When I began working on this article, I phoned my former physician, a specialist in adolescent medicine, and I was a little surprised that she remembered my name but not my diagnosis. In all fairness, my illness was a textbook case. I had faced many common risk factors, starting with a "fat list" on the bulletin board at my ballet school. The list named girls who needed to lose weight and by how much. I was never on it. But the possibility filled me with so much dread that at the start of the summer, I decided I had to get into better shape. I did sit-ups and ran every day before and after ballet classes. I stopped eating sweets, fats and meat. And when I turned 15 in September, I was as lean and strong as I've ever been.

Scientists know that environment contributes heavily to the development of eating disorders. Many anorexic and bulimic women are involved in ballet, modeling or some other activity that values low body weight. Men with eating disorders often practice sports that emphasize dieting and fasting, such as wrestling and track. And waiflike figures in fashion and the media clearly hold considerable sway. "The cultural ideal for beauty for women has become increasingly thin over the years," Berkowitz notes. In keeping, among the millions now affected by eating disorders every year, more than 90 percent are female.

Like me, most young women first develop an eating disorder as they near puberty. "Girls start to plump up at puberty," Estherann M. Grace of Children's Hospital in Boston says. "And this is also when they start looking at magazines and thinking, 'What's wrong with me?' " Recognizing that anorexia nervosa often arises as girls begin to mature physically, psychiatrists recently revised the diagnostic standards. "It used to be that one of the criteria was that you had to have missed a period or suffered from amenorrhea for three months," says Marcie B. Schneider of North Shore University Hospital. "And so we missed all those kids with eating disorders who had not yet reached puberty or had delayed it." Now the criteria include a failure to meet expected growth stages, and more 10-, 11- and 12-year-olds are being diagnosed.

Puberty is a stressful time—and stressful events typically precede the onset of psychiatric conditions, including eating disorders. Maybe I would have stopped dieting had my parents not separated in the summer, or my grandmother had not died that fall, or I hadn't spent my entire winter vacation dancing 30-odd performances of the *Nutcracker*. Maybe. I do know that as my life spun out of control around me, my diet became the one thing I felt I could still rein in. "Anorexics are terribly fearful of a loss of control," Grace says, "and eating gives them one area in which they feel they have it."

Most people under stress will overeat or undereat, Grace adds, but biology and personality types make some more vulnerable to extremes. Anorexics tend to be good students, dedicated athletes and perfectionists—and so it makes some sense that in dieting, too, they are highly disciplined. In contrast, bulimics and binge eaters are typically outgoing and adventurous, prone to impulsive behaviors. And all three illnesses frequently arise in conjunction with depression, anxiety and obsessive-compulsive disorder—conditions that tend to run in families and are related to malfunctions in the system regulating the neurotransmitter serotonin.

I most definitely became obsessed. I read gourmet magazines cover to cover, trying to imagine the taste of foods I would not let myself have—ever. I cut my calories back to 800 a day. I counted them down to the singles in a diet soda. I measured and weighed my food to make my tally more accurate. And I ate everything I dished, to make sure I knew the precise number of calories I had eaten. By November, none of my clothes fit. When I sat, I got bruises where my hip bones jutted out in the back. My hair thinned, and my nails became brittle. I was continuously exhausted, incredibly depressed and had no intention of quitting. It felt like a success.

Sitting Down for Treatment

The first barrier to treating eating disorders is getting people to admit that they have one. Because bulimics are often a normal weight and hide their strange eating rituals, they can be very hard to identify. Similarly, binge eaters are extremely secretive about their practices. And even though seriously ill anorexics are quite noticeably emaciated, they are the least willing of all patients with eating disorders to get help. "Anorectics are not motivated for treatment in the same way as bulimics are," Halmi comments. "Because anorexia gives patients a sense of control, it is seen as a positive thing in their lives, and they're terrified to give that up."

I certainly was—and a large part of getting better involved changing that way of thinking. To that end, cognitive behavioral therapy (CBT) has had fair success in treating people with anorexia, bulimia and binge eating disorder. "There are three main components," explains Halmi, who views CBT as one of the most effective treatments. Patients keep diaries of what they eat, how they feel when they eat and what events, if any, prompt them to eat. I used to feel guilty before meals and would ask my mother for permission before I ate. She never would have denied me, but asking somehow lessened my guilt.

CBT also helps patients identify flawed perceptions (such as thinking they are fat) and, with the aid of a therapist, list evidence for and against these ideas and then try to correct them. This process let me eventually see the lack of reason in my belief that, say, a single cookie would lure me into a lifetime bender of reckless eating and obesity. And CBT patients work through strategies for handling situations that reinforce their abnormal perceptions. I got rid of my scale and avoided mirrors.

Working in collaboration with researchers at Stanford University, the University of Minnesota and the University of North Dakota, Halmi is now comparing relapse rates in anorexics who have been randomly assigned to treatment with CBT or the SSRI drug Prozac, or a combination of both. Unfortunately, the dropout rate has been high. But earlier evidence has suggested that Prozac—which had not yet been approved when I was sick—may benefit some patients, helping them to at least stop losing weight. "Essentially every young woman with anorexia is also dealing with depression, and so SSRIs help alleviate some of the somatic symptoms associated with that," Grace says.

Not everyone believes SSRIs do much for anorexics, particularly those who are not desperately ill. But SSRIs have proved effective in people with bulimia. In conjunction with James Mitchell, director of neuroscience at the University of North Dakota, and Scott J. Crow, professor of psychiatry at the University of Minnesota, Halmi has just completed collecting data on 100 bulimics who received cognitive behavioral therapy for four months. Those who still did not improve underwent further therapy and drug treatment with Prozac. "When it comes to bulimia," Berkowitz tells me, "it is clear that both psychotherapy and pharmacology are helpful."

Swallowing the Truth

New treatments for eating disorders could benefit millions of adolescents—if they can get them. Most face a greater challenge getting help today than I did 13 years ago. "One of the big topics now is how to survive in this era of managed care," Schneider tells me. "You have to be at death's door to get into a psychiatric hospital," Berkowitz says, "and once a patient is stabilized, the reimbursements often stop. This is not an inexpensive disease to have." I went through a year of weekly therapy before I reached a stable, if not wholly healthy, weight. In comparison, Berkowitz notes that the insurance policies he has encountered recently often pay for only 20 sessions, with the patient responsible for a 50 percent co-payment.

"It's absolutely sinful," Halmi says. "It is a disaster for eating-disorder patients, particularly anorexics." She points out that relapse rates are much lower in adolescents who receive treatment long enough to get back up to 90 percent of their ideal weight; those who gain less typically fare worse. But insurance rarely lasts long enough. "It used to be you could hospitalize a kid for three or four months," Schneider says. "Now you can at most get a month or so, and it's on a case-by-case basis. You're fighting with the insurance company every three days." The fact that it may be cheaper to treat these patients right the first time seems to make little difference to insurance companies, she adds: "Their attitude is that these kids will probably have a different carrier down the road."

Down the road, the consequences of inadequate treatment are chilling. Debra K. Katzman of the Hospital for Sick Children in Toronto recently took magnetic resonance imaging (MRI) scans of young women with anorexia nervosa before and after recovery and found that the volume of cerebral gray matter in their brains seemed to have decreased—permanently. "The health of these kids does rapidly improve when they gain back some weight," Schneider says, "but the changes on the MRIs do not appear to go away."

In addition, those who do not receive sufficient nutrition during their teen years seriously damage their skeletal growth. "The bones are completed in the second decade, right when this disease hits, so it sets people up for long-term problems," Grace asserts. These problems range from frequent fractures to thinning bones and premature osteoporosis. "I talked to one girl today who is 16. She hasn't been underweight for that long, but already she is lacking 25 percent of the bone density normal for kids her age," Schneider says. "And I have to explain to her why she has to do what no inch in her wants to—eat—so that she won't be in a wheelchair at age 50."

Because drugs used to treat bone loss in adults do nothing in teens, researchers are looking for ways to remedy this particular symptom. "[Loss of bone is] related to their not menstruating and not having estrogen," Grace explains. "But whereas estrogen does protect older women against bone loss, it doesn't seem to help younger ones." She and a coworker are now testing the protective effects of another hormone in young girls. Halmi also emphasizes that estrogen treatment for patients with eating disorders is a waste of time. Instead "you want to get them back up to a normal weight," she states, "and let the body start building bone itself."

All of which brings us back to the concept of normal weight—something many women simply don't want to be. A recent study found that even centerfold models felt the need to lie about their heights and weights. Christopher P. Szabo of the Tara Hospital in Johannesburg reviewed the reported measurements of women in South African editions of *Playboy* between February 1994 and February 1995 and calculated their apparent body mass indices. Even though these models all looked healthy, 72 percent had claimed heights and weights that gave them a body mass index below 18—the medical cutoff for malnourishment. "Maybe 5 percent of the population could achieve an 'ideal' figure, with surgical help," Grace jokes. "I'm sorry, but Barbie couldn't stand upright if she weren't plastic."

I remember all too well thinking that I would look fat at a normal weight. Sometimes I still do worry that I look fat. But I take my perceptions with a grain of salt. After all, I haven't exactly proved myself to be a good judge in that regard. Somehow I've come to a point where I don't need to measure my self-worth in pounds—or the lack thereof—provided I'm happy and well. I gave up a lot—ballet, friendships, a sense of community and security. But in return, I got my health back.

Diet Drugs

As Fen-Phen Alternatives Emerge, Safety Questions Go Unanswered

The diet industry isn't taking this one lying down. Literally days after fenfluramine (Pondimin) and dexfenfluramine (Redux) were pulled from the market, a number of alternatives were already in the promotional mill.

The financial stakes are high: Each year, according to *The Wall Street Journal*, Americans spend a reported $5.6 billion on diet aids. But the safety stakes are high as well.

Pick Your Poison?

Here are some remedies that are being promoted to fill the "fen-phen" void:

Phentermine

Background: The "phen" in the fen-phen combination is still on the market. Phentermine (sold under the brand names Ionamin, Adipex, Fastin, and others) was originally approved for short-term use as a weight-loss aid.

Concerns: Despite the fact that it has been on the market for many years, the safety of long-term phentermine use technically is still unclear. In addition, there is little safety information regarding its use in the latest diet combinations (see below). Known side effects of phentermine include nervousness, insomnia, and hypertension.

Ephedra

Background: Traditionally, ephedra (*Ephedra sinica,* also known as ma huang), has been used to treat respiratory disorders. Two of its alkaloids—ephedrine and pseudoephedrine—appear in prescription and over-the-counter decongestants and bronchodilators. Over the past few years, ephedra has become a staple of the weight-loss scene, and many supplements now marketed as "natural fen-phen" contain the herb.

Concerns: Ephedra is a potent herb. Its use has been linked to a wide range of side effects, from dizziness and agitation to increases in blood pressure, abnormal heart rhythms, heart attacks, strokes, seizures, and brain hemorrhages.

New regulations proposed by the U:S. Food and Drug Administration would limit the dose of ephedrine alkaloids to 8 mg (milligrams) per single dose and 24 mg per day, for a maximum of seven days. Moreover, ephedra products would not be allowed to make weight-loss claims.

Prozac

Background: The antidepressant Prozac (fluoxetine) slows the reabsorption of serotonin in the brain. Because of the connection between higher serotonin levels and increased feelings of satiety—and because of reports that some patients who take Prozac experience a drop in appetite and modest weight loss—the drug is being prescribed with phentermine in the weight-loss remedy known as "phen-Pro."

Concerns: There have been no studies demonstrating that the "off-label" combination of Prozac and phentermine is effective or safe, and the drug company that makes Prozac has warned that it doesn't endorse the drug for weight loss. Known side effects of Prozac include headaches, insomnia, nervousness, anxiety, nausea, and dizziness. So far, there's no information regarding heart valve changes similar to those seen with fenfluramine and dexfenfluramine.

St.-John's-wort

Background: St.-John's-wort (*Hyper-*

icum perforatum) is used to treat mild to moderate depression. The herb may affect the reabsorption of serotonin in the brain, although its chemical actions aren't completely understood. As another version of "natural fen-phen," St.-John's-wort is being taken separately and in combination with phentermine.

Concerns: As most studies of the herb have lasted eight weeks or less, there's no information on long-term safety, nor is there any information on the herb's effectiveness as a weight-loss treatment or its safety when taken with phentermine. Known side effects of St.-John's-wort include fatigue, dizziness, skin rashes, and increased sensitivity to sunlight.

Chromium

Background: Chromium, an essential trace mineral, is needed for normal insulin function. In foods, it's found in whole grains, black pepper, and some vegetables; in supplement form, it's commonly touted as a fat-burning and energy-boosting aid.

Concerns: Chromium metabolism and safety in humans remain poorly understood, and studies have yet to support the use of supplements to help people lose weight, build muscle, or boost energy. The mineral may have merit in diabetes treatment, but that's still under investigation.

Tryptophan

Background: The body uses tryptophan, an amino acid found in protein foods, to manufacture serotonin. An over-the-counter version is being used as a weight-loss aid, both alone and in combination with phentermine.

Concerns: There's no solid proof of the synthetic compound's effectiveness or safety in weight loss, whether it's used alone or with phentermine.

Unit 3

Unit Selections

Key Points to Consider

- Abortion is a volatile issue. Should government mandate "disclosure" of alleged risks?
- Contraception is often seen as a "woman's problem." Do you agree or disagree? What role should men play in contraception?
- Sexually active women are at risk for STDs. What are some of the ways a woman can minimize her risk of contracting one?
- If you could design a new contraceptive, what would it be? What factors would you take into consideration in designing it?

DUSHKINONLINE Links

www.dushkin.com/online/

14. **A Forum for Women's Health**
    http://www.womenshealth.org
15. **Women's Health Interactive**
    http://www.womens-health.com

These sites are annotated on pages 4 and 5.

Gynecological and Reproductive Health

For a long time gynecological and reproductive health issues were what most people thought of when asked about women's health. While the definition of what is covered by women's health has expanded, gynecological issues are still a cornerstone of the discussion of women's health. In this section we have tried to provide discussion of a range of gynecological concerns from everyday pain to the burning national question of abortion.

The first hurdle is the difficulty that science has in accepting that women's sexuality may be different from men's. The lack of scientific research, it can be argued, keeps women from receiving the best health care available. In "Women and Sex: On This Topic, Science Blushes," Gina Kolata reports that while more women report sexual difficulties than do men, research is difficult, though much needed.

For women who are sexually active, the dual problems of contraception and prevention of sexually transmitted diseases (STDs) are an ever-present concern. Some STDs, such as AIDS, are life threatening. Others, such as herpes, can cause long-term problems and can be transmitted prenatally. Awareness of symptoms and prevention is critical for all women.

Even those women who are in long-term heterosexual, monogamous relationships need to think about contraception. The rate of unplanned pregnancies among women in their 40s is the same as for women in their 20s. Julia Califano's article, "Rethinking Birth Control," provides updated information on both old and new methods of contraception. She includes information on new methods and new forms of old methods, as well as discussing how each acts against STDs.

Over 9 percent of the reproductive-age population in the United States is affected by infertility. In "For Infertility Treatments, Now You're Covered, Now You're Not," we turn to the topic of how insurance status affects the provision of services.

Very few women's health issues provoke the strong response that abortion does. For this issue we have included a new article, "The Truth about Abortion and Women's Health," by Sharon Lerner, which reviews the research literature on the consequences of abortion and finds that recent legislation requiring "disclosure of those consequences" may not be grounded in science.

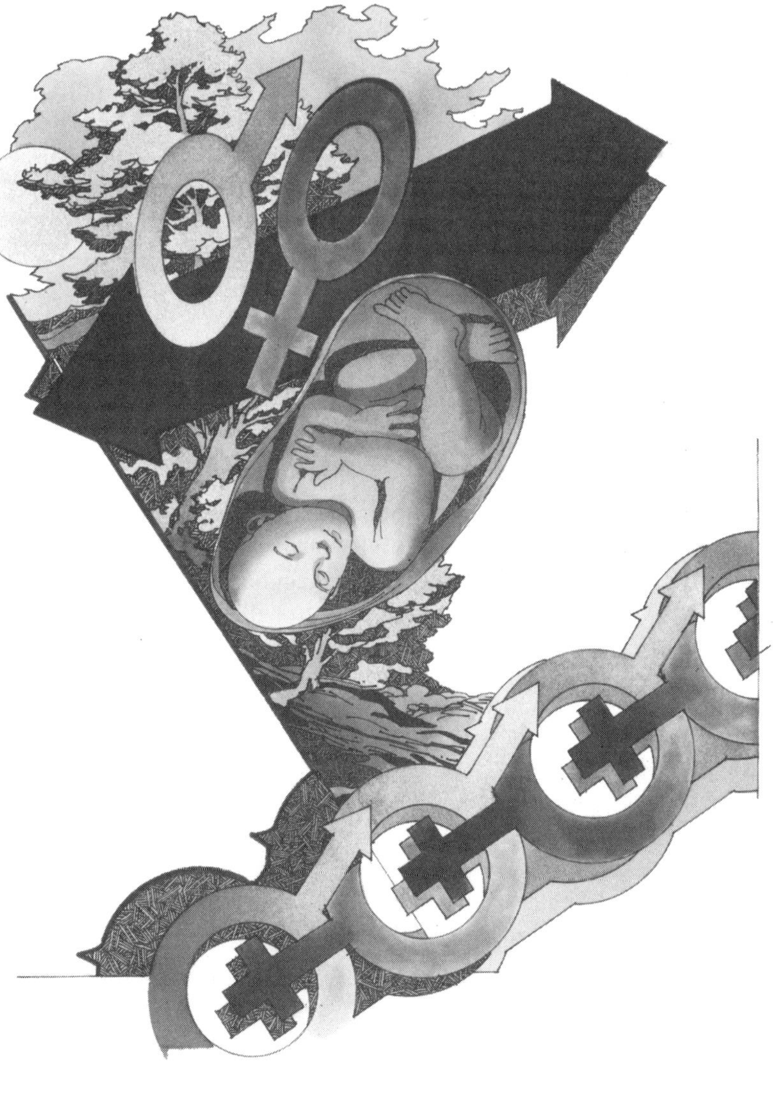

Women and Sex: On This Topic, Science Blushes

By GINA KOLATA

DR. JULIA HEIMAN, a psychologist who directs the reproductive and sexual medicine clinic at the University of Washington, wanted to know whether women become sexually excited by talk of love and romance, or are they turned on by explicit talk of sex itself?

So Dr. Heiman asked college students to wear a tamponlike device that detects blood flow to the vagina. While they wore it, the young women listened to romantic tape recordings and to erotic ones.

Dr. Heiman got her answer: if blood flow to the vagina is an accurate measure of sexual excitement, women, like men, are sexually excited by erotic talk, not romance.

That was in the early 1970's. Yet even now, when most fields of medicine have been transformed, Dr. Heiman's studies are still state of the art.

With the recent introduction of Viagra, however, the impotence pill made by Pfizer, the world has changed.

Suddenly there is a pill for men who have trouble getting and maintaining erections. Almost as suddenly, drug-company scientists, wondering whether Viagra or something like it can enhance sex for women, are asking academic scientists what is known about women's sexual responses.

The answer is not much.

"For most medical professionals, a woman's genitals are still 'down there,'" said Dr. John Gagnon, a sociology professor at the State University of New York at Stony Brook. At their mention, Dr. Gagnon added, "Everyone averts their eyes in horror."

Even worse, he said, is finding out what gives women pleasure and how to enhance their pleasure. Men worry that "if she enjoys it too much, will she do it with someone besides me?" Dr. Gagnon explained.

No one disputes the evidence that many women are unhappy with their sex lives. Dr. Sandra R. Leiblum, a psychologist at the Robert Wood Johnson Medical Center in New Brunswick, N.J., noted that "every survey invariably finds that many more women than men complain of sexual difficulties."

Dr. Leiblum cited a major survey in the United States that found a third of women respondents—but only a sixth of men—saying they are uninterested in sex. One-fifth of the women—but only one-tenth of the men—said sex gave them no pleasure.

Dr. Leiblum said she thinks most sexual complaints in women are psychological. Most women can have orgasms easily by masturbating, she said, "when they don't feel pressured to perform, and when they don't feel concerns about how they look or how they are formed or how they smell."

BUT it is also much easier and more socially acceptable to study psychological problems than the physiology of sexual responses in women.

"There is a huge resistance" to understanding women's sexual responses, said Dr. James H. Geer, a professor of psychology at Louisiana State University and an inventor of the tamponlike device that Dr. Heiman, his graduate student then, used in her studies. Dr. Geer and his colleagues developed that device without financing, he said, which is typically how studies of female sexuality are done.

As a result of this reluctance, the simplest questions have no answers. Half a century ago, when Dr. Alfred C. Kinsey surveyed the sex lives of Americans, he proclaimed that men and women have basically the same sexual responses, except that men

Gina Kolata reports on science and medicine for the New York Times.

are more influenced by psychological factors.

Dr. John Bancroft, the director of the Kinsey Institute at Indiana University, said that scientists now know that "Kinsey was wrong about psychological differences." Yet, Dr. Bancroft added, "Whether he was wrong about physiological similarities remains an open question."

For example, Viagra increases blood flow to the penis, enabling men to have erections. By analogy, some doctors have suggested that Viagra might also increase blood flow to the clitoris and enhance a woman's sexual response. And yet, Dr. Gagnon noted, the idea that women suffer from inadequate blood flow to the clitoris has no experimental evidence. "If there were women with inadequate clitoral swelling, how would we know that?" he asked.

Researchers who want to directly measure sexual responses in women are stymied by a lack of a good method, Dr. Heiman said.

Some critics have said that her studies, involving blood flow to the vagina, focused on the wrong organ. Why did she avoid the clitoris? Because no one has figured out how to study the physiological changes in the clitoris during sexual arousal, Dr. Heiman said. It is not easy to fit the clitoris with a measuring device. "The clitoris is so sensitive that simply touching it could trigger a response," she explained.

Women often complain of having difficulty lubricating, so some researchers tried to measure the secretion of vaginal fluids while women watched erotic movies or listened to erotic tapes. The researchers used tampons, weighing them before and after the women were stimulated.

But the tampons turned out to be too crude to measure the amount of vaginal secretions. So far, no one has found a reliable way to measure vaginal fluids secreted during arousal, and no one knows how much fluid is enough and how much is insufficient.

PFIZER, meanwhile, is hoping to bypass the morass of ignorance regarding women's sexual physiology and simply ask, Does Viagra improve women's sex lives?

Dr. Frances Quirk, who works for Pfizer at its research center in Sandwich, England, said that the early studies of Viagra in men concentrated solely on ways to measure the drug's physical effects on erections. But the company soon redirected its efforts, Dr. Quirk said. "One of the big breakthroughs was in understanding that patient assessments and perceptions can yield valuable information," she said. "This is probably even more important for women."

Borrowing from the same method, Dr. Quirk and her colleagues developed a questionnaire that asks women how often they have sex, how confident they are as a sexual partner and how well and how quickly they respond to sexual stimulation. They tested their survey with 1,160 women living in Britain. The results, Dr. Quirk said, appear to show a relationship between women's symptoms of sexual dysfunction and worries about the future of their sex lives.

For example, 34 percent of women who said they had difficulty becoming aroused said they worry about the future of their sex lives, whereas just 5 percent of those who had no such difficulty with arousal had this worry. And 13 percent of those who had difficulty lubricating—as compared with 8 percent who had no such problem—were anxious about their sex lives.

Now, sex researchers say, the moment of truth is looming.

It was easy to justify Viagra in men because the drug, as Pfizer keeps emphasizing, does not increase desire. All it does is help a man who already has the desire for sex to achieve an erection.

But the primary complaint among women is the lack of desire. For society to sanction research on sexual dysfunction in women, Dr. Heiman said, "People would have to view women's sexual desire as an important issue."

On the other hand, drug companies are not the Federal Government. They can go ahead with sex research if there is a problem that needs to be treated and a market for a drug.

"One could say that having a lack of information on women's sexuality is just fine with the general culture," Dr. Heiman said, "but it may not be so fine with the drug industry."

What Women Need to Know about Sexually Transmitted Diseases

Left undiagnosed, STDs can be deadly. Fortunately, many people can be helped

by Laura A. Koutsky, Ph.D.
University of Washington

Half of all women will acquire one or more sexually transmitted infections during their reproductive years. Despite this dramatic statistic, most people think sexually transmitted diseases, or STDs, are rare. This misperception arises, in part, from the fact that people are often embarrassed to talk about sex, sexuality and gen-italia. But frank discussion is needed. Every year 12 million or so new cases of STDs are reported in the U.S. The most common are chlamydia, gonorrhea and syphilis, which are caused by bacteria. The most widespread viral STDs are human papillomavirus (HPV), genital herpes, hepatitis B and human immunodeficiency virus, or HIV (the virus that causes AIDS). Among the consequences of these myriad STDs are ectopic pregnancy, infertility, preterm delivery, neurological disorders, arthritis, cardiovascular problems, cancer and even death.

This hidden epidemic primarily afflicts young people. Two thirds of STDs in the U.S. take

Genital Human Papillomavirus

Human papillomavirus, or HPV, is a particularly insidious sexually transmitted disease (STD) because it is largely asymptomatic, can cause cancer and is virtually ubiquitous. More than 50 percent of sexually active adults have been infected with HPV—and less than 10 percent of them develop the warts that can help people identify an infection. As with other STDs, the incidence of HPV is highest among 18- to 28-year-olds. Most disturbing, perhaps, is the fact that condoms have not been shown to prevent transmission effectively, because HPV can occur in areas not covered by a condom—such as the base of the penis, the scrotum and the labia.

Of the more than 100 types of HPV, at least 35 infect the skin or mucosal surfaces of the genitalia (other types cause plantar warts and common skin warts). Although two types of HPV—HPV-6 and HPV-11—are most frequently detected in genital warts, these types are rarely found in invasive cancers of the cervix, vagina, vulva, penis and anus. Most such cancers seem instead to originate with infection by HPV-16, HPV-18, HPV-31 or HPV-45.

Genital HPV infections are primarily acquired through sexual intercourse. Unlike other viruses such as HIV and hepatitis B, HPV is not transmitted through blood and bodily fluids but rather by direct skin-to-skin contact. Although it is uncommon, warts on the fingers can carry genital HPV-6 or HPV-16, and in some cases, warts can develop in and around the mouth. All sexually active people—whether heterosexual or homosexual—are at risk of gen-

The American Social Health Association (ASHA) is a non-profit organization that provides information on HPV and other STDs. ASHA also sponsors the National STD Hotline (800-227-8922) and offers pamphlets and educational materials on STD-related topics. For more information, visit the organization's World Wide Web site at http://www.ashastd.org or write to the American Social Health Association/HPV, P. O. Box 13827, Research Triangle Park, NC 27709-3827.

place among people under the age of 25. This finding is not surprising: more than 60 percent of high school seniors report having had sexual intercourse, and 27 percent say they have had at least four partners. In 1971, 39 percent of young women between the ages of 15 and 19 reported having had more than one sex partner; in 1988 that figure reached 62 percent. There is no indication that this trend will reverse soon. Although our society does not condone adolescent sexual activity, the fact remains that teenagers are sexually active and that they are acquiring STDS with some painful consequences.

This situation is especially disturbing because in many cases it is preventable. Although incidences of incurable viral STDs, such as HPV, appear to be similar everywhere, the incidence of curable bacterial STDs among U.S. teenagers and adults is higher than it is in other industrial countries. Syphilis, for example, afflicts 4.3 out of every 100,000 Americans annually—nearly three times the rate for Germans and almost 11 times the rate for Canadians. This discrepancy is caused in part by cultural differences in sexual behavior and by economic differences, but it also results from the fact that Americans have less access to diagnosis and treatment than do people in Germany or Canada—countries that provide universal health care. Indeed, one quarter of American adolescents and young adults do not have health insurance.

In developing countries, where health care resources are extremely limited, the situation is more dire. STDs, including syphilis, chlamydial infection, gonorrhea and pelvic inflammatory disease—an upper reproductive tract infection that can result from various STDs—constitute the second leading cause of healthy life lost for women between the ages of 15 and 44. Cervical cancer caused by genital HPV is the most common cancer and the principal cause of cancer-related deaths among women in these resource-poor countries, where Pap tests are not widely available.

Although they affect both men and women, STDs are disproportionately damaging in women and adolescent girls. The biology of the female genital tract lends itself to asymptomatic infections. Unlike the male urethra, which often becomes painful within days of exposure to gonorrhea or chlamydia, the cervix (which is particularly susceptible to infection in younger women) may be infected for long periods without causing any discomfort. At least 25 percent of women with gonorrhea experience no symptoms, for instance, as opposed to less than 10 percent of men. Many women, unaware of the presence of an STD, do not seek medical attention—a delay that can have serious consequences. Untreated cervical gonorrhea and chlamydial infections can ascend into the uterus and fallopian tubes, causing pelvic inflammatory disease and setting the stage for ectopic pregnancies and infertility.

Some STDs are largely asymptomatic in both sexes—most men and women with HPV or herpes infections never become aware of them. Even so, women often suffer more damage to their health from these STDs: HPV infection, for instance, is more likely to cause cancer in women than in men [*see box below*].

Routes of Transmission

For many STDs, particularly the bacterial ones, people who repeatedly acquire and transmit infection play an important role in establishing and sustaining the prevalence of disease. Such people are considered to be high-frequency transmitters—in epidemiological terms, they are called a core group. This group typically includes people who are commercial sex workers, their clients and their partners, as well as men and women who have unprotected intercourse with multiple partners.

The impact of people in a core group appears to vary for different diseases. Syphilis requires the participation of a great many transmitters to achieve an annual incidence rate of 1 percent. HPV, however, can have an annual incidence rate of more than 5 percent in populations that include a tiny core group or even no core group at all. This difference may be explained by several factors. First, HPV appears to be more easily transmitted than *Treponema pallidum*, the bacterium that causes syphilis. Second, asymptomatic diseases are harder to control: more than 90 percent of genital HPV infections are asymptomatic;

---

ital HPV infection with each new sex partner. Indeed, genital forms of the virus are not uncommon among lesbians.

Most newly acquired genital HPV infections do not announce themselves, and often people with genital HPV infection never become aware of its presence. HPV infection can be detected through certain tests for HPV DNA. Because of the high prevalence of this STD, any kind of general screening test for HPV would reveal infection in a huge proportion of sexually active adults. But the clinical importance of detecting asymptomatic infection in areas other than the cervix is not yet clear; penile cancer, for instance, is extremely rare.

The significance of genital HPV infection of the cervix, however, is quite certain. Precancerous lesions can form within a year of initial infection. Because early detection of cervical cancer is crucial for prevention and treatment, women should have regular Pap tests, which can detect HPV-related precancer, early invasive cancer and cancer of the cervix. Women should know that Pap readings are most accurate if they are done midway between menstrual periods. Gynecologists also recommend that women avoid vaginal creams, foams or suppositories the week before the exam and that they do not douche, have sex or use tampons the day before.

Women with abnormal Pap test results are referred for colposcopy. During this procedure, the cervix is treated with a mild vinegar solution and then examined for flat, whitish lesions. If these lesions prove to be precancerous or cancerous, they must be removed.

Genital warts in men and women can be surgically excised, frozen off or topically treated with medication, but the virus probably remains present in the body: it cannot be eradicated. For this reason, treatment of asymptomatic infection is not recommended.

In the near future, vaccines may be able to prevent HPV transmission. Our research group is testing an HPV vaccine that consists of the outer protein shell, or capsid, of the virus, which should stimulate the body's immune response, thereby preventing infection or disease. Similar vaccines have been effective in animals. If all goes well, an HPV vaccine may become available in the next decade.

—*L.K.*

ADRIENNE WEISS

Sexually Transmitted Disease	Percent of Women Who Show No Symptoms	Possible Long-Term Complications in Women	Effective Treatment or Vaccine Available?
Chlamydia	More than 75	Pelvic inflammatory disease, infertility, ectopic pregnancy, chronic pelvic pain	Antibiotics available; no vaccine
Gonorrhea	25–75	Pelvic inflammatory disease, infertility, ectopic pregnancy, chronic pelvic pain	Antibiotics available (although antibiotic-resistant strains exist); no vaccine
Syphilis	25–75	Cardiovascular problems, neurological disorders, damage to other organ systems	Antibiotics available; no vaccine
Chancroid	25–75	Unknown	Antibiotics available; no vaccine
Genital human papillomavirus	More than 90	Cervical, vulvar, vaginal and anal cancers	No*
Genital herpes	More than 50	Unknown	No*
Hepatitis B	25–75	Chronic liver disease, cirrhosis, liver cancer	No*; vaccine available
Human immunodeficiency virus	25–75	AIDS	No*
Trichomoniasis	25–75	Unknown	Antibiotics available

* Available treatments can reduce symptoms and complications but do not clear virus from the body. *SOURCE: Laura A. Koutsky and the Institute of Medicine*

only about 50 percent of syphilis cases are. And, finally, current therapies usually do not rid the body of HPV infection, but penicillin can cure syphilis.

Whether STDs originate with a member of a core group or not, they are generally more efficiently passed during vaginal and anal intercourse than they are during oral intercourse. (In rare situations, an STD may be transmitted from a mother to her infant during pregnancy or delivery.) Furthermore, some STDs appear to be more easily transmitted from a man to a woman than from a woman to a man. For example, between 60 and 90 percent of women engaging in unprotected intercourse with men who have gonorrhea will become infected, whereas only 20 to 30 percent of men who have unprotected sex with infected women will contract the disease.

In the case of HIV, more data are needed to determine whether infection moves as readily from women to men as it does from men to women. It is clear, however, that HIV is somewhat more difficult to transmit during sexual intercourse than

It's All Connected: The Importance of Addressing Young Men's Health

The waiting room is almost full, and it is only 4:30 P.M. Still half an hour to go before the clinic opens. The young men started arriving at 3:00, a few accompanied by their girlfriends, and they sit in rows facing a screen, watching a sexy music video. That is, until their viewing pleasure is interrupted by a slide show that opens with a graphic portrayal of the difference between an uncircumcised and a circumcised penis. The uncomfortable silence does not faze the social worker. "Any opinions on why they are different?" she asks. And the evening at the Young Men's Clinic at the Columbia University School of Public Health's Center for Population and Family Health in New York City is off and running.

For the next several hours, men and boys from the primarily Dominican, largely poor neighborhood of Washington Heights meet with doctors and nurse practitioners—as well as medical students from the New York and Presbyterian Hospital—to have HIV tests, physicals and exams for genital warts, herpes and other sexually transmitted diseases (STDs). "We use the slide show not to scare them but to open up discussion. We are trying to get them to challenge their beliefs," says Bruce Armstrong, associate professor of public health and co-founder of the clinic. About 80 percent of the young men who come in are sexually active, 40 percent have made a partner pregnant, and 17 percent have an STD; almost none of them receive health care anywhere else.

"It's teaching without preaching," adds Tschaka Tonge, one of the physician's assistants. "We talk to them about lifestyle. I ask the young gentlemen, 'Do you really need another girlfriend? Can you afford this?' We try to get them to rethink their choices."

In a small examining room, Tonge talks with a young man from Nigeria who says he needs a physical for college. Tonge knows some Yoruba and tries to get his patient to talk about his health and sexual activity: Has he been tested for tuberculosis? Where'd he lose his two front teeth? When did he become sexually active? Does he use birth control and, if so, which kind? Sabitu Ladejobi, who says he found out about the clinic from a flyer, is terse at first but slowly warms to his purple-shirted, dreadlock-sporting, hip-looking P.A.

The night of Ladejobi's visit is a particularly busy one. Not only is the free clinic—which is open only on Friday afternoons and Monday nights—filled to capacity as usual, but a group of Latin American public health experts are visiting. As one of a handful of places worldwide that offers preventive care for young men and that does not ignore their role in family planning, the Young Men's Clinic is increasingly being looked to as a model program.

Men have traditionally been left out of family-planning initiatives. Some of this bias has been purely practical: women have the babies, and most forms of birth control have been designed for them. Other aspects of the discrepancy have been incidental. "Put yourself in the mind-set of a young man who comes into a clinic and sees 50 women and a video on 'Your First Pelvic Exam' in the waiting room," Armstrong explains. "From the young fellow's point of view, the family-planning clinic is perceived as being for young women—even though that is not the policy."

New data on STDs and male sexual behavior, however, are beginning to inform other STDs. The presence of syphilis, chlamydia, gonorrhea or chancroid may facilitate transmission of HIV. Rates of HIV infection are increasing faster among 15- to 44-year-old women than they are among any other group in the U.S.

The Challenge of Prevention

Women are at a distinct disadvantage with regard to protecting themselves against STDs. Synthetic condoms, which are the only available reliable barriers to infection, are generally in the control of the man. (The female condom does not seem to have become wildly popular; *see* box "It's All Connected: The Importance of Addressing Young Men's Health.") Nevertheless, sexually active women can reduce their chances of suffering the consequences of STDs. To do so, they should use a condom during intercourse with a new partner or with a regular partner who is unwilling to be monogamous. Sexually active women should undergo annual pelvic examinations and Pap tests, as well as screening for gonorrhea, chlamydia, and HIV, if recommended by their health care provider.

Relying on over-the-counter products is no substitute for seeing a physician or nurse practitioner. Although douching is popular among some women, there appear to be few situations where it is medically required. Women with gonorrhea or chlamydia may actually increase their chances of developing pelvic inflammatory disease by douching. Women should also be aware that vaginal discharge does not always mean a yeast infection—rather it can be the sign of a more dangerous infection. Public health officials have recently become concerned that over-the-counter yeast infection treatments are encouraging women to diagnose and treat themselves, thereby delaying a trip to the doctor for a more serious problem, such as gonorrhea.

Despite this dismal state of affairs, there is hope. Researchers are working to develop vaccines for viral STDs, including HIV and HPV. A vaccine for hepatitis B is already available. And targeted behavioral intervention programs have proved successful in other countries. For instance, in Thailand, a government-sponsored and widely advertised effort to promote condoms among the general population and to enforce the universal use of condoms among sex workers has contributed to a dramatic decline in the incidence of STDs there.

There is growing awareness in the U.S. that the medical and public health community has not been effective in warning people about the rise in incidence of STDs or the possibilities for prevention and treatment. This ineffectiveness is clearly reflected in a 1993 survey, which found that 84 percent of women felt they were at no risk of contracting an STD. As many public health experts and a recent Institute of Medicine report note, the secrecy and uneasiness surrounding discussions of sex in the U.S. undermine this country's ability to address STDs. Without open discussion, education, outreach and intervention, the threats to young people will only continue with tragic consequences.

LAURA A. KOUTSKY, associate professor of epidemiology at the University of Washington, has studied the epidemiology of STDs for more than 10 years. Her research concerns genital human papillomavirus infection.

---

family-planning strategies. In the late 1980s the first National Survey of Adolescent Males provided some of the only information on the attitudes and sexual behavior of 15- to 19-year-olds. The survey recently found that between 1988 and 1995 the use of contraceptives during first intercourse increased from 62 to 73 percent; condom usage, in particular, rose significantly.

The survey's authors also found that, contrary to stereotype, 90 percent of men believe they should talk to their partner about contraception before intercourse, protect against pregnancy and take responsibility if they do father a child. These findings, as well as a review of male-oriented programs, were recently published in an Urban Institute report, "Involving Males in Preventing Teen Pregnancy."

Public health experts say the shift to include men is part of a larger social transformation catalyzed by the current fatherhood movement, the 1988 Family Support Act—which requires noncustodial parents to be financially responsible for their progeny—and the 1995 Clinton administration effort to design federal programs that include and promote the involvement of fathers. Developing "the role of men as being nurturing, caring and responsible in reproductive health matters has taken a while in many ways," Armstrong remarks. "It was just a short time ago that fathers were not allowed into the delivery room."

But perhaps most responsible for the changing approach is the alarming prevalence of STDs. According to the Alan Guttmacher Institute, 12 million such infections occur annually in the U.S.—among the highest numbers in the industrial world—and teenagers account for 25 percent of all cases. Judith N. Wasserheit, director of the Division of STD/HIV Prevention at the Centers for Disease Control and Prevention, notes that men have been the focus of STD programs in the past, largely because most STDs are more symptomatic in men. But in the past decade or so, more data have made clear the long-term consequences of asymptomatic STD infection in women—including infertility, cervical cancer, miscarriage, stillbirth, premature delivery, and mental retardation and blindness in newborns. Now, Wasserheit says, "there is a very interesting confluence with the family-planning community's saying we need to do more for men, and the STD community's saying we need to do more for women."

"Although you are talking about women's health, men are very much interwoven," concurs Anidolee Chester, education coordinator at Planned Parenthood in Providence, R.I. "If you get them to have some sense of responsibility, you will see improvements in women's health." Chester and her colleagues recently started a program for men, modeled after the Young Men's Clinic.

Armstrong and his colleagues say the clinic's success comes from their efforts to make every moment a "teachable" one and to listen without judging. "There is a stereotype that young men are healthy, not concerned about health, and hard to engage and maintain as patients," says Alwyn T. Cohall, medical director at the clinic and director of the Harlem Center for Health Promotion and Disease Prevention. "We have debunked all of these myths."

—Marguerite Holloway, contributing editor

The female condom's manufacturer, the Female Health Company, reports that the plastic vaginal sheath is 79 to 95 percent effective as a contraceptive and can reduce the risk of contracting HIV by 97 percent.

Arm Yourself against STDs

Humanity's battle against sexually transmitted diseases (STDs) is limited by the weapons at our disposal. The bacteria and viruses that cause STDs are spreading faster than modern technology and education can sequester their populations. Although there are effective methods available for preventing infection, it is estimated that at least 300 million people are infected every year throughout the world with the most common STDs—gonorrhea, chlamydia, syphilis and trichomoniasis.

In addition to abstinence, there are three principal approaches to blocking the transmission of STDs: physical barriers, chemical barriers and vaccines. These techniques are in different stages of development and have various degrees of reliability.

Physical barriers

Physical barriers, such as synthetic condoms, prevent the organisms that cause disease from entering the body. Condoms are the only method of birth control on the market today that has proved effective in fighting most STDs. (They have not been shown, however, to block the transmission of human papillomavirus, or HPV.)

In addition to the male condom, there is a female condom available—sold under the brand name Reality. A package of three female condoms costs about $9, roughly the cost of 12 male condoms. But current studies by Family Health International are evaluating whether female condoms could be reused, notes Nancy Alexander, an expert on contraception at the National Institutes of Health. According to the manufacturer, The Female Health Company, the female condom has proved effective in preventing the transmission of gonorrhea, chlamydia, syphilis and trichomoniasis—and if correctly used can reduce one's risk of getting HIV by as much as 97 percent. Alexander says that an independent study of the female condom's effectiveness in this regard has not yet been conclusive and is currently under way at the University of Alabama.

Because of its large size, the female condom has been somewhat unpopular since it went on the market in the U.S. in 1993, but the company says that sales are up and that the idea is catching on. The female condom consists of two rings connected by a polyurethane sheath. The small, inner ring covers the cervix, stretching the sheath to line the walls of the vagina. The larger ring at the other end of the sheath remains outside the woman, protecting the vaginal lips from contact with skin or bodily fluids.

Other barrier devices for women that rely on a combination of physical and chemical methods to block STDs are not as effective against infection, because they do not prevent fluids from entering the body. These methods include diaphragms and cervical caps.

Chemical barriers

Chemical barriers, such as spermicides, do not block the exchange of bodily fluids at all—but actively kill the viruses and bacteria that can cause disease on contact. Spermicides are not proved to be effective in preventing most STDs, however—not because they cannot kill the organisms but because they cannot kill all of them.

To be effective, a chemical barrier must be applied to cover every place that bodily fluids might travel during sex, a task that is nearly impossible. Yet there is some evidence suggesting that spermicides are an effective defense against chlamydia and gonorrhea, Alexander says. And although some researchers are developing spermicides that will be able to target specific viruses or bacteria, any chemical barrier will still be limited by its inability to protect all sexually exposed areas.

Vaccines

Perhaps the greatest hope for defense against STDs lies in vaccines, which activate the body's immune system to attack the organisms that can cause disease. The only STD vaccine available is for the viral infection hepatitis B. The Centers for Disease Control and Prevention and the American Academy of Pediatrics recommend the vaccine for all newborns, children and sexually active people.

Several vaccines are being tested to fight HIV, but so far none has been effective. The search for a vaccine is hampered by the fact that investigators do not yet understand how—or even whether—the human body can resist the ravages of HIV.

The quest for a vaccine for HPV—the virus associated with 90 percent of cases of cervical cancer—has just begun. Still, researchers are hopeful because animal vaccines against analogous infections, such as bovine papillomavirus in cows, have been effective.

Despite the promise of STD vaccines, Alexander predicts that they will not be available for another 20 years. The process is slow because vaccines have to be tested on humans—and precautions must be taken to prevent the spread of disease while testing the effectiveness of the treatment.—*Krista McKinsey, special correspondent*

The other epidemic

Genital herpes rages among women and devastates some newborns

BY BETSY CARPENTER

Fifteen years ago, genital herpes had the sexually permissive in a panic. One in 10 adults was thought to be stricken with this ancient, incurable venereal disease and its accompanying blisters and sores. Suddenly, "free" sex seemed very costly; here was a consequence of a one-night stand that the pill couldn't avert and penicillin couldn't remedy. Then herpes seemed to vanish, eclipsed in the public's mind by the swift, deadly rise of AIDS.

But the virus didn't go away: It surged to create an epidemic. According to a study published last month in the *New England Journal of Medicine,* since the late 1970s, the proportion of Americans infected with the herpes simplex type 2 virus (HSV-2) has increased by almost one third. Today, 45 million people over the age of 12 carry it—about 1 in 5. Women generally are more susceptible to sexually transmitted diseases (STDs), so the numbers climb even higher for women. One in five white women is infected, versus one in seven white men. One in two black women has the virus, compared with one in three black men.

To Anna Wald, medical director of the Virology Research Clinic at the University of Washington in Seattle, "Herpes has become a major public health problem." In addition to causing sufferers periodic pain and discomfort, genital herpes is potentially devastating to newborns exposed during delivery. Herpes has also been shown to confound the lives of people with suppressed immune systems, such as burn victims and transplant patients. Recent studies show that people with herpes are more susceptible to a variety of STDs, including HIV—the virus that causes AIDS.

Dangerous myths. Several misconceptions about herpes are fueling the epidemic, according to public-health experts. Most Americans think the virus is uncommon, for instance, afflicting 1 percent or less of the population, says Peggy Clarke, former president of the American Social Health Association in Research Triangle Park in North Carolina. "People just don't know how likely they are to pick it up [from a prospective partner] unless they take precautions."

Many people also hold the mistaken belief that the herpes virus that infects the mouth is benign (herpes simplex type 1 or HSV-1) and that the one that infects the genitals is malevolent (HSV-2). There are differences between the two: HSV-1, which is far more prevalent, infecting about 7 in 10 people, often is acquired in childhood and usually infects the mouth; HSV-2 is typically acquired sexually and usually infects the genitals. But the two are clinically indistinguishable and can inhabit each other's territory. Oral-genital sex is an increasing source of infections, with perhaps 15 percent of genital sores really a manifestation of an HSV-1 infection. "People need to think of [lip] cold sores as infectious to newborns and sexual partners, too," says virologist Rhoda Ashley of the University of Washington in Seattle.

In addition, studies have shown that 2 out of 3 people with the virus don't know they are infected and potentially contagious. How can they miss clusters of itching, painful blisters? For many, a first outbreak is hard to ignore—like a bad case of the flu plus lesions. But others, especially individuals who already harbor HSV-1, often experience only a mild primary infection with HSV-2—with symptoms more like paper cuts or pimples than blisters. According to Ashley, the symptoms can be so variable that "even skilled practitioners can miss [herpes]." Some people also may be refusing to face facts. According to one study, 40 percent to 75 percent of the people with genital herpes who claim to have never experienced symptoms are able to identify them after a doctor delivers the news that they are infected.

No "safe" time. Many believe that people who carry herpes are infectious only during acute episodes, when blisters erupt. Yet infected people can shed virus particles from the genital area—and enough of them to infect a sexual partner—even when they are lesion free. Recent research with a new, sensitive test reveals that even when women with HSV-2 have no visible symptoms, they are shedding the virus "subclinically" about 1 in every 6 days. This "subclinical" shedding is generally greatest in the first six months after a person contracts the virus. The shedding rate declines slightly over the next six months and appears to fluctuate thereafter. Most people today with a first-time infection appear to have contracted it from sexual partners who were not aware of any symptoms. (Similarly, people with recurring cold sores in the mouth can transmit the virus between outbreaks.) "It's a tough message to have to tell people, but there's no 'safe' time [for people with the virus] to have [unprotected] sex," says one counselor at the National Herpes Hotline (919-361-8488).

The herpes virus can be devastating to newborns, as Barbara Wilkop of Birmingham, Mich., knows too well. Her 10-year-old son, Jimmy, has an IQ of 35 as a result of contracting herpes from his mother at birth. Jimmy can hear, but he can't understand words. He can ride a bicycle, but he can't always figure out what to do at the end of a dead-end street. He has to be reminded to zip up his pants whenever he goes to the bathroom, and he has so little impulse control that at one family gathering he bit a cousin on the shoulder. "Sometimes I get so sad," says Wilkop. "Jimmy will never get a chance to drive a car, get married, buy a house, or see his first child born."

About 1 in 3,000 infants nationally contracts the herpes virus during delivery, says David Kimberlin of the University of Alabama at Birmingham. Women who have had herpes for several years before having children rarely infect their infants during delivery, thanks to protective antibodies passed from mother to child in the womb. Only about 2 in 100 such in-

From *U.S. News & World Report,* November 10, 1997, pp. 78-82.

fants pick up the virus during birth, and, in most instances, it infects only the skin, eyes, or mouth.

Infants at high risk. But one third to one half of infants delivered to women who contract the virus for the first time late in their pregnancies contract herpes. In these cases, herpes often attacks the brain, causing death or severe neurological impairment, ranging from blindness and deafness to mental retardation. Because the consequences of infection can be so severe, obstetricians usually recommend delivery by Caesarean section if they spot even the hint of a lesion at the time of delivery. "The general rule is: 'No lesion, vaginal delivery; lesion, C-section,' " according to Larry Gilstrap, chairman of the committee on Obstetrics at the American College of Obstetricians and Gynecologists. As a result, genital herpes is one of the leading causes of C-sections nationally. Although precise figures are not available, Gilstrap estimates that herpes may be fourth or fifth on the list.

Doctors are debating whether pregnant women should be screened for herpes at their first prenatal visit to the doctor, as most are for syphilis, German measles, and a host of other diseases. Zane Brown of the University of Washington in Seattle contends that adding a blood test for herpes to the list makes good sense. "I can go from one end of a decade to the other and not see [a case of] syphilis or gonorrhea, but 35 percent of my patients have genital herpes," he says of his largely middle-class practice. It's especially important to identify high-risk couples, in which the man is infected and the woman isn't. Typically, he tells such couples to use condoms and prescribes for the men an antiviral drug, such as acyclovir or famciclovir, to suppress outbreaks and subclinical shedding, or he counsels couples to abstain from intercourse for the duration of the pregnancy.

Physicians who oppose prenatal screening for herpes argue that test results aren't that useful clinically. Even women who test positive in early pregnancy won't necessarily be shedding the virus during delivery, Gilstrap says. And a woman who tests negative at the start of her pregnancy could have picked up the virus by the end.

The opposition of many doctors to prenatal testing seems to stem from a reluctance to deal with the messy emotions that crop up after the diagnosis of an incurable disease—which herpes remains. One prominent obstetrician says that with herpes, "Ignorance is bliss. What am I supposed to say to a wife who tests positive and asks, 'Where did I get this from? I've only had relations with my husband'?"

There are dramatic reasons why all health care providers should deal with the topic. Besides inflicting health problems on infants, adults can find themselves in a fierce struggle with the virus. People with compromised immune systems are the most vulnerable. In burn victims, a herpes skin infection can spread bodywide. "Though rare, it's a well-recognized complication that can kill you," says University of Washington's David Koelle. Bone-marrow-transplant patients and people with lupus can succumb to herpes infections too, although hefty doses of antiviral drugs usually will keep the virus in check. Most AIDS patients—particularly in the disease's early stages—have sufficiently intact immune systems that lesions stay localized. But outbreaks can become the size of silver dollars or larger and be slow to heal.

Public-health experts are deeply concerned about studies finding that getting herpes sores puts sufferers at a much greater risk of contracting HIV—up to nine times as great—by providing portals for HIV to enter the body. "Especially in inner-city populations [which have a high incidence of herpes], it's plausible that herpes is fueling the spread of HIV," says Sharilyn Stanley at the National Institute of Allergy and Infectious Diseases (NIAID) in Bethesda, Md.

Despite the many health threats posed by herpes, few weapons are available to fight the disease. The diagnostic tests commercially available today are unreliable. People with active lesions can have them swabbed and cultured, but such "viral culture" tests are accurate only when lesions are newly formed and teeming with virus particles. Because many people don't get in to see their doctors until their blisters are partly healed, about half the herpes-infected people who take the test are falsely assured that they don't have the virus.

Testing the blood. Doctors can give patients with no current symptoms a blood test for antibodies to HSV. But the tests currently on the market can't diagnose a case of genital herpes because they don't distinguish between HSV-1 and HSV-2. An accurate, reliable blood test that can tell HSV-1 from HSV-2 is being reviewed by the Food and Drug Administration, however, and may be available by early next year.

Several studies of couples in which one person is infected and the other isn't have shown that transmission is not inevitable, even after years of sexual contact—although often it takes only a few months for the uninfected partner to catch the virus. Herpes is a "very serious infection," according to Penelope Hitchcock, chief of the division of Microbiology and Infectious Diseases at NIAID, but "[it] is not the most infectious disease in the world."

Still, there is no reliable way to prevent transmission of the virus. Condoms provide only partial protection because the virus can be shed from parts of the body not covered by condoms. "Condoms work pretty well for HIV [which is found in body fluids], and not so very well with HSV," says André Nahmias of Emory University School of Medicine in Atlanta. Until recently, researchers hoped that nonoxynol-9, a spermicide often used with condoms and diaphragms, would prove to be an effective chemical barrier, wiping out virus particles as handily as it does sperm cells. But recent studies have shown that nonoxynol-9 is so irritating to the mucosal membranes of the female genital tract that it may increase a woman's susceptibility to infections by damaging these protective membranes. "This is the frustration of clinicians," says Nahmias. "What do you tell people to do?"

To reduce the risk of contracting herpes, Hitchcock of NIAID recommends a few sensible precautions. If a person is not in a monogamous relationship with an uninfected person, he or she should always use condoms. If one partner carries the virus, the couple should never have sex when the partner has lesions, and they should use condoms at other times. If a partner has recurring lip sores, unprotected oral sex should be avoided. Women should abstain when they have vaginal yeast or bacterial infections, which can wipe out healthy microbes.

NIAID has begun funding a host of research projects aimed at developing new tools for stemming the epidemic. A promising area of inquiry is whether daily doses of acyclovir can help carriers of genital herpes protect their partners and infants from infection. A preliminary study published last year by Laurie Scott, then of the University of Texas Southwestern Medical Center in Dallas, and her colleagues suggests that women may be able to protect their babies from infection by taking acyclovir during the last month of pregnancy. Similarly, a study by Anna Wald and colleagues last year showed that acyclovir therapy reduced viral shedding between outbreaks in women by 94 percent. Wald says, "The transmission study hasn't been done yet, but these results do suggest that the drug may interrupt transmission [between sexual partners]."

Many herpes experts say that only a safe, effective vaccine will be able to decrease the number of people infected each year. But while many potential vaccines are being developed, all are at least a decade away.

Rethinking Birth Control

If you still believe the IUD is dangerous and the Pill is for women under 35, you may be stuck in a contraception rut. Here's a roundup of the most effective methods for midlife women.

JULIA CALIFANO

Through two years of dating, 10 years of marriage and two kids, Chris, a college professor in Syracuse, NY, relied almost exclusively on a diaphragm for birth control. Indeed, this 40-year-old would still be putting up with the hassle and mess if, at her last checkup, her doctor hadn't suggested she try an intrauterine device (IUD). Persuaded by his argument that it was highly effective, long-lasting and, for most women, nearly free of side effects, she switched. She hasn't regretted her decision. "It's such a pleasure not to have to plan ahead or get out of bed in the heat of passion," she says. "We don't even think about birth control anymore."

By the time a woman turns 35, she's moved an average of eight times, switched jobs seven times and had two children, yet there's only a 50–50 chance that she has ever thought about changing her method of birth control, according to a survey by Ortho Pharmaceutical. But the truth is she should. "A woman's contraceptive needs change as her life changes," says Anita Nelson, M.D., medical director of the Woman's Health Care Clinic at Harbor UCLA Medical Center in Los Angeles. "A barrier method may be great when you're 21 and concerned about AIDS and other sexually transmitted diseases [STD's], but it's probably not ideal when you're 35 and married with kids."

Perhaps more surprising is the staggering rate of unplanned pregnancies among women in their 40s: According to the Alan Guttmacher Institute in New York City, eight out of 10 pregnancies in this age group are unintended—the same rate as for women under age 20.

How can you tell if your current choice is still your best choice? Reassess your birth control periodically, taking your lifestyle, health, sex life and desire for children into consideration. Here's a guide to the options, plus expert advice on what to use when.

The IUD: Unfounded fear

What it is: The current IUD of choice is ParaGard, a piece of plastic with copper inside it that's put into the uterus to stop sperm from reaching eggs for up to 10 years. Another IUD called Progestasert contains hormones; it works for one year.

Benefits: Long-term, reversible, worry-free protection, and an insertion process that's only slightly more involved than a Pap smear. Progestasert also reduces menstrual cramps and the flow of monthly bleeding.

Drawbacks: The copper IUD can cause heavier than usual periods, won't protect you from STD's and shouldn't be used if you're not in a mutually monogamous relationship. Users with multiple partners are at increased risk for pelvic inflammatory disease (PID), an infection that can cause infertility.

What you may not know: Though most people still associate this device with the dreaded Dalkon Shield (an IUD that caused infection and infertility in thousands of women, along with a few deaths, in the '70s), ParaGard is considered one of the best and safest birth control options. In fact, it's the most popular form of reversible contraception outside the U.S., with 85 million users worldwide.

When to consider it: If you're in a mutually monogamous, long-term relationship and have had at least one child (for childless women there's a small risk that the device will be expelled). "An ideal time to switch to the IUD is when you've completed your family but don't want to take the irreversible step of sterilization," says nurse practitioner Kara Anderson, a medical consultant to the Planned Parenthood Federation of America in New York City.

The Pill: Now for Older Women

What it is: This oral contraceptive is a combination of two hormones, progestin and estrogen, that suppresses ovulation.

Benefits: Easy, reliable and offers a wealth of health benefits. After five

From *American Health for Women,* March 1997, pp. 66-69, 104. © 1997 by Julia Califano. Reprinted by permission.

A Field Guide to Cost and Effectiveness

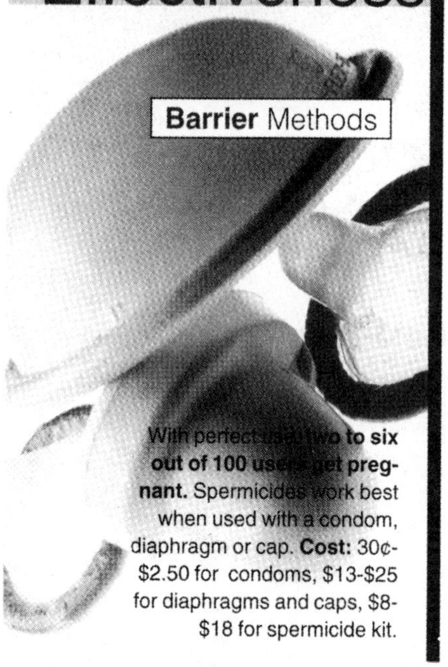

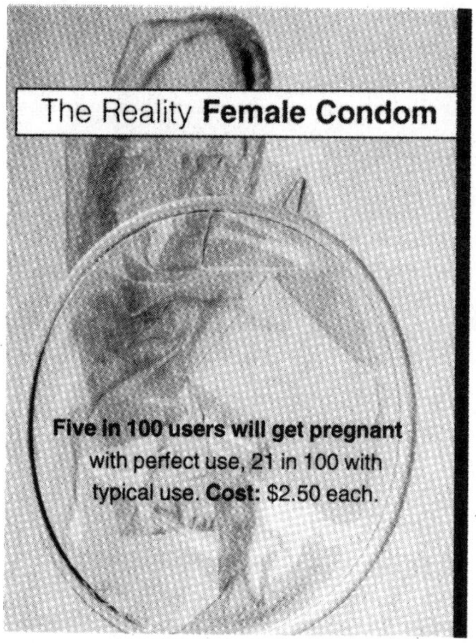

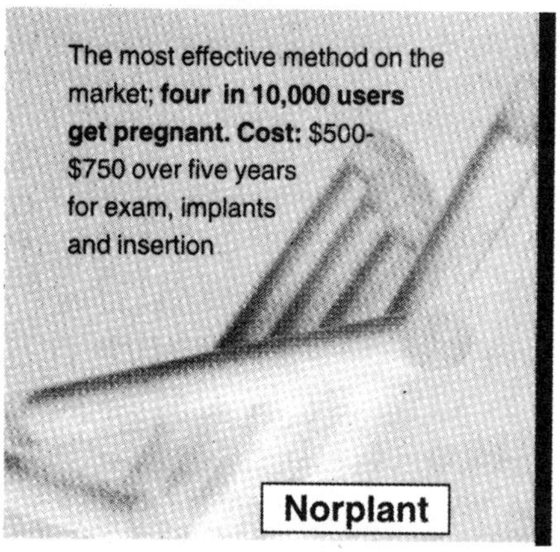

years the Pill halves your risk of endometrial and ovarian cancers, an effect that, for endometrial cancer, may last as long as 15 years after you stop using it. [Experts aren't sure how long the protective effects last for ovarian cancer.] It also reduces the risk of benign breast lumps, ovarian cysts, iron-deficiency anemia and PID.

Drawbacks: Side effects include breast tenderness, nausea, weight gain and headaches (though these usually clear up after two to three months). The Pill must be taken every day, and it doesn't protect against STD's. In addition, studies show it increases the risk of heart attack and blood clots in women over 35 who smoke. Some studies have also shown that the Pill increases breast cancer risk, though a recent analysis of 150,000 users found this risk to be negligible. In most cases, say experts, the health benefits far outweigh the risks.

What you may not know: A study at San Francisco State University found that women who use triphasic pills such as Orthonovum 7/7/7 (in which hormone levels vary throughout the course of the month) experience heightened sex drive compared with women on other types of pills.

When to consider it: If you're in a committed relationship and want a highly effective form of contraception. Contrary to what many believe, the Pill can be ideal for fortysomething nonsmoking women. It eases the transition to menopause, says David Grimes, M.D., vice chairman of the department of obstetrics and gynecology at the University of California at San Francisco. "The Pill helps regulate periods, prevent hot flashes and protect against bone loss," he explains.

Norplant: A Five-Year Plan

What it is: Six flexible, matchstick-sized capsules inserted by a doctor just beneath the skin of the upper arm. They release progestin to suppress ovulation for five years.

Benefits: It's effective and convenient—you can't mess up. Norplant is also easily reversible; after removal, any remaining drugs leave the body in about three days. In addition, experts believe Norplant may be as good as the Pill at reducing the risk of endometrial and ovarian cancer.

Drawbacks: Norplant won't protect you from STD's, and it can cause ir-

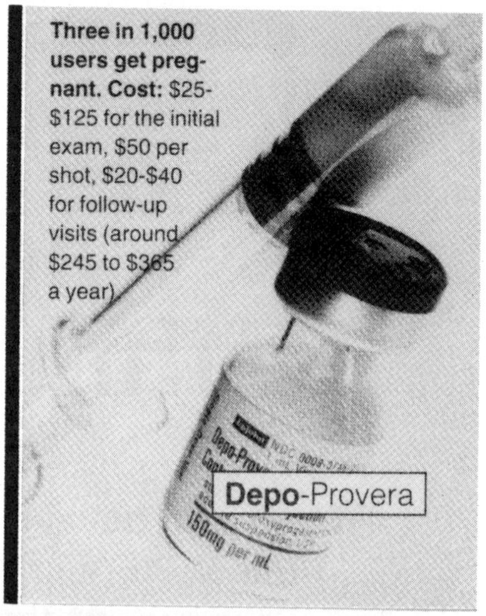

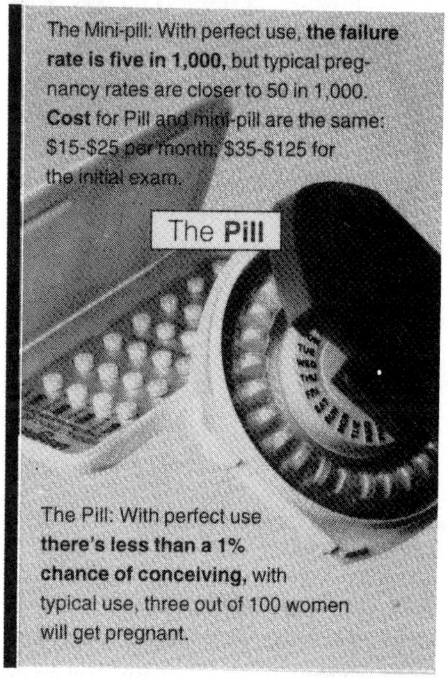

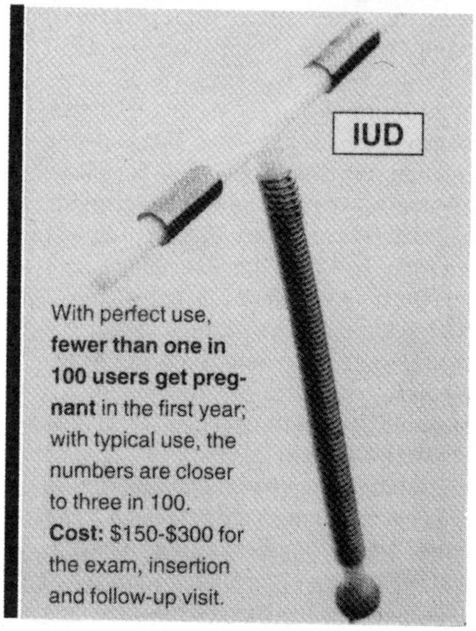

Among women who are in their 40s, a staggering eight out of 10 pregnancies are unintended—the same rate as for women under age 20.

regular bleeding during the first year. There have also been a number of lawsuits filed by Norplant users, primarily because of problems such as pain or scarring upon removal. Despite the bad press, experts say such problems shouldn't arise if you use an experienced doctor. (For referrals, call your local Planned Parenthood clinic.)

What you may not know: Norplant is very expensive if used for fewer than three years.

When to consider it: If you're breastfeeding (unlike estrogen in the Pill, progestin doesn't reduce milk flow) and plan to wait several years before having another child or if you've completed your family. You also may want to try it if you absolutely don't want to worry about an accidental pregnancy.

Depo-Provera: Convenience Without Long-Term Commitment

What it is: This injection of synthetic progestin suppresses ovulation for 11 to 13 weeks.

Benefits: Depo-Provera provides many of the health perks of the Pill, and you don't have to take it every day. After about a year, periods may stop completely, which many women consider a welcome side effect.

Drawbacks: Doctor's visits are required four times a year to get the shots, and the effects are not immediately reversible (fertility may not return for an average of 10 months after the last dose). Side effects may include headaches, weight gain, depression and heavier, more frequent periods. Depo-Provera also provides no protection against STD's.

What you may not know: Though many American women think of this method, approved here in 1992, as new, Depo-Provera has been used by more than 30 million women in 100 other countries over the past 30 years.

When to consider it: If you're nursing or trying to space out the arrival of new children, or you can't remember to take the Pill every day.

The Reality Female Condom: Women in the Driver's Seat

What it is: The Reality Condom is a floppy polyurethane tube with an inner ring at the closed end that fits over the cervix, like a diaphragm, and an outer ring at the open end that hangs outside the vagina.

Benefits: Protection against AIDS and other STD's; more spontaneity than with male condoms, since it can be inserted in advance.

Drawbacks: It has about as much sex appeal as a sandwich bag.

What you may not know: The device is reputed to squeak during use (adding a little extra lubricant can alleviate this distraction).

When to consider it: If you're not in a stable relationship or you have a partner who refuses to wear a condom.

Tubal ligation: No More Hassles

What it is: This surgical procedure blocks the fallopian tubes so that sperm and egg never meet.

Benefits: No-worry, contraceptive-free sex for the rest of your life. And, after the cost of the surgery ($1,000-$2,500), you'll never spend another dime on birth control.

Drawbacks: This procedure isn't foolproof: Though only five in 1,000 users become pregnant in the first year, surprisingly, over 10 years the failure rate is one in 50 (2%). And, as with any surgery, the procedure carries risks. Finally, depending on how it's done it can't easily be undone.

What you may not know: Sterilization is the most popular method of birth control in the U.S., chosen by a whopping 42% of contraceptive users.

When to consider it: If you're *sure* you don't want any more children.

The Mini-Pill: Fewer Annoying Side Effects

What it is: This pill contains no estrogen and a very small dose of progestin—hence the name.

Benefits: Since it contains no estrogen, the mini-pill has fewer side effects than the Pill and is not associated with any increased risk of blood clots or breast cancer. It also causes lighter than normal periods, making it a good choice for women who are anemic or who tend to bleed heavily.

Contraception **911**

Condoms break, diaphragms slip and even the most responsible woman sometimes misses a Pill. The good news is that post-coital contraceptive options are expanding. An FDA advisory panel recently agreed unanimously that the Pill can safely be used as a morning-after contraceptive. The procedure—taking two doses of two or four pills each, depending on the brand, within 72 hours of unprotected sex—reduces the risk of pregnancy by 75%, though nausea and vomiting are common side effects. Several different Pill brands can be used; check with your doctor for specifics. Note: Don't try this on your own.

An emergency IUD insertion can also be done within five to seven days of unprotected sex and is more than 99% effective. Contact your doctor or Planned Parenthood, or call the new 24-hour Emergency Contraception Hotline (800-584-9911) for a list of doctors who provide emergency contraception in your area. You'll also find a list of local providers on the Internet at http://opr.princeton.edu/ec/.

Alternatives to surgical abortion are on the way. The long-awaited French abortion drug mifepristone, better known as RU 486, is expected to be available in this country later this year. The drug blocks progesterone and causes the uterus to discard its lining along with the implanted egg. It can be used up to nine weeks into pregnancy and may also be used as emergency birth control up to three days after unprotected sex, with fewer side effects than oral contraceptives.

On the horizon: Two FDA-approved drugs already on the market, methotrexate (a chemotherapy drug) and misoprostol (used to prevent stomach bleeding), induce abortion when combined. Since research is still limited on this method, few doctors use it, but that may soon change. Planned Parenthood has received FDA clearance for a large-scale clinical trial to test the technique's safety and effectiveness.

Women who use triphasic birth control pills report experiencing a heightened sex drive.

And it doesn't require a waiting period to get pregnant after you stop taking it.

Drawbacks: It can cause irregular bleeding, offers no protection against STD's and has a significantly higher failure rate than combined oral contraceptives, particularly if you have trouble remembering to take a pill every day.

What you may not know: This method has almost no margin for error. Missing even one day can result in a pregnancy.

When to consider it: If you're nursing (which naturally reduces—but doesn't rule out—fertility); it also seems to slightly increase the quantity and quality of breast milk.

Six Reasons to Switch

If you've been using the same contraceptive since college, it's probably time to take a fresh look at your birth control options. Here are some compelling reasons to reconsider your method:

1. You've settled down with one partner. Provided neither one of you has a sexually transmissible disease, you can switch from condoms to a method you both like better and will use consistently.

2. Your health has changed. If you develop heart disease, high blood pressure or diabetes, you should re-evaluate your current method with your doctor.

3. You're breast-feeding. Consider a nonhormonal contraceptive, such as condoms, a diaphragm or a copper intrauterine device (IUD), or a progestin-only method, such as the minipill, Norplant or Depo-Provera.

4. You've completed your family. Sterilization is only one long-term option. Also consider Norplant, Depo-Provera, the IUD and the Pill.

5. You're contemplating pregnancy. If you're on the Pill, doctors recommend stopping two to three months before conceiving to re-establish your natural cycle. If you use Depo-Provera, it can take up to a year after your last shot to conceive.

6. You dislike your current method. If you hate inserting your diaphragm or can't remember to take the Pill every day, don't grin and bear it—switch.

Barrier Methods: STD Protection

What they are: This group includes condoms; diaphragms and cervical caps used with spermicidal jellies or foam; inserts and film. All prevent sperm from reaching eggs.

Benefits: They're safe, cheap and available without a prescription; barrier methods also guard against STD's. Latex condoms provide the best protection against the AIDS virus.

Drawbacks: They interfere with spontaneity and can be messy, and your partner may complain of lessened sensation during sex with condoms. Also, caps can be tricky to insert and diaphragms may increase the risk of urinary tract infections in women.

What you may not know: Lubricated condoms and spermicides help counteract vaginal dryness, a common perimenopausal and postpartum problem.

When to consider them: If you're breastfeeding, planning to get pregnant relatively soon or having sex infrequently. Condoms are the best choice if you want iron-clad protection against AIDS and other STD's. Barrier methods are also handy backups when you forget to take a Pill.

Julia Califano is a writer in Hoboken, NJ

For Infertility Treatments, Now You're Covered, Now You're Not

ANNE ADAMS LANG

IT took Carla and Bruce P. three and a half gut-wrenching years of invasive medical treatments and more than $40,000 of their savings before Carla got pregnant in April. That makes them part of a small but growing population that beat what the New York State Task Force on Life and the Law recognizes as the "disease" of infertility.

Lucky? Indisputably. First because Carla, a legal assistant, and Bruce, a real-estate broker, succeeded when the biological odds are stacked against a 41-year-old woman conceiving even with high-tech intervention. Second because Carla's new insurance carrier, U.S. Healthcare, paid for the successful round of blood tests, sonograms, laboratory work, egg harvesting, in-vitro fertilization and implanting the resulting embryos. All this was performed by one of New York City's top reproductive medical teams, which was led by Dr. Cecilia Schmidt-Sarosi and her husband, Dr. Peter Sarosi, reproductive endocrinologists.

That insurance policy saved Carla and Bruce, who do not want their last name published, roughly $10,000 that they would have paid themselves if they had approached the managed-care company just one month later. On April 1, U.S. Healthcare, now merged with Aetna, canceled its coverage of in-vitro fertilization and other high-tech fertility treatments, making it available to employers only through a rider. "Because we were one of the few programs covering IVF, women flocked to us who could not find coverage elsewhere," said Jill Griffiths, a spokeswoman for Aetna Healthcare. The policy, she said, was simply too expensive to continue.

"We contracted them in March and when I read that the company had stopped the policy, my heart just dropped," Bruce said. "But we lucked out. We got coverage on a shoestring, and we just got in under the wire."

Insurance carriers are mostly like poltergeists haunting the field of reproductive medicine. They materialize with ephemeral policies that are changed or are withdrawn in a flash. Only about two weeks ago, for example, Group Health Insurance, one of the largest carriers in New York, announced that it is withdrawing its coverage for all assisted reproductive technology.

"Unless they operate in states with mandates to cover infertility treatments, such as Massachusetts, Illinois and Maryland, managed-care and indemnity insurers have ignored fertility coverage and gotten away with it," said Dr. Norbert Gleicher, who founded the Center for Human Reproduction, a Chicago-based chain of fertility treatment centers. "That's imminently about to change."

Anne Adams Lang is a freelance journalist in New York who writes on politics and parenthood.

Dr. Gleicher, who recently contracted with Oxford Health Plans to do a joint venture with Columbia University, gave three reasons for the new interest in fertility coverage:

• Viagra. The White House decision to require Medicaid coverage of the drug that treats male sexual dysfunction, and mounted pressure on private insurance companies to do the same, has opened the flood-gates to sexual-discrimination suits. "Once insurance companies conclude they have to cover Viagra, how can they not cover female infertility drugs?" Dr. Gleicher asked.

• Legal precedent. A police officer sued the city of Chicago for violating the Americans With Disabilities Act, saying infertility is a disability. "A disability is an impairment of a body system that inhibits a major life activity," said Patricia Collins, the lawyer who won the class-action suit this year. "The only question is whether procreation is a major life activity. My position is, if work is a major life activity, I would hope procreation is as well." Judge Susan B. Conlon agreed and the city settled, saying it would follow Illinois's guidelines.

• Economics. "Smart insurance companies are recognizing that it may be in their interest to cover, even to a limited extent, infertility because it brings an underground economy in fertility services above ground," Dr. Gleicher said. He explained that doctors often perform infertility treatments, like tubal surgeries, and list them as a different, often more costly procedure so that patients can secure coverage.

In a study to be published in September, William M. Mercer, a firm of human-resource consultants, concludes that the hidden costs of infertility treatments range from 27 cents to 50 cents a month for each member of the insurance plan. "Depending on co-pay arrangements and how well the plans are managed, it would cost in the neighborhood of 40 cents to 50 cents to provide coverage," said Lisa Astor, a consultant at Mercer. "Our thoughts are that employers are already paying for infertility whether they know it or not."

There is also a wave of consumer anger over the right to reproduce that threatens to engulf lawmakers in several states, including New York. Assemblyman David S. Sidikman has introduced a bill that would require insurers to cover the diagnosis and treatment of infertility. State Senator Seymour Lachman recently introduced a similar bill.

"People who make $250,000 a year are the ones swinging the out-of-pocket costs for assisted reproduction," said Pamela Madsen, the executive director of the New York chapter of Resolve, a support and advocacy group for infertile individuals. "Maybe they have to give up the vacation. The more middle class are giving up their homes, and the working poor are out of it altogether."

MRS. MADSEN and her husband gave birth to two children using IVF and, she said: "I have four embryos at Mount Sinai waiting for me in the freezer that I can't access. I'm tapped out, mortgaged out, credit-carded out. And we were lucky. We got our babies. We still live in a one-bedroom apartment. We had a nest egg when we got married; we had health insurance, and the system wasn't there for us. We are the norm."

Even without legislation forcing coverage, assisted-reproduction technology specialists are gearing up for change. "We're seeing more and more patients going to centers, which increases the volume and lowers the price," said Dr. Mark Sauer, the director of Columbia University's division of reproductive endocrinology. "Corporate groups, for-profit groups and H.M.O.'s are learning to split the heavy overhead of a university program like research, and streamline certain operations."

Managed care, Dr. Sauer said, could act as a great leveler, making fertility treatment "possible for people without the kind of resources to go to a fee-for-service boutique practice."

Dr. James Grifo, the head of New York University Medical Center's division of reproductive endocrinology, said his group is negotiating, albeit reluctantly, with a managed-care company. "We would prefer to control our own fate," he said. The problem is that large institutions like universities have less seed capital. "It's more onerous for them to start and support these kinds of programs," Dr. Grifo said.

Economic pressure has whittled the number of large academic medical institutions where new reproductive technologies are incubated. The many that remain need high volume, said Dr. Zev Rosenwaks, a professor of obstetrics and gynecology and the director of the New York Center of Reproductive Medicine and Infertility at New York Hospital-Cornell Medical Center.

"We have over 100 staffers," Dr. Rosenwaks said. "You cannot run a program that's a good program, that has full research and all aspects of lab work without having a critical mass of patients."

THE Cornell program has grown to 750 patients a year from approximately 250 patients in 1988 to 1989. "We're constantly re-evaluating the costs," Dr. Rosenwaks added, while trying to accommodate a changing economic environment. That requires market savvy, which means he said, being patient-friendly, including securing insurance coverage for IVF.

By contrast, Dr. Schmidt-Sarosi, noting that small can be profitable, said that a successful fertility clinic doesn't need the "heavy machinery of an academic setting."

"What do I need an academic telling me how to run my clinic?" said Dr. Schmidt-Sarosi, who recently left the clinical practice at New York University to open her own practice. "Our prices are competitive and lower. I don't have the overhead of hospitals. Those of us who practice look at what is the out-of-pocket cost. We streamline, so that if a patient is going to use drugs, we do IVF faster. It's more efficient."

As for managed care, she said it will probably bring down IVF costs to $5,000 per ovulation cycle from $10,000. That could lead her to consider joining a network of small, high-quality clinics to negotiate with good insurance companies.

Other practitioners have devised a kind of money-back guarantee approach to lowering costs. At the Shady Grove Fertility Center in Rockville, Md., for example, patients pay $18,000 up front for three full IVF cycles. Embryos are frozen and transferred without additional charges. If a patient doesn't take home a baby, the money, minus a deductible of $1,250 per cycle, is returned. "Then you still have money for adoption," said Dr. Michael Levy, a founder.

Diane Aronson, the executive director of Resolve, warns that such programs could be an incentive for doctors to implant more embryos than is medically sound, to maximize the chances of pregnancy on the first round. Ms. Aronson is also concerned about the possibility of unscrupulous clinic administrators practicing a bait-and-switch in which they lure patients with the promise of a money-back guarantee only to tell them that they don't qualify for that particular program.

Defending his practice, Dr. Levy said that every program could potentially exploit the consumer. "In a fee-for-service, it's unnecessary procedures; in capitated policies with a monetary limit, it's not doing necessary procedures, and in shared risk, it's by treating patients differently than you would treat others," he said. "When we looked at our data on shared risk, we analyzed whether we transferred more embryos, and we put back exactly the same number in fee-for-service."

He added: "I'd be very happy if there was no need for shared risk. In France, where it's covered, they do five times the amount of IVF as we do. There's a lot of politics hidden in this issue."

CONSENSUS: NO LONG-TERM LINK BETWEEN the Pill and Breast Cancer

By Gary Goldenberg

MR. GOLDENBERG IS A FREELANCE SCIENCE WRITER.

Experts worldwide on oral contraceptives and cancer collaborated recently on a study designed to settle a long-standing issue: Does taking the Pill increase a woman's long-term risk of breast cancer? Their consensus is no.

"This study answers the major outstanding question we had about the Pill: Does it have any persistent effect on breast cancer long after women stop taking it? We now know that more than ten years after stopping the Pill, women are not at increased risk." So says Dr. Valerie Beral, chief of the Cancer Epidemiology Unit at Oxford University, who led the multinational effort.

"The absence of any increase ten or more years after stopping is found consistently for all groups of women studied—young women, older women, women with a history of breast cancer, women of different ethnic origin, from developed or developing countries," adds Beral. "It was also true regardless of how old women were when they began taking the Pill, how long they took it and what type of Pill they took."

The Imperial Cancer Research Fund in the United Kingdom underwrote the four-year study, which *The Lancet* published in June 1996. The complete paper constitutes a special supplement to the September 1996 issue of *Contraception*.

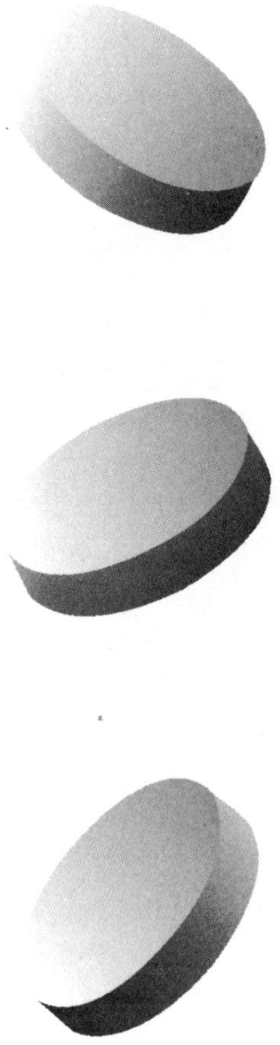

Only 29 percent of women who use birth control take the Pill, even though it is the most effective form of contraception barring sterilization.

The researchers did observe a very small rise in breast cancer among current and recent users of the Pill. But according to Oxford University researcher Dr. Gillian Reeves, who helped interpret

Good News Is No News?

The news media seriously neglected the Pill/breast cancer study, even though it had all the hallmarks of a major story: The study was the most authoritative investigation of its kind; it was published in a prestigious medical journal; it purported to settle a controversial public-health question; and it had the potential to affect tens of millions of American women.

Only after a public-relations effort by Columbia-Presbyterian Medical Center and Elsevier Science (which publishes *Contraception*) did the study receive wide coverage. (*NBC Nightly News* covered the study in 15 seconds, during which it alluded to scientists who disagreed with the findings.) To be sure, public-relations offices are a major means of getting news to the public. Still, one wonders why this study generated so little coverage directly. Is it simply that good news is no news?

"This is something that I come up against all the time," says Joshua M. Peck, a former reporter for Gannett newspapers who works for Jaffe Associates, a national marketing and public-relations firm. "If something isn't alarming or threatening to the reader, the chances of it being covered by the media moves down several notches and sometimes reaches zero. . . . The heart of this story is, 'You were worried about something, [but] there's nothing to worry about,' and to most journalistic ears that doesn't sound like a story. Give them something to worry about and you've got the front page."

Dr. Scott Ratzan, director of the Emerson-Tufts Program in Health Communication and editor of the *Journal of Health Communication*, evidently agrees.

Reporters and editors, he says, typically look for something "that upsets the status quo, where it knocks the train off the track, and that's a major problem [with] the way that health and medical news is covered." The opposite problem, he says, is making something out of nothing. "A year ago in Britain, [reporters] blew things out of proportion when they talked about [the link between] oral contraceptives and deep venous thrombosis [blood clot formation in the heart]. Well, the risk went up from 1 in 10,000 to 2 in 10,000," Ratzan notes. The misleading media coverage lead to an excess of 5,000 pregnancies, 3,000 of which ended in abortions and 2,000 of which ended in births.

The *London Sunday Times* secretly obtained a prepublication copy of the Pill/breast cancer article before its publication in *The Lancet*—and ran the story under the banner, "Pill Users Face a 10-Year Tumour Risk."

the study data, "After women come off the Pill, this excess declines, disappearing completely after ten years."

"The Pill Causes 'Diagnosis'"

"This finding does not mean that the Pill causes cancer," emphasizes Dr. Carolyn Westhoff, a birth-control specialist at New York's Columbia-Presbyterian Medical Center, who reviewed the paper for *Contraception* and wrote an accompanying editorial. "What it probably means is that the Pill causes 'diagnosis.' It may be that doctors who prescribe the Pill feel more compelled to do more breast exams, or that the sort of women who ask for the Pill are more likely to ask for mammograms. Cancer is a disease that develops over many years. If the Pill actually caused cancer, you would see a delayed effect, not an immediate one."

The finding that the cancers discovered in Pill users were less likely to have spread outside the breast than the cancers discovered in nonusers lends credence to Westhoff's hypothesis. "Women on the Pill are probably benefiting by getting diagnosed sooner, before their cancers become metastatic," she states.

Feeling the Whole Elephant

For years researchers have been giving women mixed signals about the link between the Pill and breast cancer. According to Westhoff, this inconsistency is not due to "shoddy science" but rather to the difficulties inherent in analyzing small risks and in studying a drug whose patterns of use have changed over three decades. "It has not been possible to get all the situations in a single study," she adds. "Any one of those studies will get only a little piece of the answer. It's like the [fable of the] blind men feeling the elephant." Ultimately, researchers agreed that the only way to "feel the whole elephant" was to combine and reconsider data from as many existing studies as possible. Thus, in 1992 more than 200 scientists from around the world joined to form the Collaborating Group on Hormonal Factors in Breast Cancer. The researchers combined data on more than 150,000 women from 54 studies conducted in 26 countries.

"The data presented here represent about 90% of the worldwide epidemiological evidence on breast cancer risk and use of hormonal contraceptives. What is known about the 12 studies for which data were not included would have been consistent with the main findings," Beral and her colleagues stated in *The Lancet.*

"Everybody put their egos aside and submitted all their data for this combined analysis, which has taken years to do. It's very rare that controversial areas in medicine get resolved in such a fashion," says Westhoff.

What Will the Public Believe?

The question remains: How will women react to this study? "There have been all these conflicting studies saying it depends on which Pill you're taking, what age you were when you took it, family history, length of time on the Pill, and so on," says Westhoff. "It has raised people's level of anxiety. At the very least, it has given them the idea, where there's smoke there's fire. The average person doesn't understand that science progresses by two steps forward, one step back, and 18 steps sideways. The whole issue has been bad for trust of the Pill and bad for trust of science."

Because of such confusion, only 29 percent of women who use birth control take the Pill, even though it is the most effective form of contraception barring sterilization. Most women who take the Pill are below age 26. Very few women in their later childbearing years take the Pill, apparently because they fear that doing so will lead to breast cancer and blood clots. The risk of blood clots leading to a heart attack or stroke has been limited largely to smokers over age 35; this risk has diminished with the introduction of lower-dose oral contraceptives.

"This anxiety has driven women from a highly effective form of contraception, with devastating consequences," says Westhoff, who reports that half of all pregnancies in the United States are unintentional. The unplanned pregnancy rate is even higher—77 percent—in women in their 40s. "Women need to know that we now have enough data to say that the Pill does not cause breast cancer," she says.

Women should also know that there are many reported benefits to taking the Pill, Westhoff adds. Studies show that Pill-taking decreases the risk of ovarian, uterine, and endometrial cancer; endometriosis (the extrauterine growth of mucosal tissue native to the uterus); ovarian cysts; pelvic inflammatory disease; benign breast disease; ectopic (extrauterine) pregnancy; and excessive menstruation. Taking the Pill reportedly also increases bone density.

So why didn't the media jump on this story?

The truth about abortion and women's health

Opponents of abortion now say ending a pregnancy endangers your health. Here, a hard look at the evidence

"The medical field doesn't want you to know how dangerous abortion really is." Karen McCubbin, director of the Susan B. Anthony Women's Centre in Denton, Texas, is trying to talk me out of having an abortion. I have come to this new "crisis pregnancy center" to find out what pro-life counselors are telling pregnant women these days. McCubbin has gently asked if I think having an abortion is right for me. Then, with very little prompting, she urges me to consider these "facts": "The procedure is done completely blind. The doctor is on the outside and all the instruments are on the inside, and many girls have punctured uteruses and hemorrhaging." My cervix might be torn or lacerated, she continues. I might never be able to have children afterward. I could suffer any number of other serious complications while on the operating table. The chances that my intestines could be pulled out are "good," for instance. "I don't have the numbers right here in front of me," McCubbin says, "but that's a real common one."

Or I might end up "like a drooling vegetable," she warns, handing me a copy of *Christi's Choice*, a video that describes an 18-year-old who suffered cardiac and respiratory arrest during an abortion and is now blind and brain-damaged, unable to walk, talk or care for herself. "No abortionists have to be trained in anesthesia," McCubbin explains. "I know as much about it as they do."

Like many of the 3,500 loosely allied crisis pregnancy centers in the United States, the Susan B. Anthony Women's Centre is situated right next door to a real abortion provider, Denton Women's Health Services, and advertises under "abortion alternatives" in the Yellow Pages. By offering counseling, free car seats and other maternity gear, it aims to give women an incentive to carry their pregnancies to term. But the Susan B. Anthony Centre goes far beyond simply hoping its driveway will be mistaken for that of its next door neighbor.

Through its parent organization, Life Dynamics, it also funds and distributes research on the alleged risks of abortion to women's health. It offers free legal help to any woman who feels she's been physically or psychologically damaged by abortion. Lawyers who agree to prosecute abortion-malpractice cases—Life Dynamics claims that 87 cases are pending—have access to office space at the center, as well as to dossiers on individual doctors, lists of expert witnesses and animated videos of botched abortions to present in court.

Mark Crutcher, Life Dynamics' founder and president, has said he hopes to force abortion doctors out of business by driving up their malpractice insurance rates. So far, he hasn't succeeded—rates for providers haven't budged. But by styling himself as a women's-health advocate, Crutcher has already achieved one goal: He has suc-

BY SHARON LERNER

cessfully opened a new front in the legislative war on abortion.

Despite the statistical safety of abortion—"It's about as dangerous as having a shot of penicillin and more than 10 times safer than childbirth," says Stanley Henshaw, deputy director of research at the Alan Guttmacher Institute, a reproductive health think tank—health issues are now part of the debate over the procedure. Bills requiring doctors to warn patients about a purported link between abortion and breast cancer have been introduced in at least eight states since January. And at least seven state legislatures have considered laws to require warnings about abortion-related psychological harm. The upshot: Pro-choice activists must now fend off health-related legislative actions as well as protect abortion providers and patients from violence and harassment.

Even lawmakers who are suspicious of the pro-life movement's tactics can find the health appeal hard to resist. J. Gary Pretlow, a New York state assemblyman and a member of the legislature's health committee, had to think twice about a proposal requiring doctors to warn women about the medical and psychological risks of abortion. "At first, I didn't see a problem with a doctor telling a woman the risks of a procedure he's going to do," says Pretlow. "But when I realized what forces were behind the bill, it became objectionable. They were doing this to deter women from having the procedure." The bill died in committee.

With seemingly all abortion-related health information filtered through a political lens, it's hard to know what—or whom—to believe. Here, a hard look at the evidence.

True or false? Abortion causes breast cancer

"Women who choose abortion suffer more and deadlier breast cancer." That's what Christ's Bride Ministries, a pro-life group based in Virginia, announced last year on billboards and buses from Massachusetts to Florida. A widely distributed pamphlet, "Before You Choose: The Link Between Abortion and Breast Cancer," makes a similar case. "Millions of induced abortions around the world," it reads, can account for "the mysterious jump in the breast cancer rate."

The question of whether an induced or spontaneous abortion might contribute to a woman's chances of developing breast cancer intrigued scientists long before abortion opponents seized upon it. In general, the more estrogen a woman is exposed to, the greater her breast cancer risk—that's why women who enter puberty early and menopause late have higher rates of the disease. During pregnancy, estrogen production increases sharply. Later in pregnancy, however, breast tissue "matures" in a cellular process called differentiation, which both readies the breasts for nursing and seems to offer protection against cancerous changes. Women who have carried a pregnancy to term at a young age tend to have lower rates of breast cancer than those who have never been pregnant or who delayed pregnancy until their thirties.

Some scientists theorized that women who miscarried or aborted would experience a surge of estrogen without the benefit of differentiation. But years of research failed to prove that this translated into an increased risk of breast cancer.

In 1996, Karin Michels, an epidemiologist at Harvard Medical School, analyzed more than 40 studies, spanning some 40 years, of the link between abortion and breast cancer. The studies were so inconsistent—some showed double the rate of breast cancer in women who had had abortions, others showed an opposite effect or no association at all—that Michels and her coauthors concluded that the research was probably contaminated with "reporting bias." Women with breast cancer, they noted, are concerned with discovering its cause, and are thus more likely than women without a disease to accurately report their medical histories—including a history of abortion. Since numerous other studies have shown that healthy women often fail to disclose abortions—especially if they took place before the procedure was legal—this alone could account for the different breast cancer rates in the two groups.

Most recently, a groundbreaking Danish study, published this year in the *New England Journal of Medicine*, managed to eliminate the problem of reporting bias by analyzing the actual medical records of more than one million women. It found that abortion had no overall effect on breast cancer. Says Boston University epidemiologist Lynn Rosenberg, "This is really strong evidence."

The Danish study did pique interest in a tiny subset of women—less than one percent of the million women studied—who had abortions after the first 18 weeks of pregnancy and who did have slightly higher rates of the disease. While future studies will probe the phenomenon, Michels says, "I don't give much credence to that result; it pertains to too small a group." It is also possible that women who had late abortions may have had other health problems predisposing them to breast cancer.

So little is known about the causes of breast cancer that epidemiologists are reluctant to call the issue completely settled. But the National Cancer Institute, the American Cancer Society, the American College of Obstetricians and Gynecologists (ACOG) and the National Breast Cancer Coalition have all agreed that, as ACOG notes, "Evidence is insufficient to support claims that induced abortion has an effect on the later development of breast cancer."

The political debate hasn't died down, however. "Right to know" bills requiring that abortion counseling include a warning about breast cancer have been considered in several states and have passed in two [see sidebar next page]. While the legislation usually carries a vague caveat that gives doctors an out—the information is to be conveyed only "when medically accurate"—many researchers are dismayed by this misuse of health data. "We just don't have the scientific evidence to support such bills," says Michels.

True or false? D and X abortions pose more risks to women than other methods

In what may be the bitterest—and most confusing—abortion battle yet, pro-life groups have lobbied hard to ban one particular method, which they call "partial-birth abortion" and which doctors refer to as intact dilation and extraction or D and X. Done between the sixteenth and twenty-sixth weeks of pregnancy, the procedure—which most doctors say is rarely performed—involves dilating the cervix, collapsing and emptying the fetal skull, and removing the fetus intact.

Opponents focus primarily on the admittedly gruesome technical details of the surgery, but the notion that it poses a risk to the woman has also crept into the debate. Nancy Romer, M.D., chair of the obstetrics and gynecology department at Miami Valley Hospital in Dayton, Ohio, and a member of Physicians' Ad Hoc Coalition for Truth, opposes the procedure primarily on philosophical grounds. Yet she also has "serious medical concerns" that D and X might injure the cervix and make it difficult for a woman to carry future pregnancies to term.

In May the American Medical Association (AMA) broke with its tradition of opposing legislation that interferes with a doctor's autonomy by announcing its support for a federal ban, passed by both houses of Congress in the same month. AMA spokesman John C. Nelson, M.D., called D and X a "crummy procedure" that could be easily replaced with equally appropriate, possibly safer methods for the very small percentage of abortions performed past 18 weeks.

But prominent experts in the field disagree. ACOG, among others, says that D and X is sometimes "the best or most appropriate method to save the life or preserve the health of a woman." Physicians for Reproductive Choice and Health says the contested technique is a "safer, less risky medical option during health- and life-threatening events that can occur during pregnancy," such as cancer, severe high blood pressure and respiratory, kidney, heart or liver failure.

The alternatives to D and X entail risks of their own, including those posed by induced labor and surgery. Phillip Stubblefield, M.D., chairman of obstetrics and gynecology at Boston Medical Center, believes that D and X may be the safest method of abortion in most pregnancies past 20 weeks. "Compared with other procedures, D and X decreases the fair risk you'll tear the uterine wall and injure the mother," he says.

Some women who have undergone more than one late-term abortion for a fetus with severe birth defects say there's another reason to preserve the D and X option. "It's terrible to say it was better," says a woman who had a previous second-trimester abortion by induction (in which labor is induced with injections of saline solution), "but D and X was much easier to endure. There was minimal pain."

The AMA says its decision to support the federal ban was based on last-minute changes to the bill, including one that would allow the procedure to save the mother's life. (The bill contains no specific exceptions for a woman's health, severe fetal defects or doctor or patient preference, however.) "It became clear that the legislation would pass with or without us," says the AMA's Dr. Nelson, "so we felt an obligation to make it as good as it could be."

Though the AMA denies it, rumors have circulated that the group made a deal with Republican congressional leaders. A report in *The Washington Post* linked the organization's change of heart to an eight-page list of legislative requests concerning Medicare, which was submitted the same day the group announced its support of the ban.

Many ob-gyns are dismayed by this turn of events. "I feel betrayed by the AMA," says Mitchell Creinin, M.D., director of family planning at the University of Pittsburgh School of Medicine in Pennsylvania, "just as a cardiologist would if other doctors tried to limit the decision making that goes on between that doctor and his patient."

ABORTION AND HEALTH: WHAT THE LAWS SAY

By the close of the 1997 legislative session, state legislatures had introduced or passed laws linking abortion to various debatable health risks. Where we stand:

● **BREAST CANCER** Mississippi and Montana require that women be given information about a purported breast cancer–abortion link "when medically accurate." Montana's law is being challenged in court.

Similar legislation is pending in California, Massachusetts and New Jersey.

● **PSYCHOLOGICAL HARM** Three states mandate that women be informed of the possible risk of psychological harm following an abortion: Nebraska, Pennsylvania and Utah.

Pending: California and New York.

● **FERTILITY RISKS** State-mandated pre-abortion counseling includes biased information about fertility risks in: Mississippi, Nebraska, North Dakota and South Dakota.

Similar laws face court challenges in Florida, Indiana, Kentucky, Massachusetts, Michigan, Montana, Tennessee and Wisconsin.

● **D AND X ABORTIONS** By May, both houses of Congress had passed versions of a bill to ban the late-term procedure called dilation and extraction (D and X) by doctors and "partial-birth abortion" by its opponents. President Clinton has promised to veto the bill when it reaches his desk.

Meanwhile, 17 states have enacted their own bans, although many face court challenges: Alaska, Alabama, Arkansas, Arizona, Georgia, Indiana, Louisiana, Michigan, Mississippi, Montana, Nebraska, Ohio, Rhode Island, South Carolina, South Dakota, Tennessee and Utah.

Pending: California, Massachusetts and Wisconsin. *—Kristyn Kusek*

True or false? RU 486 is dangerous for women

At the Susan B. Anthony Centre, McCubbin refers to the abortion drug RU 486 (which recently completed U.S. clinical trials but is not yet on the market) as a "human pesticide." "That's what it's actually called in the field," she told me, shaking her head. "Usually you abort the baby at home and you have to carry it to the doctor. And girls die regularly from hemorrhaging."

Life Dynamics literature makes similar use of unsubstantiated health claims. In a memo mailed to 100,000 health professionals, Mark Crutcher claimed that RU 486 has a questionable safety record in other countries and was rushed through the FDA's preliminary approval process.

It's true that RU 486 has drawbacks: The drug is used only very early in pregnancy (up to seven or eight weeks) and it has a higher failure rate than surgical abortions—just under 5 percent versus under one percent. An abortion with RU 486 routinely involves heavy bleeding, cramps, nausea and vomiting, although the FDA knows of no deaths attributed to the procedure. And although a woman would never have to carry the tiny amount of tissue passed to her doctor, a medical abortion could take place in a woman's home.

In the French studies, only about two thirds of patients aborted in the first four hours after taking the contraction-inducing drug. The overwhelming majority of women who have used the method would choose it again, but the side effects contribute to slightly higher levels of dissatisfaction when compared with surgery.

The FDA announced last September that RU 486 was a safe and effective method of abortion, based on its review of evidence from well over 200,000 medical abortions in France, Great Britain and Sweden, where it is already approved, and an additional 2,121 in trials in the United States. The review process was not rushed. "It took six months, so it was typical for a priority drug," says FDA spokesman Lawrence Bachorik.

While the FDA has deemed RU 486 "approvable," the agency will not allow the drug to be distributed until it receives information about RU 486's manufacturer and approves the drug's package-insert labeling.

True or false? Abortion causes long-term psychological trauma

Those bent on stopping abortions have focused especially on its psychological after-effects, which are arguably murkier and harder to disprove. Psychotherapist Vincent Rue, Ph.D., codirector of the Institute for Pregnancy Loss in Portsmouth, New Hampshire, argues that some girls and women who have abortions suffer from a form of post-traumatic stress disorder he calls postabortion syndrome, symptoms of which include depression, impulsive behavior, feelings of helplessness, low self-esteem, hostility and sexual dysfunction. Those who don't report such feelings, Rue has written, may be experiencing "psychic numbing."

The vast majority of psychological and psychiatric professionals disagree with Rue's assessment. "Postabortion syndrome" is not listed in the profession's bible of symptoms and diagnoses, *The Diagnostic and Statistical Manual-IV*. The largest and most recent study to dispute abortion's negative effects on mental health was published in the February 1997 issue of *Professional Psychology: Research and Practices*. Researchers looked at nearly 4,500 young women's responses to questionnaires before and after abortion. The most important influences on a woman's postabortion emotional state, they found, was her psychological state before abortion. Low income and lack of employment were related to low self-esteem. The more children a woman had, the more likely she was to suffer from depression. But having had an abortion did not appear to exacerbate preexisting psychological problems or cause new symptoms.

Nancy Felipe Russo, Ph.D., a psychology professor at Arizona State University in Tempe and one of the study's coauthors, acknowledges that an abortion—as well as an unwanted pregnancy—can be very stressful. "It's normal to feel sadness and regret as well as relief after an abortion," she says. But, Russo emphasizes, this is not the same as permanent psychological damage. "If a woman freely chooses an abortion and has friends, family members or counselors for support, she'll usually get through it just fine."

Despite the lack of scientific support, legislation requiring doctors to warn patients about the mental health risks of abortion has already passed in Nebraska, Pennsylvania and Utah and is pending in several other states.

True or false? Abortion can compromise fertility

The Life Action Advocates Web site lists an increased risk of miscarriage in its section on physical complications of abortion. What it doesn't say: Because the study cited is 17 years old, it included many women who had illegal—and thus much riskier—abortions. More recent studies of women who have had legal abortions showed they had no higher rate of miscarriage than expected among women generally.

Women who terminate pregnancies in their teens or twenties and then have trouble conceiving in their thirties may wrongly attribute their problems to past abortions. "Women often think that's the reason they're infertile. It's as if they think they're being punished," says Cecilia Schmidt-Sarosie, M.D., an infertility specialist at New York University School of Medicine. But experts say there's absolutely no evidence that an abortion without complications compromises fertility. Instead, the greatest threats to a woman's ability to have children are sexually transmitted diseases—now at epidemic levels—and advanced age.

Nevertheless, several states require doctors performing abortions to list these purported fertility dangers on informed consent forms. Such a law exists in Mississippi, where Joseph Booker Jr., M.D., is one of a handful of abortion providers. "I say the portion of the warning that's medically accurate," Dr. Booker reports, "but I really shouldn't have to say anything because it's a bunch of malarkey."

True or false? Abortion providers are poorly trained medical outcasts

Like many pro-life activists, Life Dynamics' Crutcher attacks abortion's safety by claiming that doctors who do them are outcasts from "legitimate" medical specialties. "Abortion is kind of like the last outpost," he told me. "That's where you go when your career is in shambles because of malpractice actions or just because you're a bad doctor and you can't get a practice going. Even [abortion supporter] say, 'All we get are the dregs and the washouts of the medical profession to work in an abortion clinic.' "

It's undeniable that the occupational hazards of providing abortions include vi-

Women who have trouble conceiving in their thirties may wrongly blame a past abortion

olence and harassment, and that there is a nationwide shortage of providers as a result. "Many doctors who are pro-choice have been turned away from abortion practice," says Carole Joffe, Ph.D, a sociologist and author of *Doctors of Conscience: The Struggle to Provide Abortion Before and After Roe v. Wade.* "And a tiny proportion of people who enter to fill the void are inept. But the overwhelming majority of providers are extremely competent."

In fact, antiabortion hostility may even be contributing to abortion's safety. "It's precisely because of this cultural climate that abortion is now one of the most scrutinized—and safest—procedures in medicine," says Joffe.

In 1995 the Accreditation Council for Graduate Medical Education made training in abortion techniques a mandatory part of ob-gyn residencies in hospitals nationwide. But pro-life groups quickly lobbied for—and won—a right for hospitals to opt out of providing such training. Meanwhile, Medical Students for Choice (a group founded in response to Life Dynamics' mass mailing to med students of a book of offensive jokes about abortion doctors) has branches at more than 100 medical school campuses and provides training and education on abortion to thousands of students.

Before I leave Denton, I visit Susan B. Anthony's neighbor, Denton Health Services for Women, to see what effect the new center and its bevy of protesters and lawyers are having on its work. Mary E. Smith, M.D., is the only admitted abortion provider between Dallas and Oklahoma City. She appears not to operate out of necessity. During her 24 years of performing abortions, Dr. Smith, who earned her medical degree at Temple University in Philadelphia and was trained at Kaiser Permanente in Oakland, California, has never had a safety problem. In fact, her malpractice insurance rates were just lowered because of her clean record.

No doubt her life would be easier if she let her neighbors intimidate her out of her specialty. Three years ago, posters reading "Mary Smith is an abortionist" were plastered all over town. In July, 30,000 postcards were mailed containing the same message and including Dr. Smith's work and home addresses and church affiliation. In this town of 71,000, where children of the employees of Denton Health Services play with children of pro-lifers, she worries that others will take heat for what she does. But Dr. Smith, the daughter of an evangelical Protestant minister who admits to sometimes feeling like a missionary, refuses to back out of her embattled profession. "It's the patients who keep me here," she says. "So many of them are so young and in such extreme situations. I feel like I don't have a choice."

Sharon Lerner is a freelance writer specializing in women's health.

Unit Selections

Key Points to Consider

- Describe some of the "internal pressures" that generate stress in a woman's life.
- Describe some of the "external pressures" that generate stress in a woman's life.
- Which form of pressure do you consider to be the most harmful? Why?
- Based on the readings, what advice would you give to women on how to deal most effectively with the stress in their lives?
- How does the article "The Female Brain" relate to a discussion of stress?
- Which article would you select as the most controversial? Why?

DUSHKINONLINE Links

www.dushkin.com/online/

16. **Mental Health Net: QuickFind Results**
http://www.cmhc.com/search.htm
17. **Women's Mental Health Resources**
http://mentalhealth.miningco.com/msub15.htm

These sites are annotated on pages 4 and 5.

Psychological Health

Addressing the issue of psychological health in one unit is a rather daunting task; numerous important issues clamor to be addressed. In reviewing the recent popular literature in this area, one common theme becomes readily apparent. Women are subjected to a wide array of demands and pressures on a daily basis. Some of these pressures arise from within. In "Forever Frazzled?" we explore the signs and symptoms of attention deficit disorder in adult women; "When Worry Rules Your Life" examines the effect of excessive worry on the quality of a woman's life; and in "The Dieter's Paradox" quite a different form of internal stress, termed "reactance," is examined. Reactance describes a form of self-sabotage that occurs when women try to conform to an often uncomfortable and unrealistic social standard of perfection.

Feelings of stress and anxiety can also result from a women's interaction with other people and society in general. "A War Inside Your Head" chronicles the demands on mothers to balance simultaneously career and children. In "You're Not Fat, You're Living in the Wrong Country," the author sheds light on the terrible pressure placed on women to conform to some cultural standard of beauty regardless of the effect on her health and self-esteem. "I Chose to be Sterilized at 29" relates the story of a young woman who chooses to oppose social convention and voluntarily refuses the possibility of motherhood.

Also explored in this section is coping with the negative effects of stress. "Treat Depression with More than Drugs" advocates both drugs and talk therapy as effective treatment options for this terrible illness. "Don't Face Stress Alone" extols the value of social support, that is, support from family and friends, in dealing with life's ups and downs. In "Give Your Body Time to Heal," Ann Japenga outlines the body's incredible ability to heal itself if given the time and opportunity.

Finally, the discussion of psychological health ends with a more global perspective. "The Female Brain" explores the differences in the psychological and emotional makeup between the sexes by exploring the differences in brain function.

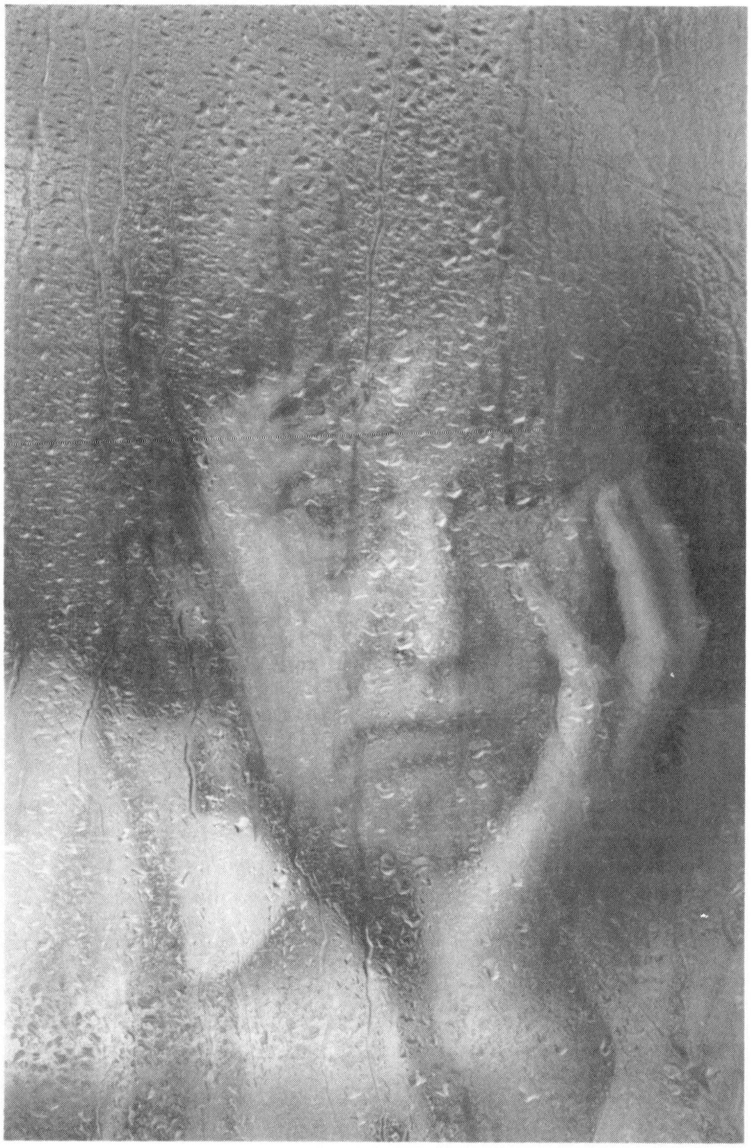

Forever Frazzled?

After years of feeling torn in a million directions, I finally got a diagnosis. And it wasn't stress

By MAYA BOLTON

Recently I had to cut short a telephone call to handle some urgent business. The distraction lasted only a few minutes, but by the time it was over I'd forgotten about the call. By chance something jogged my memory, and I called my friend back—but not until the following day.

Unfortunately, that kind of disconnect is not unusual for me. Walking around my house in the morning, I find myself narrating reminders: "Turn off the iron," or, with a slap to my forehead as I'm heading out the door, "Keys!" Shortly after arriving at the office I often have to return home to retrieve a notebook or a file.

For years friends, family members, and colleagues kindly chalked up these lapses to my being a little "spacey." I have, they would tell me, plenty of charming qualities to compensate. But lately it seemed my absentmindedness had gone out of control.

More and more people were getting insulted by those neglected phone calls. My tendency to procrastinate was reaching pathological proportions. And in the office, where I edit documents, my "eye" was becoming remarkably inconsistent. Even my boss had noticed. Eventually, at wit's end, I sought the advice of a psychologist.

After a lengthy conversation about my personal history, he offered a surprising hypothesis: Perhaps I had the adult version of attention-deficit disorder, or ADD. But aren't people with ADD hyperactive? I asked. The official name of the condition is, after all, attention-deficit/hyperactivity disorder, and as anyone who knows me will attest, I operate in anything but high gear. Even when the brain is working fast and furious, this body barely budges. That was even more true of me during childhood, when ADD is generally diagnosed.

It seems, however, that there are two distinct types of the condition: the more familiar one, called predominantly hyperactive, and one that's gaining recognition, predominantly inattentive. People with the latter variety are notably absentminded, the daydreamy types who quietly tune out at meetings or in class. Often they go undiagnosed because their symptoms are so subtle. The majority are female.

Perhaps, the psychologist suggested, I was suffering from ADD number two.

Over the next few weeks as I talked to people I knew about ADD, I heard skepticism and even contempt. "You can focus," one colleague told me. "ADD people can't focus." (She was wrong. ADDers *can* focus—just not consistently.)

"You've simply got too much on your plate," a friend said. (She had a point. I was working on many projects at once. Was I merely overextended?)

"Oh, ADD," moaned someone else. "Isn't that the disorder du jour?"

It seems that it is. Since 1990 diagnoses of ADD have more than doubled, and the curve seems to be getting steeper. Books on the topic are selling briskly. At conferences with themes like "Living the ADDventure," vendors hawk ADD-pride paraphernalia, special ADD date books, and coaching services for the terminally scattered. In some places high school and college students who have ADD can get extra time on standardized tests because of their disability.

The boom in part reflects a rise in diagnoses among children. But a portion of the newly diagnosed are adults. In 1990 Alan Zametkin, a psychiatrist at the National Institutes of Health, published evidence from positron-emission tomography scans that ADD was associated with at least one physical marker in the brain: lower levels of activity in the prefrontal cortex, from which planning and self-control proceed. Other researchers have suggested the condition tends to run in families.

The findings haven't settled a raging debate about how common adult ADD

From *Health*, July/August 1998, pp. 46, 48. © 1998 by Time Publishing Ventures, Inc. Reprinted by permission.

really is. Some critics charge that psychologists are too quick to diagnose it without the proper testing. But even skeptics agree that at least some of the newly identified are the personality type described by the psychologist I saw and could benefit from treatment.

So I decided to go for the more rigorous evaluation. During the three-hour session I took numerous tests of comprehension, memory, and problem-solving skills. The capper was a particularly frustrating one called the TOVA (Test of Variability of Attention), which consists of watching an orange square appear and disappear on a computer screen. When the square appears below the screen's center, you do nothing. When it appears above, you hit a button. Simple, right? Wrong. Despite humming and even biting my lip to stay focused, I ended up making an incredible number of errors.

It turns out my childhood history was also riddled with signs of the disorder. I recalled that often when I asked my mother a question, she'd first want to know precisely how long she had to answer. She knew at some point I would get that glazed look—distracted by other concerns, impatient to move on. At school I was a classic underachiever; lost in my thoughts, I had difficulty concentrating on the subject at hand.

Looking at the overwhelming evidence, both the doctor and I ended up convinced that mine was a classic case of attention-deficit/hyperactivity disorder, inattentive type. My reaction when she told me her opinion further convinced me: I cried, both fearful of the implications of the diagnosis and relieved to find an explanation for the problems that have plagued me all these years.

> I worry: Will people at my job think attention deficit disorder is just my excuse for flaky behavior?

And what next? There are any number of behavioral approaches to treating ADD, such as workbooks and coaching programs designed to help people focus. But for the underlying attention problem, particularly for someone like me who does detail-oriented work, the doctor favored a low dose of Ritalin, the chief medication used to treat ADD.

Though I can't begin to address the controversy surrounding this drug, particularly about its use on children, I can testify that a minimal dose works wonders for me. It keeps my editorial eye focused for three to four hours at a stretch. I feel less scattered, and I've noticed a definite improvement in my moment-to-moment memory. (And all these benefits come to me without side effects.) When I went back to take the TOVA on medication, I got a perfect score.

Still, even though my behavior has improved, I worry. If people, particularly coworkers, knew about my diagnosis, might they consider me one of the shirkers, someone who just wants an excuse for flaky behavior? That fear is why I've used a pseudonym for this story.

And I can't say ADD *isn't* a fad diagnosis. But to tell you the truth, in my case the treatment was so liberating that I don't really care.

When Worry Rules Your Life

Can simple anxiety be a mental illness? Seems extreme, but finding help could be the best move you ever make

By INGRID WICKELGREN

Last fall Andrea Richards* took a solo trek through the backcountry of Vermont. The trees were magnificent, the stars filled the night sky, and Richards couldn't stop thinking she was about to die.

One sleepless night on the trail, the 31-year-old consultant to nonprofit organizations penned in her journal a detailed description of a man she'd met earlier that day, so whoever found her body could identify her killer. "I spent five days convinced that I was going to be murdered," Richards says.

True, solo hiking isn't free of hazards. Still, when Richards got back to her Boston-area home, she had to wonder whether her anxiety was normal. An avid backpacker, she'd been well prepared for the rigors of the trail. And when she talked to female friends who'd taken similar trips, she found that none had experienced anything like the terror she'd felt.

Worry shaped most of Richards' life. After a minor dispute with her landlord, she'd fret for weeks that she'd be evicted and wind up homeless. A small problem in a routine project at work would bring on insomnia at home. In graduate school she had gone an entire year without getting an unbroken night's rest.

It was Richard's sleeplessness that tipped a doctor off to her problem: generalized anxiety disorder, or GAD, a mental illness characterized by chronic overwhelming worry that affects 10 million people in this country. The illness isn't as dramatic as panic disorder, in which sudden palpitations, trembling, and breathlessness can convince a sufferer that death is imminent. But GAD can be devastating. Richards's worrying hurt her health—she developed an abnormal heart rhythm and painful facial spasms—and strained her marriage, not least because she was too tense to want sex. "I never felt happy," she says. "There was always a cloud looming."

This name has been changed.

Of all the ills that prey on the mind, GAD is one of the most common. Fortunately, it's more easily treated now than ever before. While psychiatrists used to rely exclusively on drugs to treat the disorder, and psychologists on counseling, experts of all stripes are now likely to mix and match to find the most useful combination for each patient. Yet only about 25 percent of people with the disorder seek care. Millions of sufferers go without simple therapies that can make a tremendous difference.

In most of us, of course, anxiety is not a signal that a visit to the doctor is in order but a helpful reminder to finish a job before the deadline or drive carefully in a downpour. Anxiety becomes an illness, though, when it balloons far larger than is warranted by the risk at hand, impairing concentration and blunting motivation—paralyzing you instead of egging you on to constructive action.

Doctors as well as patients sometimes have difficulty distinguishing normal nervousness from a disorder in need of treatment. Experts use a checklist: Have you worried excessively about everyday problems more days than not in the past six months? Over that time have you been bothered on most days by restlessness, fatigue, trouble concentrating, irritability, muscle tension, or insomnia? Do you find worry hard or impossible to control?

"Even when things are going objectively well, people with generalized anxiety have this nagging sense of impending doom," says Mark Pollack, an anxiety expert at Massachusetts General Hospital. Like many people with GAD, Richards felt she worried all the time—literally. (When she kept a log, the figure was a mere 70 percent.)

Scientists believe that some people are born with a susceptibility to anxiety disorders, perhaps because of an imbalance in the neurotransmitters that brain cells use to communicate with each other. Parents may also pass their nervousness on to their children by example; it now seems clear that habits of thought actually influence how much neurotransmitter is released and when. So however a person comes by the disorder, treating it means adjusting levels of brain chemicals. Those adjustments can be made through medication, by changing thought and behavior patterns, or with a combination of approaches.

The drug Prozac is well known for its apparent ability to raise levels of the neurotransmitter serotonin. Serotonin-reuptake inhibitors, as Prozac and its relatives are called, are often used for anxiety disorders; they cause milder side effects than tricyclic antidepressants, the old standard. Valium-like medications have a role to play as well, because while antidepressants may take weeks to kick in, sedatives are immediately calming. And an antianxiety drug called BuSpar is the only drug approved specifically for GAD. Like the serotonin-reuptake inhibitors, it causes few side effects.

As for psychotherapy to treat anxiety, that's come a long way since Freud. Rather than searching a patient's past for the roots of the problem, therapists are likely to teach what are known as cognitive-behavioral strategies. A relaxation technique like consciously slowing and steadying one's breathing, for instance, helps relieve physical symptoms such as headaches and fractured sleep, and short-circuits the cycle of tension by signaling the mind that the body is relaxed. Therapists also focus on the thoughts that feed worry. Patients are taught to interrupt "what if" thoughts—those nattering voices that forecast disaster—by considering whether a doomsday scenario is really likely to come true. And most recently therapists have begun to urge their patients to face unrecognized concerns. For instance, Richards's apprehension about her landlord might reveal a feeling that at her age she ought not to be a renter at all but rather the proud owner of a home filled with children.

Learning cognitive-behavioral techniques typically takes only about 15 visits to a therapist, though it requires a lot of practice at home. "There's work to it, but when patients start to improve they feel like they did it themselves," says David Spiegel, medical director of the Center for Anxiety and Related Disorders at Boston University. "That's important for long-term improvement. Pills can undermine that sense of mastery."

Self-help groups can also be useful, providing information and companionship, and sustaining the resolve to stick with treatment. They're especially valuable for people who don't live near an anxiety center (such clinics are mostly in major cities). "Patients in support groups often know more about new research and therapies than their primary care doctor does," says Michael Liebowitz, director of the Anxiety Disorders Clinic at the New York State Psychiatric Institute.

Richards was fortunate to find doctors who knew plenty. Even before she attempted the hike in Vermont, she'd started taking an antidepressant. But her fear on that trip proved to her that she needed something more. Once back home, she discovered the anxiety center at Boston University. Now, when worry strikes, she uses deep breathing and settles in to dissect her concern. Does she have good reason to think her landlord is mad at her? Is there actually another reason for her disquiet? Each day she calms herself with yoga or a long walk.

So peace of mind for Richards is hard work. But success could not be sweeter. "I finally feel like this is a great life," she says. And now, as proof—or perhaps a test—of her newfound tranquillity, Richards has set out on another gutsy adventure: a trip around the world.

THE DIETER'S PARADOX

You decide to cut back—and immediately start eating more. Why is that?

BY MARY ROACH

IN A SMALL BARE ROOM in the University of Toronto's psychology department, a cruel experiment is taking place. The subject, a woman on a diet, has just received a painful shock. She has been told that her weight is 147.

"Oh!" Her gaze is clamped to the numbers on the scale. "Wow." What she doesn't know is that the researchers have deliberately set the scale five pounds high.

Now for the cruel part. The experimenter leaves the room and returns a minute later wheeling a metal cart of the kind used in operating rooms. On the cart are instruments of torture: three plates of freshly baked cookies. The woman's eyes go wide and glassy. It's that holiday-party look: glee tinged with panic. The cookies are small but precipitously heaped. There must be a hundred. The researcher tells the subject that this is a taste test, and that she is to sample the three kinds of cookie and fill out a questionnaire about their qualities.

The woman and the cookies are left alone. The task can be accomplished with a single bite of each type of cookie. The woman eats ten cookies.

Witness the dieter's paradox: The more worried you are about how much you've been eating, the more you eat.

Earlier today I took a turn in the cookie experiment. I ate only one of each type of cookie. I'd just eaten a muffin and wasn't especially hungry. Two years ago, when I was on a diet, the muffin wouldn't have mattered. I would have eaten ten, maybe 20, cookies. I once ate three-quarters of a pound of Entenmann's chocolate chip cookies. More often I would eat a few and empty the rest of the box into the trash, only to dig some out later, and then rebury them, this time with coffee grounds and carrot peelings on top. I went so far as to buy a cheap tabletop lockbox and insist that my boyfriend at the time keep his tortilla chips and shortbread cookies in it. It failed to stop me. Like a depraved little monkey, I soon figured out a way to jimmy the lock.

The only difference between now and then, as far as I can tell, is that then I was trying to lose weight and now I'm not. As soon as I stopped focusing on my weight, I lost my passion for cookies. And shortbread and chips and ice cream and cheese danish. Food is just food. I eat it when I'm hungry.

Why is this? And how do you get from Point B, monkey with a lockbox, back to Point A, normal human being? Janet Polivy's offices, downstairs from the cookie room, should hold some answers. Polivy is a professor at the University of Toronto and a well-known authority on the psychology of eating more than you want to eat. In 25 years of studies like this one, she and her graduate students have tempted women with forbidden foods just the way Jody in human resources or Aunt Eunice in Wichita Falls tempt their coworkers and neighbors with Christmas cookies and tins full of fudge. Some women so tempted cannot resist starting to eat and cannot stop once they start, Polivy has found. Others enjoy a cookie or two, then stop. And the overeaters, Polivy has concluded, tend to be the ones *most* committed to the idea of eating less.

That's the paradox. We're meeting for lunch at noon so she can explain it.

THE COOKIES at the campus cafeteria are three times the size of the experimental cookies. A woman in a purple suede vest at my table is eating two of them, back to back. She isn't thin.

Janet Polivy doesn't see anything wrong with the eating habits of the woman in the purple vest. Polivy *is* the woman in the purple vest. "I always have two cookies for dessert. You can ask anyone who eats lunch with me."

From *Health,* November/December 1997, pp. 96-99. © 1997 by Time Publishing Ventures, Inc. Reprinted by permission.

There was a time when she wouldn't have been able to quit at two. "When I was a teenage dieter, I could sit down and eat cookie after cookie."

Stop right there. How come? What has changed?

"Because I was depriving myself of them. Psychological deprivation is a very large factor in this. If you think to yourself, I can't have cookies, or Never again will I eat a cookie, what is it you're going to crave?" Polivy breaks off a bite of a Macadamia Delight. "Cookies."

Polivy describes a psychological phenomenon called reactance. "Human beings," she says, "don't take kindly to having their freedom taken away." If you put restrictions on someone in any dimension—food, sex, spending money—then what that person will want most is the prohibited thing. "That's what a diet does," she says. "It takes away your freedom to eat whatever you want." Deprivation leads to obsession.

One of the earliest studies to document this was done in the 1940s by a psychologist named Ancel Keys. He put a group of men on a diet, cutting their calorie intake by 25 percent, to lose a quarter of their body weight. Over six months the men became increasingly preoccupied with food. They hung pictures of food on their walls and dreamed up elaborate menus for meals they'd cook when the study was over. One or two made career plans to become chefs.

I witnessed this sort of thing in my mother when, owing to an intestinal blockage, she was being tube fed. Literally all foods were denied her. Her dreams were a nightly food fantasia of gallivanting hamburgers and chocolate pudding volcanoes. When my brother introduced her to his new girlfriend, Lisa, my mother, in her semistarved delirium, understood the name to be Pizza.

But my mother and Key's dieters were practically starving. Someone trying to drop a few pounds is, more often than not, merely frustrated. Is it the same?

Polivy thinks so. She says the effects of psychological deprivation that she sees in the dieting women with whom she works are strikingly similar to the effects of physiological deprivation. "Food is all they can talk about." Polivy heaves a short sigh. "Dieters can be very boring." And it is this single-mindedness, she says, that makes dieters overeat.

By its nature, dieting requires you to ignore your feelings of hunger. The trouble with this, says Polivy, is that you also start ignoring your feelings of fullness. Soon your body isn't in control of your eating. Your diet is. And a diet, as anyone who's been on one knows, is an erratic taskmaster, liable to walk off the job at a moment's notice. Combine something that makes you nervous about eating (standing on an inflated scale) with momentary exposure to food (the cart of cookies) and all bets are off.

Polivy calls it the what-the-hell effect. Once a weight watcher's resolve has been broken she figures, What the hell, I've blown it; I'll start over tomorrow. And proceeds to devour everything in sight.

In one study Polivy divided subjects into two groups according to whether or not they were trying to eat less. Those in both groups were fed a "preload" of two milk shakes and then set loose to do a taste test of three ice creams. The nondieters behaved logically, consuming a few bites of ice cream after the shakes. Not so the dieters. The preload broke the diet, triggering the what-the-hell effect and prompting a binge of sometimes mythic proportions. One milk shake–loaded woman ate another pint of ice cream.

Clearly dieters such as these aren't eating by their body's cues. Instead, Polivy says, they end up feeding themselves by all manner of arbitrary rules. I didn't have dessert yesterday, so today I get two. If I skip lunch, I get to eat as much as I want this evening. "I hear this all the time," she says. "'All I ate today was an

A Practical Guide to Holiday Eating

Say no to sweets during the winter merrymaking? It may sound sensible, but Janet Polivy says it's bound to backfire. After 25 years of studying the psychology of dieting, she's concluded that deprivation usually leads to overeating when the first plate of gingerbread cookies comes into view. She advises making yourself happier and possibly slimmer this year by following a different strategy: Eat when you're hungry, then stop.

Seems too easy? Here are Polivy's golden rules for making it work.

ENJOY THE PARTY. If there's a holiday gathering in the afternoon, plan to arrive slightly hungry, to eat what's served—and to relish every bite. "You have to recognize that there's going to be all kinds of cakes and candies and God knows what all, and factor that in," Polivy says. "If you say you're not going to let yourself have *anything*, then a) you're going to be miserable, b) you're going to wind up bingeing, and c) you're going to gain weight, and you won't even have enjoyed the food." Find simple ways to compensate for the calories: Have a slightly smaller lunch or, better yet, schedule a longer-than-usual workout.

EAT ANY FOOD YOU DESIRE. Rather than forbid yourself to touch a certain treat, indulge yourself. But wait until late in a meal, when you're just short of full, to give in. "If what you love happens to be pizza or pasta, then start the meal with a big salad. If desserts are your weakness, eat them where they belong: as dessert. Then eat it slowly, and savor it, and stop when you're full." People don't gain weight from chocolate cake just because it is high in fat, she says; they gain weight because they eat three pieces.

MAKE YOURSELF A NEW KIND OF NEW YEAR'S RESOLUTION. For 1998, vow to eat according to your appetite instead of some prescribed plan. Dieters usually end up putting on pounds and feeling inadequate and out of control. And don't worry about your weight. Wherever it settles, you can live with it, no doubt happily. *—M.R.*

Once a dieter's resolve has been broken she figures, I've blown it; I'll start over tomorrow. Polivy calls it the what-the-hell effect.

apple and a yogurt. I'm entitled.'" Invariably it backfires. "By the time you get home," Polivy says, "you're so starving you could eat the refrigerator." Dieters are also more prone to emotional eating. In a study of depressed women, Polivy found the nondieters tended to lose weight during the time they were depressed, while those trying to cut back gained weight. Polivy has a two-part explanation for this: Deprived of food, they valued it more, and hence turned to it for comfort. Having lost touch with feelings of satiety, however, they ate more than their fill of warm fuzzies.

To refamiliarize dieters with their own physical hunger, Polivy has them do group eating exercises. They bring in a meal and divide everything in half, eat half the meal, and then stop and pay attention to what's happening inside their bodies. If they're still hungry, they cut what's left in half and repeat the exercise. Beforehand many fear they won't be able to hear what their bodies are saying over the roar of their chewing. The exercise, Polivy reports, often convinces them they can eat according to their hunger.

Others, like New York psychotherapists Jane Hirschmann and Carol Munter, coauthors of *Overcoming Overeating,* think there are evolutionary reasons weight watchers break diets with binges; unconsciously, they're trying to stock up before the expected next diet begins. To this end, Hirschmann and Munter advocate stocking the house with huge quantities of the foods once placed off limits: a hundred lockboxes, locks sprung. "Once you've demonstrated to yourself that there's never going to be a day when you can't have cookies," Hirschmann claims, "you find you don't need cookies in the same way. Many people calm down very quickly. In a matter of a few weeks, the bingeing stops."

When they succeed, programs like Hirschmann's and Polivy's do two things. First, they get people off the seesaw of abstaining and gorging. They also help many people lose weight. Polivy is an example: "My weight had been artificially elevated by my attempts at dieting. I'd starve myself all day; when I finally sat down to eat I would eat way past the point where I was full. Whereas when I eat when I'm hungry, I don't overeat."

This is not to say you'll end up at your dream weight. "Some people," advises Polivy, "are going to have to accept that constitutionally they were meant to be fatter rather than thinner." This bitter fact is the nub of the dieting problem for most women, she says, because flab is not easy to accept. She herself is 5 foot 8½ and between 160 and 170 pounds (she hasn't weighed herself in years). If she could magically drop ten pounds, would she? "Magically? Yes." Then she thinks for a moment. "But not with a diet. I'm happier now than when I was a dieter. When food stopped being an issue, my life became a lot easier."

So did mine. But I didn't quit dieting through revelation; I quit through giardia. The parasite left me eight pounds lighter, and I no longer wanted to lose weight. I stopped monitoring myself, and food lost its grip on my thoughts. "Here's the scary thing," Polivy says when I tell her the story. "If someone told people, 'All you have to do is have giardia and you can lose eight pounds,' and then sold bottles of it, do you know how much money that person would make?"

Back home that evening, I watch my weight-conscious fiancé succumb to Häagen-Dazs after a meager dinner of fat-free, taste-free chicken and rice. I point out that he could have had a dinner he actually enjoyed, eaten slowly until he was full, and then been satisfied with a few spoonfuls of ice cream. In the long run he'd end up happier, saner, and probably thinner.

"You're absolutely right," he says. And finishes the pint. He knows I am talking as a giardiasis beneficiary, not as someone who learned the lesson the hard way. Still, the message appears to register. The next night his daughter, Lily, is trying to decide if she wants a third slice of pizza. "Are you still hungry?" he asks her. Lily says no. "Then don't eat it."

The slice of pizza stuck around till midnight. At which point I ate it. Because I was hungry.

Mary Roach is a contributing editor.

A War Inside Your Head

Stay-at-home mothers criticize working moms for neglecting their kids, while office-going moms disparage stay-at-homes for getting some sort of retro free ride. As a new mother looking for a place in between, she entered the battle zone unprepared—and struggled to find a way out

By Tracy Thompson

"Do you see her? Do you see her? I kept asking David. The sterile drapes blocked my view. "No," he'd say. Then, finally: "I see her head." There was no sound in the operating room except for the doctors muttering to each other. And then: a tiny gasp.

I think she must have been too amazed to cry. I was. At 8:06, there were seven people present. At 8:07, there were eight. Just like that. The emotional force of this ordinary event obliterates the intellect. You try out the words, to see how they sound, and it is as if you are experimenting in ancient Farsi. "We have a daughter," you say. "I am a mother now." You look at her: She is fabulous. It does not seem real.

My old life was gone—blown away more completely than if a bomb had destroyed my home and my workplace and everything I owned. The universe narrowed to three: me, my husband, this child. I am a new person, I thought, as raw to this world as if my skin had been peeled away. Emma is here.

I was at Ground Zero of the Mommy Wars. By then, I'd already gotten my draft notice.

In my eighth month of pregnancy, I had gone to a party in honor of a friend who had written a book about the war on drugs. In his irreverent way, Danny took me around the room introducing me to guests as "my friend Tracy, a pregnant crack addict." "Actually, I work for The Washington Post," I would add, hoping to clarify things, and people would say, "Really? What do you cover?" and then I had to say, "Nothing at the moment, I'm on maternity leave." And there conversation would stop. After this happened three or four times, I began to get the distinct impression that it would have been better, conversationally speaking, to have come to this affair as a pregnant crack addict.

Six weeks after Emma was born, I encountered one of my old news sources at a social gathering downtown. "Hey," he said. "Haven't seen your byline lately. What are you working on?" Nothing, I said; I was taking a year's leave to stay home and be a mother.

"Oh." A pause. A very *long* pause. "Do you have children?" I asked—a question I never even thought to ask before—and he answered me, but his eyes were searching the room. Within 60 seconds, he'd eased away and found somebody else to talk to. That was when I started to put two and two together. Showing up at a Washington social gathering as just a mom is like showing up in your underwear: revealing and chilly.

This sudden social demotion is the way many women get inducted into the Mommy Wars, my shorthand for the cultural and emotional battle zone we land in the minute we become mothers. It is a war fought inside your head, on soccer fields or in PTAs in the wary undercurrent between working and stay-at-home moms, in the car when you leave your child for another long day at day care, at play groups, at work and in your own bedroom in those lights-out talks with your spouse. It involves many different social and moral and financial issues, yet it often boils down to a personal question: How does this child fit into my life, or should my life now fit around this child?

The seriousness of this question is, quite often, the inverse of the seriousness with which society now regards you. One woman I know, who used to practice corporate law

From *The Washington Post Magazine,* February 15, 1998, pp. 13-17, 27-31.

with a prestigious K Street firm, recalls being asked the usual what-do-you-do question by a female partner at an equally prestigious New York firm. Upon finding out my acquaintance was now a stay-at-home mom, the other woman simply turned her back and walked away. Another lawyer-turned-full-time-mom says that used to happen to her, too, but she learned to fight back. "Now I say, 'I'm in-house counsel to a small family firm,' and people can talk to me." Before her children were potty-trained, she used to add that her specialty was "environmental cleanup." This being Washington, that could jump-start a conversation.

In retrospect, I don't know why I was so shocked at suddenly finding myself in the middle of a cultural battlefield. Everybody told me a child would change my life, and I had no trouble believing it; I'd seen it happen with friends. I knew this little person would change my body, my marriage, my work habits, my finances, all in unsettling and profoundly emotional ways. I expected a roller coaster, and that's what I got: first euphoria, then loneliness. In the mornings, my husband, David, would leave for work, the neighbors' cars would pull out of their driveways, and I would be left with this new person, she of the inscrutable and never-ending needs. I would think of the newsroom, crackling with gossip and inside jokes, and then Emma would start crying again: I traded that for *this*? One day I was a big city newspaper reporter; the next, I was wearing stretch jeans and comparing diaper prices at Wal-Mart. In my old life, I'd written a book; in my new life, I was just one of those generic maternal units referred to by the nurses in my pediatrician's office as "mom."

Perhaps it was a question of the context in which my motherhood was unfolding. I was 41 when Emma was born, happily married, with a husband who is a physicist. I was a veteran of nearly two decades as a working journalist, the last nine years of which had been spent in Washington, the Valhalla of the working woman: According to the Department of Labor, 67 percent of all women in this region work, more, even, than in New York City. And Washington reveres mothers who go to the office. It's the city of Hillary Clinton, perhaps the country's most famous working mom, who juggled law and politics with raising a daughter; of Madeleine Albright, who learned Russian while rocking her babies to sleep; of Supreme Court justices Ruth Bader Ginsburg and Sandra Day O'Connor, whose careers barely paused when children came along; of Marian Wright Edelman, who created the nation's leading advocacy group for children while managing three sons; of congresswomen and countless others, black and white, of lesser fame, who have managed to change diapers, make lunches, help with homework—and put in a full day at the office.

My first ambition, after the ballerina dream got ditched, was to avoid becoming the heroine of *Marjorie Morningstar,* a 1955 bestseller I read as an adolescent, in which Marjorie dreams of becoming a Broadway actress but instead winds up living a mundane life on Long Island as Mrs. Milton Schwartz, housewife and mother of three. *Please, God,* I thought when I was 16, *don't let that happen to me.* And then one day I found myself living in Washington with a job that entailed staying at home and spending a lot of time dealing with baby vomit and dirty diapers. Is it any wonder that few people thought of what I did as important anymore? And how could I blame them?

That this attitude thrives in a culture that frets endlessly about the welfare of its children is just one example of the doublespeak we are drowning in on this subject. We say we value motherhood, but in fact what we value is jobs with power and paychecks, especially in status-obsessed Washington. We structure the workplace to give women money and feedback and perks they would never get at home, and then we expect them to say they'd rather be at home with the kids. We say men and women are free to swap roles, that greater involvement by men would solve some of the childcare problems, but unwritten rules of the workplace penalize fathers who take extended parental leave, and stay-at-home dads are considered weird. Experts tout the cognitive benefits to children of mothers staying at home while their children are very young, yet the solutions to the "child-care crisis" political leaders come up with mostly have to do with creating more government-subsidized and corporate day-care slots. We say teenage pregnancy is bad because young girls are too immature to handle the heavy responsibility of children, but every year thousands of teenage girls imported from abroad are given virtual full-time care of somebody's offspring. Feminists say they value sisterhood, but behind the scenes, stay-at-home mothers often criticize office-going moms for neglecting their kids, and working mothers often disparage their at-home counterparts for getting some sort of retro free ride. We say mothers on welfare should work, but when they do go to work, we give them dirty, crowded nurseries for their children, or nothing at all. Meanwhile, upper-middle-class moms who work are somehow blamed if tragedy strikes their child while they're at the office.

Given this kind of dissonance, it's not surprising that we are always looking for hidden agendas. And while the number of working mothers with young children continues to surge, there is an undercurrent of venom on this subject these days that seems new. When British au pair Louise Woodward went on trial in Massachusetts last year for shaking 8-month-old Matthew Eappen to death, the nation was transfixed not so much by the horrendous nature of the crime, but by the debate that sizzled around a much murkier issue: the morality of a mother who had left her young children in the care of a 19-year-old to pursue her career as a doctor. (Somehow, Matthew's father never came in for the same opprobrium.) "It seems the parents didn't really want a kid," said one caller, cruelly, to a Boston radio talk show. "Now they don't have one." Hearing that, I remembered a story I covered for The Post in 1990—a sentencing hearing in D.C. Superior Court for a nanny who, in a fit of rage, had killed the 9-month-old girl in her charge by beating her head against the wall because the baby wouldn't stop crying. The infant was the firstborn of Lawrence and Amy Banker, who are both lawyers. I remember watching Amy Banker in the courtroom, and wondering how anyone could survive that kind of loss. Now, I suddenly wondered: Were people saying that kind of thing seven years ago? "No, thank God," Amy Banker says. "Nobody breathed a word like that to us. All we got was sympathy."

Somehow, in the 1990s, the issue has stopped being just child care and started being the ethics of parenting choices as well. In 1994, 8-week-old Brenton Scott Devonshire, of Ashburn, died while in the care of his Dutch au pair, who admitted prosecutors had enough evidence to convict her of shaking him to death and eventually pleaded guilty to a misdemeanor charge. Yet, it was Brenton's parents who found themselves in the spotlight, quite literally. Stephen Devonshire remembers walking out of the courthouse one night and being blinded by television lights, hearing a voice from behind those lights shouting, "Your parenting skills have been called into question. Do you have any comment?" After a Post article appeared referring to their house as "spacious," they got at least one anonymous letter—maybe more, Sharon Devonshire tries not to remember—telling them they'd obviously placed a higher priority on having a nice house than on caring for their child, that it served them right their baby had died.

What was it like to be on the receiving end of some of our cultural anger and angst? Sharon Devonshire and her husband have become media spokesmen on the subject of "shaken baby syndrome," the name for what killed their son as well as Matthew Eappen. The Devonshires seem more baffled than angry about the hate mail. "People were just looking to find fault," Sharon says, and she seems disinclined to probe the mindset of those letter writers any further. She kept the letters for a while, but eventually threw them away. "I thought, 'Why am I saving these? This is sick.' "

But the truth is, those anonymous letter writers are onto some thing, in their own malicious way. What motherhood boils down to, quite frequently, is a series of choices, and sometimes they are quite agonizing. The only thing worse than making those choices is not having a choice at all.

Ana Kinney is someone with no choice. A tall woman of 38, with long, cascading dark hair and an upbeat manner, Ana is the daughter of Cuban immigrants. She lives with her husband and two kids, 4-year-old Alexander and 1-month-old Josefina, in a small house in Columbia, where they moved after Josefina was born and their one-bedroom apartment in Alexandria began to seem like a holding cell. It was a stretch, but they found a place they felt they could afford and were surviving—until Ana's husband, Hal, lost his job when a business venture with a friend went sour. Since then Ana, a hairdresser, has been the family's main breadwinner.

Hairdressers at the better salons generally keep only about half of whatever the client pays, plus tips. On her best days, Ana has made $400; on her worst a mere $75. Because hairdressers are independent contractors, they get no health insurance, no 401(k), no sick leave. When Alexander was born in 1993, Ana was able to take three months off by saving up vacation days and using Hal's holiday bonus. By the time Josefina arrived in April 1996, there was no cushion whatsoever: Ana was back at work when Josefina was 2 weeks old because they needed the money. "I was breastfeeding, and it was very important to me, but I had to give it up at six months with her," she says. "That was devastating. I had no quality time with her. I hardly got to hold her when she was a baby."

Finding child care has been agony. Because Ana and Hal work irregular hours (he has found part-time work at night as a gym manager), they faced unaffordable before- and after-school surcharges at every day-care center they investigated. At the moment, Hal stays home with the kids during the day; in the past they have relied on some of the recent immigrants who live in their area. Mostly, their hires have been disasters: One older woman beat Alexander, Ana says, and another woman fed the children nothing but plain boiled macaroni and ignored the kids until Josefina's diaper rash became one big open sore.

Since Hal's job ended, they've had no medical insurance. When Josefina and Alexander get sick, their pediatrician gives them samples from her medicine closet, and charges a reduced fee. Ana hasn't been to a doctor herself since Josefina was born. The past year has put a major strain on the marriage, too. Eight months ago, Ana recalls, she and Hal were "at each other's throats." Divorce was in the air. And then one night there was an extraordinary heart-to-heart talk at the kitchen table, just the two of them, and from that talk emerged two people more strongly committed to each other than before. Hal, a tall, dark-haired man with an athletic build and an easy smile, gets watery-eyed when he recounts the same story.

The more I hear about Ana's life, the humbler I feel. Being tortured about the choices before you, I realize, is a luxury.

What would Ana's ideal life be? "I'd work out of my home, doing my bridal consulting business," she says promptly. It's clear she's given this extensive thought. "I'd work here maybe two days a week and use this place as my base. I'd still be a working mom, but I'd have the joys of going on vacation and not having to worry about money." Could she ever imagine being a full-time stay-at-home mom?

She laughs. "I wouldn't know where to begin."

I had never thought of myself as a full-time stay-at-home mom, either. But it was lovely, being at home. "You're so lucky" my friends in the newsroom would say, and even if some of them thought of maternity leave as a kind of vacation, they still had it right when Emma was about 2 months old, I found a new-moms support group, and it was a lifesaver. I met new people; Emma made it past the newborn stage and became a settled baby; and, like countless mothers before me, I discovered this new job could be fun. I spent a lot of time every day lying on the floor next to her, making nonsense sounds, watching her discover her toes. I'd put my face up to hers, and she would try to bite my nose, making little baby pants the whole time—*Hah!... hah!*—and squeals of delight. Some mornings, I would steal into her room and find her quietly awake, amusing herself. When she saw me, her whole body would go rigid with anticipation—mouth a perfect O, arms and legs outstretched, waving: *Pick me up! Come play!*

Once Emma and I had recovered from her birth and my Caesarean section, I turned into a low-rent Martha Stewart. I loved cooking. I even loved folding laundry, making neat, sweet-smelling piles out of what had been a mound of dirty clothes. My house was clean, windows open to those first glorious days of spring. It reminded me of my childhood, when life was ordered and time seemed expandable and the house smelled of broiling pork chops and the dinner table was set with a cobalt-blue bowl of nasturtiums in the center. A whole new world was opening up to me, and it had a new cast of characters; several of the women in my support group were becoming close friends.

What struck me about these women was how kind they were to one another—kinder than I was to other people in my head, lots of times, and far kinder than I usually am to myself. On a couple of occasions someone in the group wept over some problem, and there was no orgy of pity, no competing to see who had a bigger problem, no wallowing in "what-are-the-childhood-roots-of-this." Just a piece of tissue and a moment of genuine sympathy, and then collective brain-storming: What would help here? Motherhood was an intense and all-consuming job, I was learning; it was easy to get mentally backed into a corner, too stressed to think. We helped one another out that way.

I never wept in that group, though I sometimes felt like it. Mostly, what made me want to weep was an increasingly urgent question: what was I going to do with the rest of my life now that Emma was here?

David and I had easily agreed that I'd be the one to stay at home for a while; I wanted to, and he was just reaching cruising speed in his career. But I needed to work. I needed to do this not just for the money, which was becoming tight without my salary, but also because work had defined me for the last 20 years. Being a writer was almost as intrinsic to my identity as my gender. Yet the kind of writing I had always done had meant long hours in a downtown office, tramping around the city. How could I reconcile the demands of that life with the delight my days with Emma had become? It was a problem we talked about often in support group; the consensus was that dealing with a colicky infant was a piece of cake compared with figuring out how to pick up your old life where you left off.

The most obvious answer to my dilemma, though by no means the easiest, was to persuade The Post to give me another unpaid leave to write another book—at home. I had had no trouble getting my first book published, and if sales didn't exactly set the charts on fire, the experience convinced me that I could at least make a little money.

That spring, I set to work on a book proposal about motherhood after 40. "I thought the market was pretty much saturated with books about motherhood," said my friend Danny, the war-on-drugs author. I paid no attention to the warning; my agent was enthusiastic. I spent weeks reading, refining my ideas, figuring out whom to talk to, coming up with a rough outline of what I hoped to accomplish. As I pushed Emma in her stroller on long walks through the neighborhood on those sunny June days, I revamped and rewrote in my head. The day that I finally shipped off the proposal—my future and Emma's in a plain manila envelope—I stopped on my way to the mailbox to rub it on her little bald head. "For luck," I said.

I had prepared myself for the possibility that I wouldn't get a terrific advance; I told myself all I needed was something. What I never expected, in my eager innocence, was to fail utterly. But I did. Not a single publisher made so much as a low-ball bid. I had put all my psychic eggs in this particular basket, and managed to narrow the future down to one of two melodramatic possibilities: a successful book, or a dreary life of getting up at 6 a.m., hauling Emma off to some faceless day care, returning home exhausted at 7 p.m. after fighting the rush-hour traffic, getting to spend maybe half an hour with her before she went to bed. Now that Plan A was gone, it was July, and Plan B loomed like an execution date.

The day the last hope of the last publisher died, David came home to find me sitting disconsolately on the living room floor. Emma, then 8 months old, was playing nearby. "Talk to me," he said, and all my self-doubt and fears and anguish came pouring out. I saw exactly two bleak options: either consign my daughter to long days at some impersonal day-care center, or give up my cherished career. No rational thought about other options could penetrate that fog, at least initially. So I sat for a long time on the floor, sobbing, David holding my hands. After a while, Emma came scooting over to us on her bottom and started lightly patting my leg. David said later that if he hadn't known better, he would have sworn she was trying to comfort me.

I framed my dilemma in melodramatic terms, as is my unfortunate nature, but there are times when it really does boil down to this: Only one person's needs can be met in this situation, so who's it going to be? That's how Cheli Figaro thought of it: "It was me, or it was him."

At the time, she was a new mother with a colicky, high-need baby. She and her husband, Michael, had recently moved to Prince George's County from New York, so she had no friends nearby. Her husband had a demanding job as an Air Force doctor, and between the two of them they had not a single relative within 250 miles to lean on.

Before her son, Brandon, was born, she had thought she would return to the office quickly. That's what society seemed to expect, and as an African-American woman she felt that expectation doubly. Black women had always worked outside the home, had done so in the face of formidable obstacles, and were proud of it. "Very few women in my generation or my mother's generation were stay-at-home moms," she says. "My husband's grandmother had seven kids and never missed a day of work." Cheli also had a considerable investment in her career: A degree from Columbia Law School could take you a long way. At the time of Brandon's birth, she was a staff attorney at the Commerce Department, and had worked as a corporate lawyer for a big firm in New York. A decision to get off the career ladder at this point would probably mean playing catch-up with her law school classmates from here on out. "But I asked myself: when I'm 90 years old and dying, what choice could I live with? What am I going to feel least guilty about?"

On one recent day, Cheli is moving around in the kitchen of her modest town house in Bowie. Brandon, now 4, is sitting at the table contemplating a bowl of spaghetti noodles, which he is too sleepy to eat. His mother, 34, an athletic-looking woman dressed in black jeans and a red turtleneck, her hair in neat braids, fields telephone calls from the real estate office where she works a few hours a week, sees her husband out the door, cajoles Brandon into at least drinking his juice and manages to keep talking, all more or less at the same time. The kitchen is adorned with a plaque that reads, "Cheli's Bed & Breakfast: Open 24 hours, year round. Caterer, chauffeur, laundress, moneylender, seamstress, psychologist, tutor, nurse, etc. Gifts and other recognition greatly appreciated."

In retrospect, the groundwork for her decision to stay home had been laid when she and her husband bought this town house instead of a larger single-family home. It was a conscious decision to keep their options open, to live below their means, in a neat but modest development where the front yards are approximately the size of a walk-in bath and the neighbors are just a wall away. Sometimes she gets house envy. "All my friends are in nice homes," she admits, "and that's rough."

What Cheli has done might look to some like an abdication of a promising career; a clear case of downward mobility. So why does she make this sacrifice? What does Brandon get from a stay-at-home mom that he wouldn't get any other way?

As she drives him to Watkins Park for a weekly science class for preschoolers, Cheli answers: "The main benefit is to me," in knowing all the minutiae of her son's life, becoming part of a community of stay-at-home mothers, many of them black women like herself whom she discovered in that first lonely year at home. "Brandon gets the benefit of knowing his mom. No matter how much your caregiver loves your kid, no one is going to love him like mom and dad. Mary Poppins doesn't exist."

Still, the sacrifice looks substantial. The science class this week is about recycling, and the kids' project is to make Christmas ornaments from recycled and found objects. As Cheli and Brandon struggle to affix some glitter to a spiky sweet gum ball, she mutters, "I'm out of my comfort zone here." And I wonder: What would her law school classmates at Columbia think of her now? "I don't know," she says. "But I have a better life than they do.... Hopefully, I'll live a long time. There will be time to catch up. And if I die young, I'll know I spent the most important years with my son.

Later, en route to a meeting of Cheli's at-home-mom network, a group of black women who call themselves Mocha Moms, she thinks about this issue some more. Brandon's wide awake now, interrupting his mother with questions: Are we going to play group now? (Just as soon as we go home and pick up some things.) Can I play with Austin? (Yes.) "I don't dwell on what the benefits are to him," she says, "because I have too many friends who work full time—and, frankly, it's not PC. I won't preach."

What does rankle, though, is the perception of some people that stay-at-home moms are some kind of pampered, privileged class. "You have to have some serious self-esteem to do this," she had said over breakfast. "You have an infant who's not going to pat you on the back. You get all the scut work." So when she hears parents say they can't afford to stay home with their children—as if money were no consideration for the likes of her—she has an answer ready in her head: "People make choices. You know what? If you hadn't bought that big house for $300,000, you wouldn't have to work."

> **'But I asked myself: When I'm 90 years old and dying, what choice could I live with? What am I going to feel least guilty about?'**

Some people look at those houses and see the American dream. Cheli sees "golden handcuffs."

For the working poor, for single parents, the choices are limited or nonexistent; for the truly wealthy, maybe, or those who knew, just knew, that motherhood was their only calling, the choices are easier. It's the rest of us who wind up making the judgment calls. Many working mothers who say they "have to" work could, strictly speaking, stay home. They could move to a less expensive house or even rent an apartment; they could shop at thrift stores; they could forgo vacations and new cars. Their children might also have to forgo that private school, a home computer, those enriching summer camps—but it could be done, if money were all we were talking about.

But, it is not. Work isn't just about money. Men and women do get yoked to their jobs, and what began as a choice may easily be come a mind-dulling necessity. In the best of circumstances, though, work reflects other values every bit as all-American as motherhood, and chief among them is ambition. Ambition to be something—to make your mark on the world. Work can be, should be, something that gives meaning to the arc of a person's life.

The trouble comes in reconciling ambition to reality. I heard a story once about Leonard Bernstein's father, who had balked at first at paying for his son's music lessons.

Maybe, 40 years from now, you'll realize your time would have been much better spent playing jacks with your 4-year-old.

Much later, when his son was a renowned conductor and composer, somebody asked Mr. Bernstein about his early reservations, and the old man shrugged. "How was I to know he'd grow up to be Leonard Bernstein?" he said.

Put the shoe on the other foot, and you have the mother's quandary. Can your child do without your constant presence so that you can go to grad school, work on that important brief, crash that deadline? Of course your child can. And later on, when your work yields great rewards—even fame—people will congratulate you for making the right choice. You could be a Madeleine Albright, walking proof that you can be a devoted mom and have a brilliant career.

Or you could just spin your wheels. Maybe your ambition exceeds your talent; it's been known to happen. Maybe, 40 years from now, you'll realize your time would have been much better spent playing jacks with your 4-year-old than attempting to write that godawful novel, but so it goes. You took a gamble and it didn't pay off, and who knows how much your children missed out on? How were you to know you'd grow up to be Mrs. Milton Schwartz?

But that's the point: You don't know. All you can do is take what you do know and plod ahead. That's the conclusion I came to as I emerged from that bleak period, after my book proposal sank without a trace. I asked myself: What's important to me right now? The answers: Emma and my work and my marriage, in no particular order because they were all so interdependent. Do I want to be a full-time stay-at-home mom? Not forever. Was I ready to go back to a full-time job downtown? No. Maybe next year. But at 9 months, she needed me utterly—and I needed to be with her.

All I had to do, then, was invent some way I could stay at home a little longer and earn enough money to get by, while still staying attached to my career. In this, I found, I had a lot of company.

Jayne Lytel distinctly remembers the day she went back to work after her son was born. Her boss at a trade publication, which had hired her to create a newsletter for the financial services industry, called her in to tell her that her job had just moved to Manhattan, and that she could either move with it or quit. She quit. It wasn't even a tough decision. Her son, Lucas, was only 3 months old at the time, and if finding good day care for him had been hard, leaving him there had been harder. She had some severance pay, and a husband whose job as an online business consultant would keep the roof over their heads. So at 42, Jayne decided the next phase of her career would be at home.

In doing so, she joined a group of women the Department of Labor is having a hard time tracking.

According to the department's statisticians, Jayne falls under the broad category of working mother—one of a group of women whose numbers have swelled every year for roughly the past 20. In 1997, 65 percent of women with children under 6 worked. Thus, the public perception that the "working mother" is the norm.

What, then, is a "stay-at-home mom"? Jayne would call herself one, and so would I. So, in fact, would every woman in my eight-member new-moms support group, a group that includes two technical writers, one journalist, a nutritionist, a sign language interpreter for the deaf and a schoolteacher. All but two of us are doing some kind of work on a freelance or part-time basis at home. But, because we are working and getting paid for it, the Department of Labor counts us as being in the labor force—just as if we were punching a time clock and working 50 hours a week in an office.

The department's mandate is to keep track of people who work, regardless of how they choose to participate in the labor force. By its definitions, I've never left the work force: People who are on leave—like me—count as being employed, because we have jobs to return to. Women on maternity leave count, as do people on sick leave, seasonal workers, people who work without pay for a "family-operated enterprise," and women who provide child care in their homes for other mothers, among other categories.

This way of counting the labor force—which doesn't distinguish well between part-time and full-time, home-based and office centered—is an increasingly bad fit with the real world. More people are using untraditional arrangements to structure their workweek. The line between work and home is being blurred by voice-mail pagers and portable faxes and laptop computers. Upheavals in the corporate world, combined with "family friendly" company policies that exist mainly on paper, have created an incentive for people like Jayne—with the skills and savvy and confidence—to become self-employed entrepreneurs and resign from the ranks of the commuting hordes.

This could explain why conversations at my play group center as much on software and modems as they do on teething and ear infections, and why every parenting magazine in my pediatrician's office has at least one article on running your own home business. Put simply, the term "stay-at-home mom" is much more a matter of self-definition than of government statistics—and there are a lot more out there than you might think.

One conclusion to be drawn from all of this is that the more divisive Mommy Wars stories—from the stay-at-home mothers who gripe that office-going neighbors never pull PTA duty and the working moms who get irate when their kid and nanny can't join a moms-only play group—will remain a social undercurrent, but perhaps a less virulent one. These corrosive battles do happen, I know; a book agent friend who has a son a year older than Emma tells me about trying to deal with the other mothers in her son's daycare center, who are all stay-at-home-moms. "They all know each other, and they're home all day, and I work," she says, sounding disheartened. "And I feel that there is this door that is closed to me." It gnaws at her; these seemingly trivial social interactions determine who her child's first friends will be.

But, increasingly, such combatants will have a hard time choosing uniforms: Today's working mother may, like me or Jayne, be tomorrow's stay-at-home mom, and vice versa.

So, will the future bring us millions of moms cycling in and out of the labor force as they please? Yes and no. The millions of working mothers who, like Ana, make their money in the service industries will still find themselves at the mercy of clients and corporations; only the technologically elite will be able to surf the waves of change. And even then, it will take a lot to succeed. Jayne Lytel will be able to walk up to the second-floor office in her Northwest D.C. town house and pursue a career as an Internet columnist for women's magazines because she has extensive experience as a financial journalist and as the creator of an online newsletter. She also has a husband with a stable job to provide a financial cushion. "It's a seller's market out there," she says, curled up in an over-stuffed chair in her living room as Lucas, who is teething, contentedly gnaws his fingers in a bouncer at her feet. "There's a big demand for people with my skills. I'm not worried about finding work." There's just one major downside, she said: no co-workers. The new world of stay-at-home working moms is, at the moment, looking pretty lonely. But I wonder how long it will stay that way.

Marian Gormley is convinced change is on the way. She is the part-time public relations director of Mothers at Home, a nonprofit organization founded in 1984 by three stay-at-home moms in Northern Virginia. Mothers at Home publishes Welcome Home, a monthly magazine with a circulation of

13,000, and employs a paid staff of 25 people—all, naturally, part-timers. It is one of roughly half a dozen national organizations for stay-at-home mothers that have sprouted in the last 10 to 15 years. In some circles, Mothers at Home has an anti-feminist reputation, which Gormley says is unfair, and which may simply be a reflection of what feminist writer Anne Roiphe calls "this hard uneasy tension between motherhood and feminism."

Mothers at Home has no polling data, but its anecdotal evidence indicates that attitudes toward stay-at-home mothers are changing profoundly, says Gormley. The Internet enables women to work at home and still maintain a moment-to-moment connection to the outer world. Changes in the workplace will result in most workers switching jobs five or six times in a career, meaning women who cycle in and out of the work force to have babies will no longer be a special group. More women are having babies later in life, which means the creation of a group of mothers who have achieved enough clout in their careers to demand flexibility from their employers. These women are a select few, says Gormley, but she thinks there's bound to be a trickle-down effect.

When Brenda Barnes, the president and CEO of Pepsi-Cola North America, left her job to stay home with her kids, some people saw the adulation she received as part of a backlash against working women and the feminist movement. Gormley sees a woman using her freedom to make a choice—and that, she says, is what feminism is supposed to be about.

"For some women," she continues, "work is easier. Home is hard. Raising children today, trying to keep marriages intact, trying to find downtime for yourself—it's not easy. And when women make the choice to be at home, you have to redefine success." Those words undoubtedly will enrage thousands of office-going mothers who do not think their lives are one bit easier. But they also remind me of a colleague who, on the day she was supposed to return to work from maternity leave, made it as far as the Red Line subway platform, turned around and went home. And I wonder: How did we get here? It's not as if having babies is some astounding thing that just recently began to happen; it's not as if the phenomenon of working women has just been hatched. So how did we wind up here—so harried, so pressed, making momentous life choices between the 8:11 and the 8:17 train?

The solution to my work/home dilemma, which had tormented me for so many months, arrived one day through the office grapevine: There was about to be a job opening on The Post Magazine. I immediately made a phone call. One week later I had an informal agreement to spend the next year writing articles for the Magazine, working from home. There was one drawback: I would not get paid as much as I'd hoped. David and I were dipping now and then into our savings, we had long ago eliminated luxuries like the health club membership and fancy meals out, and when I went to Nordstrom these days it was to use the baby-friendly ladies' room, not to shop. Clearly, we couldn't continue on this financial course forever. But the money was enough to make it feasible for now—and, most important, there would be lots of time with Emma. I got my formal leave from the newspaper extended, and it was done. Not a permanent solution, but a huge weight lifted nevertheless, and one I felt incredibly lucky to have found. I drove home that day laughing.

One night not long after this, I received a visit from the spirit world.

Or maybe it was just my subconscious being interesting. At any rate, it was a dream, and in it I found myself standing in some public place; the surroundings weren't clear. When I happened to look off to my right, I saw three rather frumpy middle-aged ladies, two of them white and one black. There was nothing out of the ordinary about them. They might have been waiting for the bus, except for one detail: They were standing in midair, about three feet off the ground.

"You're angels, aren't you?" I asked, when I noticed this, and one of the three ladies turned and nodded curtly at me, as if to say, *Yes, but please keep your voice down.* Then she said, "You will see us again in your life, but for now we want you to continue on your journey, which is important." And then they left.

What a strange dream, I thought when I woke up. (I don't normally dream about angels.) But it was clear to me my subconscious was just trying to tell me to keep going. There was no point in trying to find some big answer to the question of how to fit life and child and work into one perfect piece again. "Women's careers don't go in straight lines," Madeleine Albright once told a Time magazine interviewer. "They zigzag all over the place."

And maybe that's the best image. Motherhood these days is like zigzagging around in bumper cars, except ours have kiddie seats. We're all behind the wheel—Ana, who worked too hard to breastfeed her baby as she wanted; Cheli, who made her choice not knowing how much harm it might do her career; Jayne, whose solution is probably going to be lonely; me and a million other women, struggling to figure out a way to be good mothers and still stay connected to work we love. The fun-house music keeps getting louder and faster, and the moms in the bumper cars keep going in tighter little circles, and though some cars are fancier than others, we are all prisoners of the apparatus, which is a culture that treats children as sentimental objects or consumers or inconveniences—as anything but people. And I wonder: How do you stage a bumper car revolt?

You're not fat, you're living in the wrong country

***A fuller figure** is desirable in more than 80 percent of the world. In certain societies, women take **drastic steps** to fatten up—some are even **force-fed** so they can find a husband.* Marie Claire *reports from four cultures where **large women** are envied*

Florence Okumgbe sits in her Fattening Room, trying to eat the piles of food her grandmother, Monday Moses, has set before her. After four weeks of constant eating, Florence is expected to emerge fat and voluptuous, with plump curves.

According to the tradition of the Nigerian Warirke people, putting on weight improves a girl's marriage prospects. Florence has been selected, along with 14 other young women in Ogoloma, to take part in a tradition, called the *Iria*, which will encourage them to get fat and attract a suitable husband.

Each girl stays in a room which has been set aside as the Fattening Room. For four weeks they are expected to do nothing but eat. Parents want their daughters to find the best husbands possible, and being fat will enhance their chances.

For the next month, Monday devotes herself to preparing her granddaughter's favorite food and making *rappas*, short sarongs that Florence wears in the Fattening Room. She also wears heavy copper bands (called *ikpala*) around her legs. They clank as she walks; their purpose is to prevent girls from straying from the Fattening Room or having sex. "If a girl makes love, the ikpala make so much noise—like cow bells—that everyone will know," Monday explains.

Florence enjoys her stay in the Fattening Room, though she develops sores as the ikpala tighten around her fattening legs. "Food is brought to me all the time, and I sleep a lot. When I wake up I am taken to the toilet and my rappa is changed." She welcomes the break from her normal household chores. She can only leave the Fattening Room to bathe in the lake.

Unlike previous generations, Florence does not want to get fat. "I do not want people to say I am clumsy. Some men do not like fat women, and some don't like skinny women. I like to be average so I look good in whatever I wear."

But she is clearly plump enough, because a chief's son asks Monday if Florence will be his wife. Monday reluctantly turns him down. "I told my grandmother I will do Iria on one condition—that I will not get married after it," Florence insists. "I will complete my education first. I want to be a teacher. I know the sort of man I want to marry. I would like a Christian, someone who will listen to me and say sorry if he does something wrong." *—Christine Aziz*

Curves stir men's desires

Sexiness in the land of Kama Sutra is undergoing a revamp. Satellite TV has beamed *Baywatch* and rock-chick chic to India for the past five years, and Hollywood videos have been the rage since the mid-1980s. Now that Indian youth has discovered that thin is in, erotic fantasies are altering and family conflicts can result.

Tara* has her plump mother, Sudha, in despair. Since she started working as a receptionist in Delhi, Tara's dropped 25 pounds. "Her cheeks are sunken," moans Sudha. "She must eat to look healthy." Like many mothers, Sudha has three chubby rolls bulging over the folds of her sari. She's proud that she looks prosperous. Her daughter flatly refuses to carry a lunch box of her mother's fried bread, chicken curry and buttery lentils to the office. "My mom wants to fatten me up to please some future mother-in-law," Tara sighs, lighting a cigarette. On her lunch break, she goes to a gym and runs on the treadmill instead.

**Name has been changed*

But slim women may never be full-blown sex symbols in India. Popular Hindi films feature lineups of busty girls doing hip thrusts in unison. Movie posters often are enhanced by sign painters who stroke on broader backsides to widen the appeal of new films in certain neighborhoods.

"Once men hit their 30s, there is a difference between what is stylish and what stirs desire. Most Indian men still respond more to a full-bodied woman than to young girls in tight jeans," Sheba Chhachhi maintains. Sheba, now 39, is a Delhi-based artist whose multimedia works have been exhibited in Paris and London galleries. She is a strikingly voluptuous woman.

"In my 20s I was really big, and lots of men would tell me that they liked my figure very much. The idea of what is attractive is not only visual. The pleasures go beyond just image: The eye gives way to the touch. A soft belly, chubby knees, fleshy clefts in unexpected places . . . all delicious."

One physician, speaking at a 1994 international conference for orgasmologists in New Delhi, organized by Dr. Prakash Khotari, put it down to physiology. Sexually experienced men often prefer weighty women after they notice that such women's vaginas are tighter. (If a woman loses 10 pounds, her diaphragm size increases; if she gains weight, it gets smaller, because there is more flesh around the opening.)

Bhaskar Bhattacharyya is a Delhi TV executive who routinely must assess the appeal of women on the small screen. "Curves are a must," he says. "Skinny women have nothing to squeeze. Plump women look more wanton, like they have the time to lounge and be indolent. Shapes vary. Tamil Nadu women are little dumplings with large almond eyes. The ideal Punjabi woman is big and well-rounded, with a prominent rear end. Only a very few westernized guys want a disco dolly in a miniskirt for more than a one-night stand." *—Jan McGirk*

Force-fed before marriage

Mani wants to attract a desirable husband. To do so, she will try to force-feed herself, not an easy task for a Tuareg girl in one of the world's driest regions. Mani lives in northern Mali, where recurrent droughts have had devastating effects on the herds. The traditional Tuareg diet—high in meat, milk and butter—has been hard hit by the droughts, as cattle are few and lean. Mani's parents can not provide the food she needs to reach her ideal size.

The Tuareg are pastoral nomads who live on the edge of the Sahara, herding cattle, goats, sheep and camels. They do little manual work themselves, because they retain ex-slaves, or Bella, to labor for them. When slavery was abolished in the 1950s, many Bella chose to remain with their masters in return for food and shelter.

Yearning for status drives the Tuareg man, and the ultimate trophy is a fat wife who obeys him. Her size symbolizes wealth —plenty of milk and meat from a large herd of healthy cattle. It also conforms to the ideal of a woman who does no work, relying on her Bella to do it all. A noble Tuareg woman spends most days sitting in the shade of her tent. Lethargy is encouraged, and some of the women are too obese to exert themselves even if they tried.

Ahmed is one of the richest Tuareg men in Mali. He owns extensive herds and a fleet of Land Cruisers. His sisters are vast—dangerously so—and lie on their beds all day. Not even the prospect of food raises them: They eat Roman style, propped up on one elbow, or are spoon-fed like babies by a Bella attendant. Only the regular call to prayer brings them to their knees, a feat that is agonizing to watch, as they heave over in a futile attempt to touch their foreheads to the ground.

But most women are like Mani, unable to find the food they need to build up their weight. "I want a good husband who has plenty of milk and who will bring me presents of beautiful cloth and beads," she muses.

The ultimate status symbol is a weighty women, but fat is not considered beautiful so much as highly desirable. A man is turned on by the messages a wife give to his peers—messages of wealth, not physical charms. A parting gesture from Ahmed sums it up: "These are my prizes," he boasts, waving at the sisters who are each twice his size, "and one day they shall find suitable husbands." Their reputation has spread far, and Mani dreams of similar proportions. "If I were like them, I would have all the choice in the world!" she grins. But it is the dry season and her father's small herd produces less than half a bowl of milk each morning. She watches the precious ration disappear down her breastfeeding mother, and waits for her own time to come.

—Sarah Snyder

Forbidden to diet

Tucked between the Sigatoka River and the steep cliffs of Fiji's verdant south coast, the village of Sigatoka is almost idyllic. Bamboo rafts float along, steered by women who pass their days with a fishing line in their hands. Mereisi Tuituba, 21, is considered "Sigatoka's most beautiful girl." She lazes through balmy afternoons on her terrace. In between naps, she plays with her year-old daughter. As with most women in Fiji, when Mereisi was pregnant her family coaxed her to eat as much as possible. As a result, she gained more than 50 pounds. "I was always a little more than average in my build," Mereisi says. "And then I got pregnant. Now I am big but I feel good. You don't have to be slim to be beautiful."

Mereisi's husband agrees. "She is very beautiful, now more than before," Eveni gloats. Even at almost 200 pounds, Mereisi embodies Fijian beauty. Joanna Rokumatu, the 67-year-old female chief of Sigatoka village, says, "Mereisi is how Fijian women should look."

In Fiji, body weight is a symbol of how well your community takes care of you. As in many South Pacific island cultures, social events are celebrated with elaborate feasts, where gifts of food are exchanged. Community wealth is measured by a family's ability to share food, personal generosity by the amount placed on the table.

With such a social emphasis on eating, a full-figured body is not only a reflection of how well your village cares for you, it is a measure of beauty. A cardinal feature of physical attractiveness in Fiji is the shape of a woman's calves, which are thought to be the sexiest part of the female body. The worst insult you can offer a woman is to say she has thin legs.

But young Fijian women are beginning to feel caught between two cultures as they become exposed to the Western world. With American culture transmitting across the airwaves, Fijian girls are witnessing the American concept of beauty.

"The more girls watch television, the more likely they are to diet," Chief Joanna explains. She believes it is her responsibility to maintain village traditions, and this means discouraging such behavior, which she believes is harmful to Fijian society.

"Dieting is not the Fijian way. What if we didn't sit down to eat together in the evening? What if we stopped farming, stopped fishing? We can't allow these things to happen," declares Joanna. "Television is the source of many problems." *—Sara Hare*

reality check

■ Peter J. Brown, a professor of anthropology at Emory University, explains the cultural preference for larger women: "Where food is scarce, fat carries prestige: Men like to show that they can afford to pamper their women. In societies of plenty, like America, the 'perfect body' is impossibly thin. Either way, achieving the beauty ideal requires both effort and money."

While many cultures see premarital plumpness as sexually attractive, in some societies weight gain after marriage reflects fidelity—a mother should not be too concerned with her appearance. As a matter of fact, it is only in societies where a woman's prestige is not based on her role as a mother that thinness is considered ideal. But regardless of what a given society considers a perfect figure, an almost universal characteristic of the women in it is dissatisfaction with their bodies. Equally prevalent is the lack of concern most men express about their weight.

I chose to be sterilized at 29

I've never had any maternal instincts.

*Dana knew that she never wanted to have children. Last year, she made an **irreversible decision** that has eliminated the possibility forever. She explains to Denise Dowling why she did it*

Everyone told me that one day my biological clock would go off and that my feelings would change, but living in a house with a white picket fence, a husband and two kids has never been my dream. I thought more about what I would achieve, both in my career and my personal life. I work as an account executive at a Silicon Valley firm that specializes in Internet startups, and to me, success is having a job I really love while being able to enjoy life and spend time with my family and friends.

My older brother has two children and I love them to death. I'm very happy visiting them . . . and then going home. When my nephew was an infant, my brother took a photo of me holding him, which was a big joke to the people who know me. I enjoy kids, as long as they're other people's. When I was younger, people often asked, "Don't you want to babysit to earn some extra money?" "Hell, no!" was always my response.

I don't think there's anything wrong with me for not wanting children. In fact, there are a lot of people who probably should have thought more about whether they would make good parents. I think some marriages break up because couples have children too quickly instead of taking the time to really create their own bond.

I really hated the Pill, which I'd been on since I was 18. It gave me headaches, made my hands swell and raised my cholesterol. I didn't like putting something in my body that tricks the system, but I didn't feel there was another reliable option. Although I'd heard a lot of negative things about the IUD, I started to look into it a year ago. I went to Planned

Parenthood, and they told me they normally don't give IUDs to unmarried women because there can be complications that cause sterility. I told them I had no intention of having children. Eventually, they agreed to fit me for an IUD, but in the end it turned out that my cervix was too small and would have rejected the device. That's when I began seriously considering having a tubal ligation.

I had three counseling sessions before they would proceed with the tubal. The clinic has a rigorous set of questions to ensure your reasons are valid and that it's not something you might regret later on. They consider it permanent. I was told, "Don't even consider having this operation if you think you'd ever want to reverse it," because the success rate is so low. It varies depending on the doctor, but about one in every 200 to 1000 reversal operations succeeds.

The counselor asked me to consider different life-changing scenarios and how they could affect my decision. I was asked about my boyfriend and what would happen if I ended up with someone else. I was more concerned about the medical aspects than the emotional ones. I wanted to know what the operation was like, whether there would be residual problems or scarring and how it would affect my menstrual cycle.

A tubal ligation is a really quick outpatient procedure. I went to the hospital in the morning and was home by noon. The doctor inflated my stomach with carbon dioxide to pump it up so the instruments wouldn't injure another organ. Then he made two incisions, one by my belly button for the scope, and the second near the hairline. That one is for the instrument used to cut and then cauterize the fallopian tubes. Everyone's body reacts differently, but the gas settled strangely and I was pretty sore. The instruments go through your stomach muscles, so for three days it hurt to walk. I took a week and half off work, and my abdomen was swollen for almost a month. The operation was nine months ago and I still sometimes experience a dull pain in my left ovary for the first two days of my period. The doctors thought it would subside sooner. I have no regrets about the operation, but I want to find out what's causing this pain.

There's nothing wrong with me not wanting children. I think a lot of people should've thought more before they had kids.

I talked to a lot of people before the surgery and told many people afterward. Not one of them responded negatively. And although I wasn't expecting my parents to be surprised by my decision, I was relieved at how understanding they were. My father thanked me for being open with them and said, "We want your contribution to the world to be whatever makes you happy." My mom said that they respected my choices, and then asked, "Does this mean I can let your niece and nephew have the clothes I've saved from when you were growing up?"

My boyfriend has been very supportive. We've been together for two and a half years and my considering sterilization forced us to discuss our future. We've talked about marriage, but we go back and forth. I said, "If you know you're not going to have children, why don't you get a vasectomy?" But men have this thing about it—they just don't want to do it. He was quoting all these wrong statistics and saying that it's totally reversible with women, so I told him to read up on it.

In the end, he said that if we do get married, he'd be perfectly happy not having children. Some of the men I dated before him would say, "Oh, you'll change your mind about kids." It's maddening to have other people impose their thinking on you when they can't possibly know. If I ended up dating someone else and found out he really wanted children, I'd probably stop going out with him. I wouldn't want to lead him on.

Another alternative

A childless, unmarried young woman who has a tubal ligation is very much an exception to standard medical procedure. "With such an absolute decision, it is critical for a woman to weigh alternative methods of equally reliable contraception," advises Dr. Pouru Bhiwandi, a North Carolina-based OB/GYN. "I would recommend Norplant or the Paragard IUD, neither of which is permanent."

Prozac has helped millions cope. But it's hardly time to hail it as a cure—or to give up on an effective treatment like talk therapy.

TREAT DEPRESSION WITH MORE THAN DRUGS

By Deborah Franklin

FOR 21 YEARS they have sought him out, three or four people every day, each unhappy in his or her own way. There are chain-smoking salesmen too hostile to sit, sunken-eyed students unable to sleep, widows whose lips tremble, eyes brim at the mere mention of a husband three years dead. Whatever the heart-numbing loss, and perhaps especially when the agitation or fog seems to arise from no loss at all, they are referred to Victor I. Reus or others like him—neuroscientists, the leading emotional healers of our day.

Reus is a psychiatrist and professor of psychopharmacology at the University of California at San Francisco and, as such, tends to be a wizard of last resort. He is a counselor's counselor—the guy the pastor or family doctor sends you to when getting more exercise, easing back at the office, or leaning on friends isn't enough. As a medical doctor, the only brand of psychological healer in the United States permitted to prescribe drugs, he mostly gets patients looking for exactly that. And thanks to a recent boom in transformative pills to ease depression, Reus quite often does have something chemical to offer.

But lately he has noticed that many patients come to him not just depressed, but confused.

"I hear it again and again," Reus says. "They'll sit down and say, 'Look, I've been to other docs who tell me my problem comes from a chemical imbalance in my brain, and they want to give me a drug. But no one has ever actually *tested* me for an imbalance, and that is where I want you to start.'"

At which point Reus has to break it to the peeved patient as

HEALTH BREAKS THE NEWS

Prozac is not a lifelong solution for most depressed patients, Peter Carlin concluded in January of this year. Perhaps, he wrote, some alternatives deserve a chance.

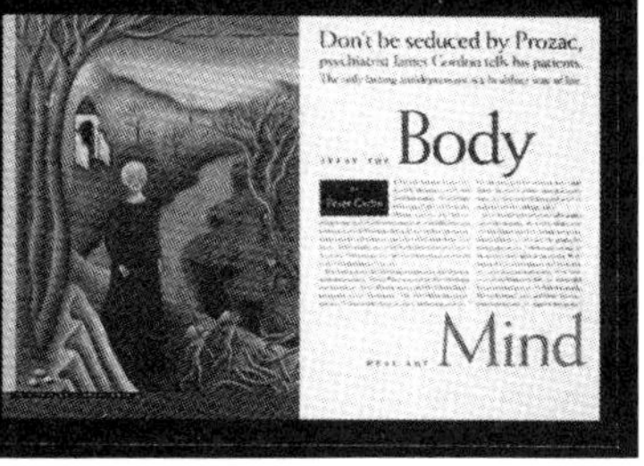

gently as he can: "I could spend a lot of your money taking pictures of your brain, and chances are there will be nothing wrong with it that we can peg your symptoms to," he tells them. "I can measure levels of serotonin in your blood or cerebral spinal fluid, and still that won't tell me anything useful. After all that testing, I'll be in the same position as every other doctor: I can recommend psychotherapy and one or another drug that has helped other people with your symptoms, and then we'll just have to watch and see how you do."

Really? The news, Reus says, always comes as a bit of a shock. This is the Decade of the Brain, for Freud's sake, and faith in biological precision is riding high. "Getting inside someone's head" these days is less often about analyzing thoughts and feelings than snapping pictures of them with the help of PET scans that illustrate in brilliant color the parts of the brain that rev up or shut down during a funk, and MRIs that offer up photographic slices of gray matter without ever cracking a skull. Besides serotonin, researchers have identified more than 60 other chemical messengers, or neurotransmitters, up from just a handful a few decades ago. Today it is undisputed that severe mental illness is rooted in a chemical mix-up of some sort—whether prompted by an inborn miswiring of the brain or by a virus, environmental toxin, or psychological trauma that has somehow knocked a person's brain chemistry out of whack. "Good-bye Oedipus," an article in a recent issue of *Time* magazine declared. "The three-pound organ that rules the body is finally giving up its secrets."

Depression, once seen exclusively as a stumble of the spirit, has been recast in the popular imagination as just another physical imbalance, like diabetes or iron-poor blood. "My wife has depression," General Colin Powell mentioned at a press conference in 1995. "It is not a family secret. It is very easily controlled with proper medication, just as my blood pressure is." *Next question?*

That's fine, of course. Surely any drug that safely enables even a fraction of those suffering from depression or other mood disorders to resume full lives should be celebrated. When a life has been wrenched to a standstill by pain—whether by the shrill torment of daily migraines or the deeper growl of fierce depression—the immediate goal is to make it stop.

But trouble begins when, like a garbled message in the party game telephone, word comes down that the chemical imbalance underlying depression is simply a serotonin deficiency, with Prozac and other serotonin-boosters the obvious cure. The cold, hard truth is that even when these drugs work, no one really knows how or why.

That single, widespread misconception—that the new drugs cure depression the same way vitamin D prevents rickets, or vitamin C fixes scurvy—feeds a host of all-too-practical problems, ranging from the discounting of a drug's serious side effects to the assumption that what's needed is a lifelong prescription. Saddest of all, the misplaced faith may lead us to spurn treatments that work just as well—or even better.

> Talk therapy—the very human encounter between a patient and a trained counselor—has essentially the same success rate as drugs.

OF ALL THE DEVELOPMENTS that have primed Americans to think of lasting anguish as a simple chemical deficiency, none has been as seductive or pervasive as Prozac. Since the drug was introduced in 1987, the global market for it and other selective serotonin-reuptake inhibitors (SSRIs)—including Zoloft and Paxil—has mushroomed to around $4 billion. In just the last two years, the number of prescriptions for these drugs has jumped by 20 percent, and the list of ailments for which they are often prescribed has stretched to include anxiety, bulimia, obsessive-compulsive disorder, premenstrual syndrome, and obesity. Eighteen million Americans—about one in every eight adults—has at one time or another been put on Prozac, out of 24 million people worldwide. And today it's not the psychiatrist but the family doctor who writes far and away the most prescriptions. These generalists, who tended to shy away from the older antidepressants, have been much freer with the SSRIs because they require fewer daily doses, less monitoring, and seem to have a higher margin of safety.

The theory behind these drugs has been repeated ad infinitum: Prozac is said to lift spirits by boosting the brain's stores of serotonin, a ringleader among the chemical messengers that communicate emotion and other information from cell to cell. That idea is based on computer modeling and animal studies showing that all SSRIs slow the process by which serotonin is vacuumed up from the tiny clefts between brain cells. If serotonin is allowed to linger, pooling between the cells, the feel-good message passed along is presumably stronger than it would have been without the drug.

But just because Prozac both boosts serotonin and makes some depressed people feel better doesn't mean too little serotonin caused their depression, any more than headaches are brought on by an aspirin deficiency. Any neuroscientist, if pressed, will agree that the mechanisms of depression are much more complicated than a simple flick of the serotonin switch. "This myth that you can isolate and treat depression with some sort of medical version of a surgical strike, we now know, is totally bogus," says Reus.

For one thing, SSRIs help only about two-thirds of depressed patients. That's the same success rate as (or even slightly lower than) the older antidepressants—the so-called tricyclics and MAO inhibitors—which differ chemically from SSRIs and seem to interact with a much broader sampling of the brain's chemical messengers. And even when SSRIs are effective, there

QUIZ

HOW BAD ARE YOUR BLUES?

IF YOU'RE PRONE to feeling down-and-out, the test below can help you determine whether you're experiencing ordinary bouts of sadness or something closer to full-blown depression. Read each statement and circle the number that reflects how often it applies to you. Then tally the numbers and put your total below. Remember, this is a rough evaluation; only a professional can make a definitive diagnosis.

Never . . . . . . 0 Occasionally . . . . . . 1 Often . . . . . . 2 Nearly always 3

I have lost interest in relationships, sex, work, and other pursuits.

0 1 2 3

I feel inconsolably sad.

0 1 2 3

I find it hard to concentrate.

0 1 2 3

Everything seems hopeless to me.

0 1 2 3

I let projects, responsibilities, or personal hygiene slide.

0 1 2 3

I feel overwhelmingly tired and lacking in energy.

0 1 2 3

I have trouble making even simple decisions.

0 1 2 3

I have experienced a dramatic shift in my appetite.

0 1 2 3

I have noticed a major change in my sleeping habits.

0 1 2 3

I think I might be better off dead.

0 1 2 3

. . . . Total

IF YOU SCORED OVER FIFTEEN, you could be suffering moderate to severe depression and should consider seeking help. If you have suicidal feelings, you should consult a mental health professional right away.

Finding Help

See your physician. Some disorders, such as thyroid disease, can cause symptoms that mimic depression; so your first step should be to get a thorough physical exam. If your doctor suggests taking antidepressants, consider consulting a therapist first to explore the question further.

Make lifestyle changes. Exercise, stress management, and closer ties to friends can help lift mild depression. Deeper, more persistent bouts require more help.

Consider talk therapy. A trusted friend, doctor, pastor, or rabbi may be able to refer you to a state-licensed psychologist, psychiatrist, or social worker. Popular types of therapy include interpersonal, which focuses on resolving relationship conflicts; cognitive, aimed at correcting negative behavior and thinking patterns; and psychodynamic, which explores underlying drives and desires. Often just a few sessions can get you through a rough patch and help you develop some coping skills for the future. For more information on treatment options for depression, call the National Institute of Mental Health at 800/421-4211.

is generally a several-week time lag between the moment the first dose is swallowed and the point at which the drug begins to take effect. If a simple increase in serotonin directly eased depression, researchers agree, patients would start feeling better within a matter of hours or days, not weeks.

Further muddying the waters, a little-known drug from Europe called tianeptine takes the opposite tack from Prozac—it *depletes* pools of serotonin from between the same cells—and yet is quite an effective antidepressant.

Nor is any serotonin-enhancer likely to radically change you or society—despite what you may have heard. In his 1993 best-seller, *Listening to Prozac,* Rhode Island psychiatrist Peter Kramer startled and captivated readers with his reports of the way SSRIs seemed to transform his patients' personalities. Highly sensitive patients taking Prozac became more resilient, he reported, and rigid folks became more flexible. Prozac is to the shy personality, he warned, what silicone breast implants are to flat-chested models and anabolic steroids are to Olympic swimmers—a form of cosmetic, chemical enhancement that shifts the definition of acceptable and normal.

"In the science-fiction horror-story version of the interplay of drug and culture," Kramer fretted, "a boss says, 'Why such a long face? Can't you take a MoodStim before work?'"

Kramer's concern now seems a bit overlathered. For starters, ten years of experience have shown that the drugs' side effects—most notably nausea, sometimes-severe sleep disturbances, and in up to 50 percent of patients impotence, decreased libido, or an inability to reach orgasm—are significant enough that most people won't stay on the pills if their only goal is to feel less inhibited. And the drugs probably are no more transformative than the antidepressants available decades ago, Reus says. In the first documented study of SSRI use in healthy, nondepressed people, he and colleagues at UCSF recently found that Paxil did produce some increase in self-confidence and assertiveness while decreasing negativity. "But the effects were fairly small," he says. "The drug certainly did not make anyone euphoric."

Why are we all so eager to see depression and maybe even shyness as serotonin deficiencies—as simple, physical problems best fixed with a pill? Maybe to get around the stigmas that have long cloaked both mental illness and mood-enhancing drugs. Robert Fancher, a New York psychotherapist, argues convincingly that we Americans, born of Puritanism, have always had a difficult time owning up to our equally strong hedonistic streak. Especially today, in the just-say-no era, reaching for a drug involving the mind—even to relieve psychic pain—carries substantial shame for some people. "That sounds too much like avoiding one's problems through drugs," says Fancher, author of *Cultures of Healing: Correcting the Image of American Mental Health Care*.

But if a drug can be pitched differently, he says, not as an escape or a psychological fix, but rather as a medicine that specifically corrects a biological flaw, the stigma magically evaporates. Insulin for diabetes, iron for anemia, serotonin for distress or shyness . . . Ah yes, we see.

It's not that neuroscientists or family doctors set out to deceive, Fancher says. Their enthusiasm for everything that modern biology *has* revealed about the brain in the last 50 years encourages them to play along, smoothing the gaps in knowledge with provisional explanations the public rushes to take up as gospel.

Lost in the hoopla is this: Just as a drug can influence the mind's chemistry, so too can every epiphany or insight prompted by a treatment that would seem, at first blush, to have little to do with brain chemistry. In a study last year of people diagnosed with another psychiatric condition—obsessive-compulsive disorder—psychiatrist Jeffrey Schwartz of the University of California at Los Angeles published brightly colored PET scans taken of the patients' brains before and after each had undergone treatment with either Prozac *or* talk therapy. The results clearly showed that the treatments not only worked equally well but produced identical changes in brain metabolism. He's now beginning similar studies of depressed patients.

Given what we're learning about how different emotions reflect and influence brain activity, Schwartz's finding makes perfect sense: If you change someone's outlook, you change their brain chemistry, too. The results of a number of recent large studies of talk therapy bear this out. The very human encounter between a depressed person and a counselor trained in any of the main schools of psychotherapy has been shown to have *essentially the same success rate as medication*—around 60 or 70 percent. People who don't get relief from one or another drug are often helped by counseling, and vice versa.

Yet, despite its proven effectiveness, talk therapy is being pushed toward oblivion. Already, health maintenance organizations and traditional insurers are chary of reimbursing patients for more than a few psychotherapy sessions. If the doctor serving as gatekeeper to further medical care can just prescribe Prozac with the stroke of a pen, the labor cost of lengthy psychotherapy can be eliminated. Simplifying the definition of depression to "serotonin deficiency" makes it easier for HMOs and family doctors to rationalize the approach. But that doesn't make it right.

"When a depressed person comes to us," Fancher says, "we don't know right away whether it's an illness itself, a sign of an illness, or a sign that the person needs to change something in his or her life." Talk therapy can help the patient discern between those sources of discomfort in a way that a 15-minute office visit and prescription for drugs can't.

"It's like if you came in with a pain in your foot," Fancher says. "You might have the pain because of a rock in your shoe or because your shoe is two sizes too small. We can give you a drug that will make you not mind the fact that your foot hurts, but wouldn't it be better to change your shoe?"

Drugs have a proper place in treatment, Fancher and most other therapists readily agree. "When depression has made somebody nonfunctional—they're missing work, say, or can't come within spitting distance of keeping up with their lives," he says, "I think you need to medicate quickly. Talking things through can only help if a patient feels well enough to talk." And even people with milder distress may find a short course of the drugs genuinely helpful.

But, Fancher says, anyone who clings to a Prozac prescription as proof that he or she is chemically deficient without the drug is making a Faustian trade. "The loss of autonomy may be the biggest risk of all," Fancher says. "If you perceive that your problem arises from a defective brain, you may start to panic if you go on vacation and your prescription runs out." Also, defining distress as a deficiency and Prozac as the cure, he says, may provide a misplaced shield for those of us whose depression arises partly from rifts in relationships or our own skewed behavior—aspects of our lives we'd do better to consciously address and try to change.

Fancher offers in illustration a male client in his late thirties whose talent, charm, and good looks had bought him years of indulgence from family and friends, despite a continuing failure to stick with a job, pay rent, or honor other adult commitments. Eventually even his nearest and dearest got tired of bailing him out, Fancher says, and as the man gradually found himself alone, he was—as you might imagine—depressed.

"He came to me for psychotherapy, and we were making some progress, but he'd heard a lot about Prozac and wanted to try it," Fancher says. "A month after he started taking the drug—about how long it takes to kick in—he decided he was fine and didn't need therapy anymore. Now he's close to 40, still can't hang on to a job, doesn't have a steady place to live, but he feels great."

Deborah Franklin has been a staff writer at the magazine since 1987.

It's no news that stress can make you sick. But recent research says the solution isn't working less or playing more. It's having someone to confide in.

DON'T FACE STRESS ALONE

By Benedict Carey

THE CURE FOR EXCESSIVE STRESS SHOULD be excessive cash. A fat pile of Microsoft common that provides for limo service and trips to the Seychelles and nannies and someone to vacuum those tumbleweed pet hairs that breed in every corner of the house. Better still, a house that cleans itself. That way we'd have time to read Emerson, learn to play some baroque stringed instrument, and sample Eastern gurus like finger food, accumulating vast reserves of inner peace and healing energy. . . .

We're fooling ourselves. Even stinking rich, most of us would often feel rushed, harassed, afraid that the maid's boyfriend had designs on our Swedish stereo components. We'd lose sleep, lose our tempers, and continue to wonder whether stress was killing us. Not because money doesn't buy

Almost half of Americans say they'd rather be alone when they're stressed. Only 18 percent would call a friend.

tranquility; it buys plenty. But because what we call stress is more than the sum of our chores and responsibilities and financial troubles. It's also a state of mind, a way of interpreting the world, a pattern of behavior.

Think of the people you know. There are those who are so consumed with work that they practically sleep with their cell phones, who go wild when they just have to wait in line at the checkout. And then there are those who breeze through the day as pleased as park rangers—despite having deadlines and kids and a broken-down car and charity work and scowling Aunt Agnes living in the spare bedroom. Back in the 1960s cardiologists Ray Rosenman and Meyer Friedman labeled these polar opposites Type A and Type B. They described Type As as "joyless strivers," people who go through life feeling harried, hostile, and combative. Type Bs, by contrast, are unhurried, even tempered, emotionally secure. In person Type As may be twitchy, prone to interrupt, resentful of conversational diversions. Type Bs are as placid as giraffes, well mannered, affectionately patient. In a landmark 1971 study Rosenman and Friedman found that Type As were about twice as likely to develop coronary artery disease as Type Bs. This was the first evidence of a phenomenon that we now take for granted: People consumed by stress often live short lives.

Often. But not always. Some Type As live long and prosper. Some Type Bs succumb to heart attacks before they turn 50. Rosenman and Friedman's theory represented a giant step in tracing a link between disease and personality. But it only partly explained why stress sometimes damages the heart. So the search has been under way to discover a more specific connection between personality and illness. In the past decade findings in fields as seemingly unrelated as sociology and immunology have begun to converge on a surprising answer. Of course it matters if your life is a high-wire act of clamoring demands and pressing deadlines. And yes, it does make a difference whether you're angry or retiring, effusive or shy, belligerent or thoughtful. But what really matters appears to be something much simpler: whether you have someone in your life who's emotionally on call, who's willing to sit up late and hear your complaints.

HUMAN EMOTIONS ARE a messy affair, fleeting, contradictory, and as hard to define as human beings themselves. So it's no wonder researchers have found themselves groping around the dim and convoluted catacombs of personality, trying to locate the core of the trouble with Type As. Some suspect the real villain may be a specific trait such as hostility, cynicism, or self-centeredness. And indeed, all of these characteristics are prevalent in many people who develop coronary disease. But none has proved terribly useful for predicting who will get sick. The search has been a little like being fitted for glasses: Lens two looks clearer than lens one at first, but then you're not so sure. Still, something's there, all right, and several studies conducted in the late eighties and early nineties have finally brought its ghostly shape into focus.

"If you look across all of these studies for a pattern," says psychologist Margaret Chesney, who has spent the past 20 years doing precisely that, "you see that the hostility questionnaires and the Type A interview and all the other measures—they're all picking up the same thing. It's this person who's often suspicious; who sees people as being in their way; who, when they meet someone new, asks, 'What do you do? Where did you go to school?'—not to make a connection but to assess the competition."

More details emerged in 1989 when psychologists Jerry Suls and Choi Wan of the State University of New York at Albany reviewed the Type A research to look for a common thread. They concentrated on studies whose authors had performed general psychological profiles as well as Type A assessments. As a rule, general psych profiles ask directly about fears, insecurities, childhood traumas, and so on, while the Type A diagnosis focuses on how pressured a person feels and how pleasantly he or she answers aggressive questions.

Suls and Wan had suspected that Type A behavior would be associated with emotional distress. But they found something strange. The Type As did show strains of insecurity and emotional isolation—but none of the anxiety and fear associated with the garden-variety neurotic. These are the sort of people who need counseling but consider therapists overpriced palm-readers. "The picture we're getting is of someone who has deep problems but doesn't admit them," says Suls. "So there are a couple of possibilities here. Either they're in denial. Or they really don't have rich inner lives. They never really think about these things."

They aren't Oprah Winfrey fans, in short. They're happy enough talking about work, fashion, sports—anything but the mushy personal stuff. "If you confront them with that," says Suls, "they get angry. They blow up." As one researcher puts it, "They never let their guard down. If you come close, they wonder, What is this person after?" Spare me the advice, Sigmund, can't you see I'm busy?

This evidence, admittedly raw, is still the subject of much debate, but it has even the most authoritative, skeptical, hard-line figures in the field talking like late-night radio shrinks. Just listen to founding father Rosenman, who has guarded the Type A franchise like a hawk, staring down dozens of psychologists whose work he deemed soft or flawed. "After 40 years of observing and treating thousands of patients, and doing all of the studies, I believe that what's underneath the inappropriate competitiveness of Type As is a deep-seated insecurity. I never would have said that before, but I keep coming back to it. It's different from anxiety in the usual sense, because Type As are not people who retreat. They constantly compete because it helps them suppress the insecurity they're afraid others will sense.

"If I felt this way, how would I cover it up? I'd distract myself, go faster and faster, and win over everybody else. I'd look at everyone as a threat, because they might expose me."

Avoiding exposure inevitably means avoiding close relationships. The person Rosenman is describing has friends, sure, but no genuine confidants, no one who's allowed so much as a whiff of frailty. That's why many researchers now believe that the symptom most common among those vulnerable to stress is emotional isolation. As Chesney puts it, "These people might have the biggest Rolodex, but they're alone. They're busy looking for more connections, charming more people. When they feel isolated they get busy. It's a defense mechanism."

The people most vulnerable to stress are those who are emotionally isolated. They might have the biggest Rolodex, but they're alone.

According to Jonathan Schedler, a research psychologist affiliated with Harvard

They Touched a Nation

THANKS TO PUBLIC FIGURES who spoke out about their illnesses, we have all grown more comfortable in the past decade confronting health problems that were long shrouded in lonely silence.
—*Rita Rubin*

MUHAMMAD ALI

It was the most arresting moment of the 1996 Olympics in Atlanta: the former boxer, arm trembling, face frozen, raising the torch to the light the ceremonial flame. Calls flooded the National Parkinson's Foundation, which adopted a torch as its symbol.

ANNETTE FUNICELLO

In 1992, when the onetime Mickey Mouse Club girl publicly revealed her diagnosis, we all suddenly knew at least one person with MS: Annette. "She is everyone's extended family member," says Arney Rosenblat of the National Multiple Sclerosis Society.

LINDA ELLERBEE

Months after the journalist underwent a double mastectomy, she produced an emotionally charged special on breast cancer. "I can be fair and honest," she says of the disease. "But objective I cannot be."

RONALD REAGAN

Ever-folksy, the former president announced he had Alzheimer's disease in a handwritten letter addressed to "my fellow Americans" in 1994. He called his gesture "an opening of our hearts."

WILLIAM STYRON

The novelist told of his depression in the New York Times and later in *Darkness Visible: A Memoir of Madness.* "The overwhelming reaction made me feel that inadvertently I had helped unlock a closet from which many souls were eager to come out."

CHRISTOPHER REEVE

"You only have two choices," says the actor whose 1995 fall from a horse left him permanently paralyzed and who has raised millions for spinal injury research. "Either you vegetate and look out the window or activate and try to effect change."

GREG LOUGANIS

Mortified that he'd hid his HIV-positive status when his head wound bloodied the Olympic pool in 1988, the diver finally told his story during an interview with Barbara Walters in 1995.

University, the tests researchers use to identify hostile personalities essentially measure something he calls interpersonal warmth. "It has to do with whether you see the people in your life as benevolent or malevolent, whether they offer nourishment or frustration," he says. "The fact is, humans are emotionally frail. We need real support from other people, and those who don't acknowledge it are going to feel besieged."

These notions could easily collapse into sentimentality. Yet scientific evidence for the physical benefits of social support is coming in from all sides. At Ohio State University, for example, immunologist Ron Glaser and psychologist Janice Kiecolt-Glaser have found that the biggest slump in immunity during exam periods occurs in medical students who report being lonely. Analyzing data from the Tecumseh Community Health Study, sociologist James House calculated that social isolation was as big a risk factor for illness and death as smoking was. And these were just the warm-up acts. In 1989 David Spiegel of Stanford Medical School measured the effect of weekly group therapy on women being treated for breast cancer. As expected, those who met in groups experienced less pain than those who didn't. But that wasn't all. The women in counseling survived an average of 37 months—nearly twice as long as those without the group support. Other researchers, including Friedman, have also lengthened some heart patients' lives through group therapy.

The reason remains anyone's guess. Perhaps, as Spiegel has suggested, being in a group makes patients more likely to take their medications, perform prescribed exercise, and so on. Patients may also benefit from advice offered in therapy, which can range from the commonsensical to the cornball: from "slow down, spend more time with your family, and don't sweat the little things" to "control your anger, read more poetry, and verbalize affection." Hardly the sort of wisdom that transforms lives.

If these interventions have anything in common, though, it is the presence of other people. This makes sense if you think of stress the way most doctors do, as a hormonal response to pressure. The body perceives a threat, mental or physical, and releases hormones that hike blood pressure and suppress immune response. According to the theory, some of us (the hostile, the troubled, the Type As) have a higher risk of heart disease or cancer because we secrete more of these hormones more frequently than the average joe. This stress response isn't easy to moderate, but one of the few things that seems to help is contact with a supportive person. In several lab experiments, for instance, psychologists have shown that having a friend in the room calms the cardiovascular response to distressing tasks such as public speaking. It's the secret of group therapy: We relax around our own. The simple grace of company can keep us healthy.

Humans are, after all, social by nature. So perhaps it makes sense that the healthiest among us might be the ones who find solace in companionship, who can defuse building pressure by opening up our hearts to someone else. As the late biologist and writer Lewis Thomas observed, human beings have survived by being useful to one another. We are as indispensable to each other as hummingbirds are to hibiscus.

And by finding ways to help each other out, the latest research hints, we forge the emotional connections that could very well sustain us. Thomas understood this. In a *New York Times* interview in 1993, just two weeks before his death, the reporter asked him, "Is there an art to dying?"

"There's an art to living," Thomas replied. "One of the very important things that has to be learned around the time dying becomes a real prospect is to recognize those occasions when we have been useful in the world. With the same sharp insight that we all have for acknowledging our failures, we ought to recognize when we have been useful, and sometimes uniquely useful. All of us have had such times in our lives, but we don't pay much attention to them. Yet the thing we're really good at as a species is usefulness. If we paid more attention to this biological attribute, we'd get a satisfaction that cannot be attained from goods or knowledge."

Benedict Carey has been a staff writer at the magazine since 1988.

It's only natural: When you hurt, you want a diagnosis and treatment—right away. But slow down. When it comes to your everyday medical care, the best doctors do the least.

GIVE YOUR BODY TIME TO HEAL

By Ann Japenga

IN THE SPRING OF 1987 I was living a Nike ad. Brimming with vitality, I routinely jetted off—reporter's notebook in hand—to kayak in ocean storms or go helicopter skiing in the Sierras. To wind down at the end of an eventful day, I'd swim laps or run along Santa Monica beach, six blocks from my house. Then I began suffering "swoops," as a friend called them, periods when for weeks at a time the color drained from my face and my body felt like it was made of clay. Once the swoops came on, I couldn't even muster the energy to stroll down to the pier for gelato.

My mother, a pediatrician, came to my house one day, laid my arm on the kitchen counter, and drew some blood. She tucked the vial into her cracked black bag. A few days later the results came back. Mononucleosis.

I was relieved. At the time I had a sunny view of medicine. A test would lead to a diagnosis; a diagnosis, to treatment; a treatment, to wellness. And now I had a diagnosis, a disease.

There was only one problem: I didn't get well. Long after the mono virus should have run its course I was still shuttling from one time-consuming doctor's visit to another, feeling irritated because I had skydiving appointments to keep.

The doctors opined that I might just be overworked or depressed, or that I might qualify for a new malady—chronic fatigue syndrome—which was untreatable anyway. I became obsessed with finding a physician who could give me a more concrete explanation. More than once I had blood drawn and checked for every disease you can name. When still no answer came, I named my sickness "the voodoo bug" and cursed the profession too incompetent to cure it.

Of course, I wasn't the only one who spent at least part of his or her thirties demanding answers from doctors. Sickness seemed a rite of passage, judging from my equally vigorous friends and coworkers' susceptibility to fatigue, chronic viruses, insomnia, infertility, depression, bad backs, and bum knees.

My peers shared the belief that tests would lead to a treatment and therefore a cure. Unwittingly, all of us had been indoctrinated by a cultural phenomenon known as medicalization. This is the tendency to see bona fide illness behind every discomfort, coupled with an inordinate belief in the ability of doctors to relieve the pain.

Medicalization has been in ascendancy for much of my lifetime, prompted by the apparent ease with which Marcus Welby and Ben Casey cured illness, researchers' announcements of high-tech "breakthroughs," and ferocious marketing of everything medical—doctors, tests, drugs, cures. By the mid-1980s there were few symptoms left that might not warrant a doctor's visit. Tired? A blood test should find something. Stomachache? Could be an ulcer or cancer; see a specialist. Backache? Time for an MRI.

But during the year my voodoo bug took hold, medicalization began to come under scrutiny. In 1986 an article published by University of Oklahoma researchers James Mold and Howard Stein in the *New England Journal of Medicine*

From *Health*, April 1997, pp. 62-67.

Docs Through the Decades
How They Lost Our Trust

WHY DO WE EXPECT so much from doctors, then suspect the worst when they don't diagnose and cure our ailments fast? Look back at the medicine depicted on television since the 1960s. For two decades these shows—which the American Medical Association screened until the late 1970s—glorified physicians and trumpeted their healing power. But no longer, says Joseph Turow, a communications professor at the University of Pennsylvania and the author of *Playing Doctor: Television, Storytelling, and Medical Power.* "The doctors have been knocked off their pedestal."—*Kathleen Moloney*

DR. KILDARE
1961–1966

Richard Chamberlain stars as part superhero, part eagle scout. (He described Kildare as "good, high-minded, loyal, kind, warm-hearted, friendly, sincere, and chaste.") "If I suffered from a deadly disease," Kildare says to a recalcitrant alcoholic, "I'd do everything in my power to help the doctors who were helping me." Though little actual treatment is shown—most action takes place in the hospital's break room and cafeteria—the patients always get better.

BEN CASEY
1961–1966

Vince Edwards stars as a brooding neurosurgeon at County General. The show is low-tech, offering only vague shots of equipment while most clinical scenes take place in a shadowy room with a bed and a table. Casey is brusque and powerful. "If you don't want medical help, you've taken leave of your senses, woman," he barks. "I'm a neurosurgeon. My job is to identify, isolate, and cure."

MARCUS WELBY, M.D.
1969–1976

Robert Young ("Father Knows Best") stars as a beloved family physician. Welby gives injections on screen—a TV-doc first—and spends hours counseling patients on autism, abortion, impotence, addiction, menopause, and homosexuality. (He has trouble believing that a gay patient doesn't actually like girls.) He makes house calls, rarely uses medical terms, and almost always—with the help of a crack specialist—heals the patient.

MEDICAL CENTER
1969–1976

Chad Everett stars as Joe Gannon, a young yet seasoned physician-turned-department-chief beset by personal and professional crises. Often hurried and abrupt, Gannon tosses off terms like aortic stenosis and mastectomy. He operates on screen and is cagey with his back-talking, eccentric patients. Still, hardly anyone dies.

ER
1994–present

In a seething emergency room, the staff—with Anthony Edwards as Dr. Mark Greene and George Clooney as Dr. Douglas Ross—practices harsh, snap-judgment medicine. ("Two-day-old male infant, full-term, vaginal delivery, found cyanotic in his crib. Resp 50, heart rate 160.") Yet for all the techy talk and shiny equipment, the doctors struggle. "We work 36 hours on, 18 off, which is 90 hours a week, 52 weeks a year," says Dr. Peter Benton (Eriq LaSalle). "For that we are paid $23,739 before taxes—and we make our own coffee."

ST. ELSEWHERE
1982–1988

At Boston's fictional St. Elegius Hospital, actors Ed Begley, Jr., Denzel Washington, and countless others mark a shift by playing up medicine's seedy side. Patients die as often as they live, doctors are mugged in the ER, blood and jokes flow, and the screen fills with people in hospital greens darting amid gadgets. One doctor gets AIDS, another becomes a rapist, a third kills himself.

CHICAGO HOPE
1994–present

In a large city hospital, Hector Elizondo (Dr. Phillip Watters), Mandy Patinkin (Dr. Jeffrey Geiger), and Adam Arkin (Dr. Aaron Shutt) wallow in ethical and personal dilemmas. This show flaunts what the old shows hid: profiteering, gore, and death. ("That bowel stinks like a cesspool. I'll never operate on anybody with a stinking bowel. Air freshener!") Doctors display heroism, then rush off to gouge a colleague. "Sometimes it feels like we spend all our time saving people we don't know," says a surgeon. "People who are ignorant and racist."

was one of the first to point out that in the rush for diagnosis patients often just frighten themselves and make their symptoms worse.

The authors told of a 59-year-old patient admitted to a hospital to have a hernia repaired. While awaiting surgery, the patient complained of mild chest pain, so doctors began a battery of tests, which increased his agitation and pain. The patient ended up in the coronary care unit with a catheter in his heart and an IV dripping nitroglycerin into a vein. The original operation had been forgotten entirely, and as it turned out, there was nothing wrong with his heart.

"The chain of events seemed to be fueled by both the patient's anxiety and the 'anxiety' of the health care system," wrote the authors. They coined a new phrase to describe how events had gotten out of hand: *clinical cascade.* And the catalyst in most of these cases, said the authors, was a medical test.

Not long after, a panel of experts released the nation's first-ever evaluation of medical tests, from Pap smears to electrocardiograms, and the results confirmed Mold and Stein's warning. Of 169 tests, only nine actually reduced the incidence of disease—and many tended to lead to faulty diagnosis, launching patients into treatments they didn't need.

In one study, 80 percent of subjects whose hearts registered "abnormal" on a treadmill stress test actually had no heart problems. In another, scans employed to test for bulging disks as the source of back pain found them in nearly half of people whose backs were perfectly fine. Yet doctors were using both tests to recommend surgery. This was alarming: People with nothing more serious than passing chest or back pain were being marched off to get their hearts repaired or spines fixed as a matter of course.

You may think you'd never let yourself fall headlong into such a tangle of unnecessary treatment. But every cascade starts with something as simple as an aching wrist, a jabbing pain, a touch of malaise. It might all start with a voodoo bug.

MY MALADY HUNG AROUND for several years. I never suffered a classic clinical cascade, but I did experience an emotional one familiar to researchers of patient-physician interaction: My visits to the doctor's office increased my worry that something was really wrong with me. The anxiety made me focus on my symptoms so much that they seemed worse. And every failed attempt to elicit relief left me resentful of money and time wasted. This made me sicker; resentment is hardly a healing emotion.

Despite my frustration, I began to notice that the swoops would run their course. If I rested and spent time with jovial friends, the bad days went away sooner. I found that no matter what the doctors did or didn't do I'd eventually be able to dust the sand off my Boogie board and hit the beach again.

I was learning something about patience, not just in health but in life. Stormy weather, broken hearts, houseguests—nothing ever seemed to go away as fast as I wanted it to. But I had to admit that it all got better over time.

Many of my friends were experiencing similar medical revelations: the bad knee that repaired itself with rest, the depression that lifted without antidepressant drugs. In fact, the majority of all complaints people bring to their doctors do resolve spontaneously, according to Arnold Relman, a former editor in chief of the *New England Journal of Medicine*. "Life is one vast collection of little aches and pains, and the vast majority of aches and pains and worries get better on their own," he says.

By my mid-thirties I was starting to believe a little less that medicine had all the answers and a little more that my body could heal on its own. But clearly I had more to learn.

Five years after the voodoo bout I skidded on wet leaves and fell on my arm, bruising the ulnar nerve. Day and night the nerve dispatched urgent messages from my elbow to my little finger. The pain kept me from swimming and typing my assignments—actually, I never could type, but now I couldn't even peck.

Once again, outrage at being deprived of my activities sent me into a flurry of consultations. This brings me to the humbling low point of my tale: the day I allowed a doctor to plunge spikes into my arm and electrify my flesh.

These were nothing so inoffensive as acupuncture needles, mind you; they felt more like crochet needles. I tried to hold still while the physician zapped electricity back and forth between the needles. My muscles contracted and my arm jerked like a marlin on a line. When it was over, the doctor announced: "They say this is the worst test in medicine."

The worst test has value for some: It can determine if a nerve is, in effect, dying. If that proves to be the problem, sometimes it can be corrected surgically. But my doctor said that even if my test revealed serious damage he wasn't optimistic he could repair it.

The episode forced me to acknowledge my own role. By demanding answers even when there was no good treatment, I was letting myself in for an excruciating test and, if I'd pushed harder, surgery that would undoubtedly have led only to complications and more intervention.

As it was, I could have saved myself a lot of misery by waiting. In a few months the bruised nerve began to heal and my hunt-and-peck was fully restored.

WHILE I WAS HAVING that lesson jabbed home, medical experts started to look beyond tests, to the treatments at the end of any clinical cascade. Most procedures developed out of tradition, and recipients weren't tested to see how they fared. The cost crisis finally prompted a review of these practices. The results again gave the lie to our blind faith in medicine.

Researchers found the usual therapies for lower back pain—ultrasound, nerve stimulation, bed rest, and surgery—to be of little use. (Chiropractic, by contrast, did help.) Among men with early-stage prostate cancer, those who underwent surgery or radiation got no better results than those who were sent home untreated. Ailment by ailment, researchers advised backing off from medical care. Because often, they learned, the most effective treatment was to do nothing.

It wasn't just big-ticket items that flunked. Antibiotics for colds? They only make it harder to treat a real virus later. Common procedures to ease vascular leg pain? Three in four patients get relief just by walking more.

In an ideal world these findings along would make us think twice before rushing to the doctor. But for years we've been conditioned to believe that our health is precarious. Human nature being what it is, it'll take more than a bunch of studies to persuade us of the reverse, that we are basically durable. This conviction can only come from a shift inside ourselves.

My own worldview has been tested recently. In ten-year commemoration of the voodoo bug, I've developed a new mystery ailment involving a persistent ache in the neighborhood of my right kidney. A CAT scan revealed nothing. When the doctor suggested more tests, I flashed back to all the dead-end doctor visits I'd endured over the years and decided then and there to invoke what I'd learned. I'm trying to have faith in my powers of regeneration, though that doesn't come easily.

To counteract my tendency to backslide, I'm trying yoga, an age-old method for getting reacquainted with the body's inherent well-being. I've tacked a poster of 908 positions on my bedroom wall, and I spend a few minutes each evening settling into new poses. You might wonder if I'm missing the boat here. While I'm busy coaxing my toe to my ear in the pigeon pose, might I be neglecting a potentially life-threatening problem?

That's conceivable. In the past decade I've witnessed not just the slow wonder of healing but out-of-control illness as well. My brother ignored a stomachache and would have died from a ruptured appendix if he hadn't been rushed to surgery. An editor friend was too busy with work to attend to a suspicious mole; during the time I spent writing this article, she died, at age 40, of melanoma.

Yes, it's always possible that the voodoo ache could be something dire. If the

ARE YOU AND YOUR DOCTOR GOOD PARTNERS?

QUIZ

THE BEST WAY TO avoid the cycle of overtreatment—where every symptom seems to require a drug or a test—is to cultivate a good relationship with your doctor. You need to be comfortable asking questions, weighing alternatives, and taking your time. Basically, you need someone who is willing to consider you a partner in your medical care. Here's a short quiz to help you determine whether your doctor fits the bill, followed by some tips on how to nudge him or her in that direction. Circle true or false for each of these statements.

My doctor never makes me feel that I'm imposing by asking lots of questions.
TRUE or FALSE

At the end of an appointment, my doctor always asks me if I have any additional questions or concerns.
TRUE or FALSE

If I ask ahead of time for a longer appointment, my doctor will usually give it to me.
TRUE or FALSE

My doctor always explains why she's giving me a particular test.
TRUE or FALSE

My doctor explains things without using medical jargon, in words I can understand.
TRUE or FALSE

If she doesn't, I can ask her to rephrase the explanation until I understand it.
TRUE or FALSE

I can reach my doctor or a nurse for advice by phone.
TRUE or FALSE

My doctor always asks what prescription or over-the-counter medicines I'm taking.
TRUE or FALSE

My doctor discusses the possible side effects of any drug she prescribes.
TRUE or FALSE

I feel calm and comforted after interacting with my doctor.
TRUE or FALSE

My doctor presents several approaches to treating a problem, in a manner that helps me decide what to do.
TRUE or FALSE

When an insurer creates difficulties, my doctor will stand up for my rights.
TRUE or FALSE

When I'm unhappy with my doctor for any reason, I feel comfortable enough to tell her.
TRUE or FALSE

.... **Total number of trues**

SEVEN OR MORE TRUES
You and your physician have an enviable partnership. You talk easily about your concerns, and it sounds as though the two of you can work together to solve any problems that arise.

SIX OR FEWER TRUES
You and your doctor need to treat a nagging ailment: your relationship. But if you had at least three trues, the prognosis is good, as long as you're willing to make an effort and approach the process with an open mind.

Getting the Kind of Care You Want

Be friendly. Even the best physicians may find themselves constrained in this era of cost-cutting and abbreviated office visits. But being busy doesn't necessarily mean a person will be unsympathetic, and sometimes all it takes to get the ball rolling is a little natural, human contact. Start by broaching your concerns the same way you would with a friend. Explain what you want—more time, more information, more compassion—and see how your doctor reacts. He or she may be perfectly willing and able to accommodate your needs.

Put it in black and white. If your doctor needs help in the communication department, write down your questions ahead of time and bring the list to each appointment, suggests Boston internist Timothy McCall, author of *Examining Your Doctor: A Patient's Guide to Avoiding Harmful Medical Care*. If you're prepared, you won't get flustered and forget what you wanted to say.

Request a longer appointment. If you'd like to have a more open-ended discussion—say you're thinking about whether to go on hormone replacement therapy or you want to consider a new treatment for your chronic headaches—ask for more time when scheduling your next appointment. Feeling rushed is frustrating and may compel you to make decisions before you're ready.

Do your homework. The more informed you are about your condition, the better you can evaluate your treatment options. Doctors aren't always up on the latest remedies for every ailment. So do some research at the library or on the Internet, then share what you learned at your next appointment.

Consider switching. If you've tried everything you can think of to improve the relationship but you're still not happy, you may want to shop around for a different doctor. In the end, you have to trust your instincts. Despite the hassle involved, you may be better off starting fresh with someone new.

This brings me to the humbling low point of my tale: the day I allowed a doctor to plunge spikes into my arm and electrify my flesh.

symptoms change or get worse, I'll jump back on the medical hamster wheel. But I'm letting go of the idea that another test is the breakwater standing between me and mortality. Gilbert Welch, a Vermont physician and researcher, says: "The public really overestimates the ability of the medical profession to significantly change the course of events in many situations."

The work of my thirties was to relinquish the childhood notion that there's always someone who can protect me, someone out there—a parent, teacher, or doctor—with the answer. The work of my forties, I imagine, will be to invite doctors back into the equation in a more realistic light. But if I no longer expect physicians to supply me with diagnoses and cures on demand, what do I expect them to do?

I expect them to behave a little more like my mother. Although she's retired now, she really was a prototype of the postmedicalization doc. At dinnertime when I was small, she was often summoned to the phone to talk to a worried parent about a sick child. My siblings and I listened in as her voice dipped an octave and she murmured, "That's normal. Normal. Nothing to worry about."

She was slow to prescribe drugs and tests, quick to reassure. Most important, her tone conveyed: This is a question worth asking, a concern worth interrupting my dinner for. No matter how many times the parent phoned back in the subsequent hours, days, or weeks, she always had time for him or her.

After all, these were her patients, and one meaning of the word *patient* is having the ability to persevere in trying circumstances. To bear discomfort graciously. To wait.

Ann Japenga has been a contributing editor since 1992.

the female brain

Research has finally proved what we've suspected all along: Women really do use more of their brains than men do. Here, the latest scientific findings about the way our minds work

By Dianne Hales

After twenty years of marriage, my husband still doesn't understand me. Why, he wants to know, am I always doing three things at once? How is it that I am never at a loss for words? And how can I recall the names of the couple we met years ago in Hawaii when he can't?

Now I know what to tell him: It's my brain. Breakthrough research in neuroscience is revealing that the root of many puzzling gender differences may lie in our heads. This is not to say, as scientists once believed, that the female brain is in any way inferior. In fact, men's and women's brains have much in common, but they are definitely not the same—in size, structure or sensitivities.

Overall, a woman's brain, like her body, is on average 10 to 15 percent smaller than a man's, yet the regions dedicated to higher cognitive functions such as language are more densely packed with neurons. While we don't yet know the implications of all these findings, one thing is very clear: "Male and female brains do the same things, but they do them differently," says neuropsychiatrist Raquel Gur, M.D., Ph.D., of the University of Pennsylvania, in Philadelphia.

According to researchers, these are the ten most important ways women's brains differ from men's.

Reprinted with permission from *Ladies' Home Journal* magazine, May 1998, pp. 128, 173, 176, 184.

1. Women use more of their brains.

"Whatever women do—even just wiggling their thumbs—their neuron activity is more greatly distributed throughout the brain," says Mark George, M.D., a psychiatrist and neurologist at the Medical University of South Carolina, in Charleston, and a pioneer in using sophisticated neuro-imaging techniques, such as MRI (magnetic resonance imaging). As George explains it, when a male puts his mind to work, neurons turn on in highly specific areas. When a woman does, so many brain cells light up that the scans look like a night view of Las Vegas. Though researchers have not yet discovered the reason for this difference, one possible—though controversial—explanation is that the corpus callosum, the bridge of fibers running down the center of the brain, may be thicker in females, allowing more crosstalk between the emotional, intuitive right hemisphere and the rational, just-the-facts left.

Because the male brain is more compartmentalized, George notes, men may be better able to focus intensely. This may explain why husbands can immerse themselves in the sports pages while the baby cries, the phone rings and the dog barks.

"Traditionally, a male's main function was to defend territory, find food, find a female," says neuroanatomist Marian Diamond, Ph.D., of the University of California at Berkeley. "He had to be able to focus in order to survive. What the female needed as a mother was to be ready to go in all directions in order to protect her young."

A woman's whole-brain modus operandi is just as valuable for the way we live today. With so many things to do, no woman could possibly get by using half her brain.

2. The female brain responds more intensely to emotion.

Three years ago, when psychiatrist George scanned the brains of men and women as they recalled a range of emotional experiences, he wasn't expecting to find any major gender differences. "When I did, they were so huge that I hesitated to report them," he recalls. His research showed that the sexes clearly respond differently during emotions, especially sadness. In his experiments, melancholy feelings activated neurons in an area eight times larger in women than in men.

"The experiences that evoked sadness in our volunteers all involved family, friends and loved ones," says George. "They were rarely about work or achievement."

Neuroscience may be confirming what psychologists have been telling us for years: Relationships matter more to women. And our brains' intense reaction to their loss may, at least in theory, increase our vulnerability to depression, which is twice as common in women as in men.

The female brain also can detect others' emotions more accurately. Raquel Gur and her husband, Ruben Gur, Ph.D., a psychologist, did brain scans on volunteers who looked at photographs of actors depicting various emotions. Both sexes knew happiness when they saw it, but the men had a much harder time recognizing sadness, especially in women. "A woman's face had to be really sad for a man to see it," Ruben Gur says. "The subtle expressions went right by them, even though their brains were working harder to figure it out. When it comes to reading emotion, men just don't get it."

3. The female brain is wired for expression, not aggression.

When they studied women and men in a state of relaxation, the Gurs noticed differences in the limbic system, a ring of structures within the brain that process the entire spectrum of human emotion. Most male brains "idle" in an ancient region of this system sometimes called the *reptilian brain*—that gives rise to active expressions of emotion, such as aggression and violence. The resting gear of most female brains, in comparison, lies in a different region—the *cingulate gyrus*, a more recently evolved

boosting your brain power

We've found that at every age, both genders can change brain structures and improve abilities," says neuroanatomist Marian Diamond. Here are some ways to go about it:

- **SEEK OUT STIMULATION. "Newness is exceedingly important," says Diamond. "But no two human brains are the same, so each person will be stimulated by different things." For some, travel provides energizing novelty; for others, painting does.**
- **USE EMOTIONAL TAGS. If you want to remember the name of a restaurant, remember how you felt the last time you were there. Do the same when adding any new information to your memory banks.**
- **PRACTICE SKILLS THAT DON'T COME AUTOMATICALLY TO YOU. For instance, if you've never had a head for figures, strengthen your math skills by using your brain—rather than a calculator—to balance your checkbook.**
- **WATCH YOUR BLOOD PRESSURE. If untreated, hypertension can cause fuzzy thinking later in life and can increase the risk of stroke and age-related memory loss.**
- **DON'T NEGLECT SLEEP. "Women often underestimate the profound effect that fatigue has on memory and concentration," says psychologist Thomas Crook. "Variations in a normal sleep cycle can diminish performance by thirty percent." The impact of sleep loss gets even worse as we get older.**
- **EXERCISE YOUR BODY. "Strong data show that physical fitness is important to cognitive function," says Crook. Regular exercise—especially aerobic workouts—may enhance mental sharpness by improving circulation of blood and oxygen through the brain as well as the body.**
- **EAT SENSIBLY. "Protein is essential [to the brain], as are B vitamins," says Diamond. "You want to enrich your brain, so you need a balanced diet." —D.H.**

part of the limbic system related to symbolic forms of expression, such as gestures and words.

Does this mean that men are emotionally more primitive than women? "The logical conclusion is yes," says Ruben Gur. "At the least, this difference may explain why men are prone to physical action, while women opt for verbal tactics. Beating somebody up comes from the old limbic brain. Saying 'I'm angry with you' comes from the new limbic. You could argue that women are one half step ahead of men in evolution in the sense that they use the newer part of the brain more in dealing with emotion."

4. The female brain has a way with words.

Girls generally speak sooner, learn to read faster and have fewer learning disorders. The reason, according to Yale University professors of neurology Sally Shaywitz, M.D., and Bennett Shaywitz, M.D., may be that they use neural regions on both sides of the brain when they read or engage in other verbal exercises. In contrast, males draw only on neural regions in the left hemisphere.

This bilateral approach may give women an advantage by allowing us to draw on the emotions and experiences of the right brain as well as the reasoning powers of the logical left brain. As adults, women tend to be more verbally adept than men: In timed tests, women think of more words that start with the same letter, list more synonyms and come up with names for colors or shapes more quickly than men. Women even memorize letters of the alphabet faster.

But the female brain's dual-hemisphere language processing provides a far more significant benefit: It helps women who suffer stroke or brain injury recover more easily. "Because women activate a larger number of neurons than men when they speak or read, they're less vulnerable if part of the brain is damaged," says George. "In medicine, we've observed that women who have strokes tend to regain more of their verbal abilities than men do, and their use of neurons in both hemispheres may be why."

5. Sexual pleasure may register in a different location in the female brain.

According to a recent medical report, a Scottish woman developed a most unusual complaint: uncontrollable orgasms that interrupted her driving, conversations and daily routines. Since these "sexual seizures" began about the same time as intense headaches, her doctors suspected the problem might lie in her brain. Tests did indeed reveal an abnormality in the right temporal lobe—a highly developed part of the brain—that was probably caused by an undetected hemorrhage several years before. Treatment with antiseizure medication relieved the woman's symptoms—and led her doctors to speculate that female orgasms may originate in a different brain location than male climaxes. In a previous report on a man with a similar disorder, doctors had pinpointed the hypothalamus, a more primitive brain region, as the site of male sexual satisfaction.

6. Women notice more than men and navigate differently.

On the road, women pay more attention than men to what they see, particularly to landmarks like the coffee shop on the corner or the church across from the playground. When retracing a route or giving directions, women rely on such landmarks—unlike men, who think in terms of direction and distance (half a mile west, then north two miles).

An innate sense of space and distance may be part of a human male's biological legacy. "I suspect that males are born with some biological component that gives them an edge in spatial tasks," says Deborah Blum, a science writer and author of *Sex on the Brain* (Viking, 1997), who notes that males consistently score higher in exercises such as mentally rotating an object in three dimensions. Once this skill may have translated into better aim when hurling a spear at a woolly mammoth; today it may explain why my husband can park a minivan in a space the size of a postage stamp.

Women's spatial skills do improve with time and experience. By middle age, women's scores on spatial tests are about equal to men's; later in life, they surpass them.

7. A woman's vision is more acute and her hearing is more sensitive.

Male and female brains perceive light and sound very differently, says neurologist Karl Pribram, M.D., director of the Center for Brain Research and Informational Sciences at Radford College, in Radford, Virginia. A woman's hearing tends to be so sensitive that she can often hear whispers that never even register to a man's ear. And her vision is so much more acute that she can tread her way along a slippery path by moonlight as he squints before taking a single step.

Sensory tests confirm that men are less tolerant of bright light but retain their ability to see well at all distances as they age. A woman's vision begins to decline between ages thirty-five and forty-four; a man's, between forty-five and fifty-four.

On the other hand, women hear a much broader range of sounds than men. Female hearing doesn't start to deteriorate until the late fifties; men start losing their ability to detect high tones in their late forties.

8. A woman's memory is sharper.

"At every age, women's memories outperform men's," reports psychologist Thomas Crook, Ph.D., president of Psychologix, a research organization based in Bethesda, Maryland, and Scottsdale, Arizona, that has tested the memories of more than 50,000 men and women. "Women have a greater ability to associate names with faces than men do, and they're also better at recalling lists of things, like groceries and details of personal experiences."

Both genders are prone to age-associated memory loss, which diminishes the ability to remember words and names by as much as

50 percent between ages twenty-five and sixty-five. However, says Crook, women's memories generally stay stronger. One reason may be that we have a unique way of filing information in our memory banks.

"The events people remember best are those that we tag with an emotion," Crook says. "Since women use more of their right brains, which process emotions, they may do this automatically."

"At every age, women's memories outperform men's"

9. The female brain ages more slowly than the male's.

A new study reported in *The Archives of Neurology* earlier this year found that the male brain shrinks faster than the female brain.

In fact, according to Ruben Gur, who has done his own research on women and men at various ages, the male brain loses tissue at almost three times the rate the female brain does. Because of this gender difference, men's brains, which are larger and heavier than women's when both are young, shrink so much that their all-important frontal lobes are approximately the same size by the time both sexes reach their forties.

Other parts of men's brains also atrophy more rapidly. "If you look at men in the age range from eighteen to forty-five, you see a steady decline in abilities, and this decline is correlated with a decline in frontal-lobe volume," says Gur. "We don't see a trend in women the same age toward any deterioration of abilities or brain volume." Among the consequences of male brain shrinkage are poorer memory, less ability to pay attention—and greater irritability. "Yes, men do get grumpier with old age," says Gur. "You can blame it on their brains."

The reason that men's brains change size so drastically may have to do with fuel efficiency. The female brain seems able to reduce its metabolic rate—that is, its use of brain glucose—over time, whereas the brains of older men metabolize glucose at higher rates than when they were younger. Women, in other words, gear down to a more fuel-efficient cruising speed as they age, while male brains keep revving the engine—possibly because of testosterone's influence. "Even though women also lose some tissue as they age, they seem to be riding herd on what's left," says Gur. This difference, he speculates, may be part of the reason that females generally outlive males.

But while women's brains are more durable, they do have one greater vulnerability as they get older: a threefold increase in risk for Alzheimer's disease. Of the approximately four million Americans affected by this form of dementia, an estimated three quarters are women. Researchers believe this may be due to the declining levels of estrogen as women age. According to preliminary tests, estrogen replacement therapy may reduce the risk of Alzheimer's and delay the symptoms of the disease in women.

10. The female brain is more intuitive.

Because of the constant crosstalk between the left brain's rationality and the right's emotionality, the female brain may make connections that might not occur to a man. Some call this skill a form of emotional intelligence; others think of it as woman's intuition.

"Intuition involves a network in the brain and the body," explains Mona Lisa Schulz, M.D., Ph.D., a psychiatrist in private practice in Portland, Maine, and author of *Awakening Intuition* (Crown, 1998). "We've learned that people use multiple areas of the brain when making decisions—intuitive or otherwise. And because women's brains are less lateralized, they may have better access to both sides of the brain. They usually don't see things as cut-and-dried, the way men do."

This can be a real advantage in every part of a woman's life—whether it's figuring out why a young child seems anxious or why office morale has slumped. "Because they're so good at seeing emotional nuances," notes Raquel Gur, "women can read what's happening quickly and ask themselves: What should I say now?"

Dianne Hales is a contributing editor of Ladies' Home Journal.

Unit 5

Unit Selections

Key Points to Consider

- How would you define chronic illness and why is it of special concern to women?
- In your opinion, what are the most serious chronic illnesses facing women today?
- Based on the readings, what advice would you give to women living with chronic illness?
- Why is the issue of personal empowerment so important in a discussion of chronic illness?
- What hope for the future would you offer someone living with a chronic illness?

DUSHKIN ONLINE Links

www.dushkin.com/online/

18. **Heartinformation Network: Women's Health**
    http://www.heartinfo.org/reviews/wmhd.htm
19. **Mayo Clinic's Women's Health Resource Center**
    http://www.mayo.ivi.com/mayo/common/htm/womenpg.htm
20. **NCI's CancerNet Cancer Information for Patients**
    http://wwwicic.nci.nih.gov/patient.htm
21. **Search Federal Health and Human Services**
    http://www.hhs.gov/search/

These sites are annotated on pages 4 and 5.

Chronic Diseases

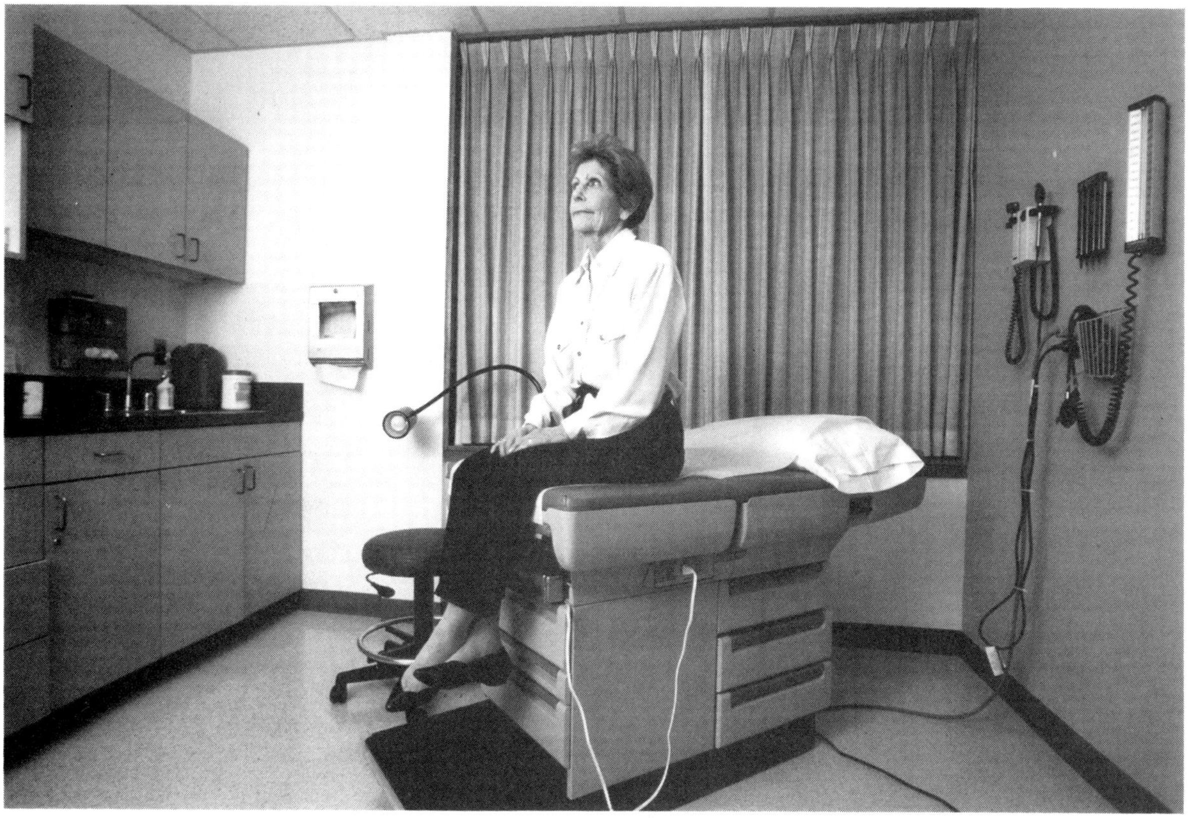

The past few years have witnessed a rapid growth in interest about chronic illnesses that affect women. Because women generally live longer than men, it is much more likely that they will be forced to deal with this issue at some point in their lives. The question becomes how well they will deal with both the physiological and psychological ramifications of chronic illness.

"Conquering Chronic Illness: Mastering the Medical Challenge, Part 1" does an excellent job of defining chronic illness, describing common examples of chronic illness, and examining the impact of chronic illness on the health care system. Part 2 of the article "Conquering Chronic Illness: Nurturing Your Emotional Needs, completes the picture by addressing the social and emotional ramifications of chronic illness in the lives of women and their families.

"The Enemy Within" focuses on a subset of chronic illnesses, the autoimmune diseases. They are diseases that result from the body's own defenses turning against itself. "Heart Disease in Women: Special Symptoms, Special Risks" not only describes the symptoms of heart disease in women but also how the presentation of symptoms differs between the sexes. Since heart disease is the number one killer of both men and women in this country today, it is important for women to realize that they too are at risk.

"Stopping the Deadliest Cancer" describes the leading cause of cancer deaths among women. Much to the surprise of the average person, it is not cancer of the breast or reproductive organs. The leading cancer killer of women is lung cancer. The topic of cancer is dealt with in a very different way in "Breast Cancer Cost Me My Job." In this case, the social and legal impact of cancer treatment is described, not the illness itself.

To provide a more balanced view of chronic illness, the issues of treatment and lifestyle adaptation are also addressed. "Closing In on Cancer" describes promising new therapies and possible cures for this indiscriminate killer. "Healing Power" provides a very different perspective on treatment and lifestyle adjustment. Here, the focus is on patient empowerment; making the most of what a woman can do, not on what abilities have been lost or diminished.

PART ONE*

Conquering Chronic Illness

Mastering the Medical Challenge

One out of every three women will develop a chronic ailment such as asthma, arthritis, diabetes, hypertension and migraines. **Our breakthrough guide** to the latest treatments and management methods will soothe your body and ease your mind ◆ By Linda Marsa

For more than a decade, asthma had a stranglehold on Nancy Sander's life. First her infant daughter Brooke developed a severe case of the disease. Two years later, exhausted from shuttling Brooke back and forth to the emergency room, Sander herself was diagnosed at age 29. "I coughed so hard on the way to the hospital that I broke a rib," says Sander, now 44, the founder and president of Allergy and Asthma Network/Mothers of Asthmatics, an information and advocacy group in Fairfax, VA.

Throughout her early 30s, Sander's life was completely circumscribed by asthma. It became virtually impossible to plan anything; even grocery shopping trips could end in a frantic race to the doctor's office. Cigarette smoke and petroleum fumes set off her symptoms, so everyday events such as dining out with friends or putting gas in the car could leave her wheezing and short of breath.

Ironically, even after Sander had been hospitalized for a life-threatening attack, her

*The second part of this two-part series begins on page 125 of *Annual Editions: Women's Health.*

From *American Health for Women,* October 1997, pp. 73-74, 76, 78, 80. © 1997 by Linda Marsa. Reprinted by permission.

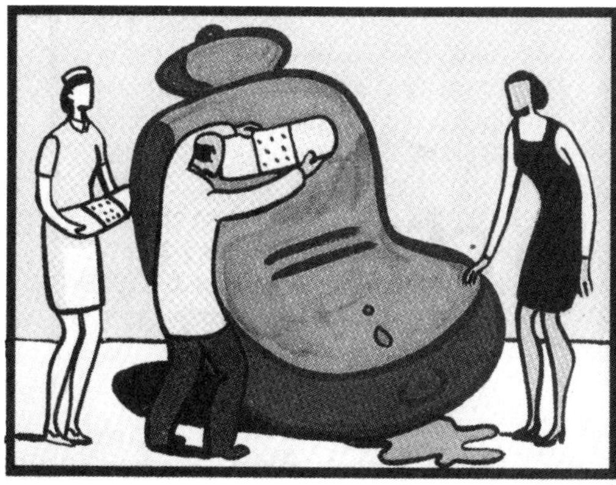

> America's health care system is probably the best in the world when it comes to dealing with crises, but it's woefully inadequate when it comes to treating chronic illness.

primary-care physician didn't provide her with the information that would have kept her out of the hospital in the first place. When she was diagnosed, the doctor said, "You have asthma," and handed Sander a prescription for an inhaler. There was little discussion of the lifestyle changes that would later help her cope with her disease. Only when her daughter was eventually enrolled in a study of asthma treatments did Sander discover sensible strategies that could effectively control her asthma. Today, she says, "there's hardly anything I can't do."

The High Cost of Chronic Illness The extent to which Sander's asthma was disabling, frustrating and, ultimately, relieved through access to information about breakthroughs in prevention and treatment is typical of the experience of most people with chronic illnesses. America's health care system is probably the best in the world when it comes to dealing with crises such as heart attacks and injuries, but it's woefully inadequate when it comes to treating ailments whose symptoms wax and wane and often last a lifetime. Acute illnesses get sympathy, while people who soldier on despite discomfort from asthma, arthritis, migraine and other chronic conditions are often viewed as complainers.

Even some physicians turn a cold shoulder. A 1989 survey conducted at the University of Michigan in Ann Arbor found that doctors have negative reactions to people with chronic conditions, because they are frustrated by the fact that such illnesses can't be cured. And as Sander's experience shows, many physicians are trained to give care in a crisis but are not yet focused on teaching patients prevention techniques.

The attention our medical system gives to chronic illness must increase dramatically if we want to avert what is shaping up to be a major public health crisis. According to a landmark 1996 study published in the *Journal of the American Medical Association,* chronic conditions afflict almost 100 million Americans, nearly half the population. Even AIDS is now classified as a chronic illness. They cost society an estimated $660 billion a year, and experts say that unless new systems of care are created, the annual tab will climb to a staggering $798 billion by the year 2030. The growing needs of people with long-term illness will put enormous pressures on a medical system that is ill equipped to deal with them.

The burden of chronic illness falls most heavily on women, who suffer more than men do from such conditions as arthritis, asthma, migraine and diabetes. As

Asthma: Breathing Easier

Seven million women between the ages of 18 and 64 are struggling for breath.

Symptoms Wheezing and tightness in the chest occur when irritants in the air cause the bronchial airways to swell and fill with mucus.

Worst-case scenario A severe attack that isn't treated promptly or doesn't respond to medication may be fatal.

Latest breakthroughs Researchers have come to understand that asthma often requires the same vigilant monitoring and management as diabetes. "People need to realize the importance of treating this as a chronic disease and to develop a plan of action," says Betty Wray, M.D., president of the American College of Asthma, Allergy and Immunology in Chicago. Federal guidelines released earlier this year advocate regular use of corticosteroid inhalants or bronchodilators to keep airways from swelling, in combination with drugs like albuterol to relieve flare-ups. Patients are also advised to monitor their lung capacity daily with a gadget called a peak-flow meter.

Several new therapies can help prevent inflammation in the first place. Two of them, Accolate (zafirlukast) and Zyflo (zileuton), were approved late last year by the FDA. Taken regularly, the pills block the production of molecules that cause lung tissues to swell and contract the smooth muscles of the airways. Similar drugs are waiting for FDA clearance. "Even some hard-to-treat patients seem to be responding," says Dr. Wray.

Lifestyle Rx Avoid the allergens that trigger your attacks, whether it's cockroaches, dust mites, pollen or animal dander, and discuss with your doctor whether you should take medication preventively if you know you're going to be exposed. Also reduce your exposure to tobacco smoke and environmental irritants. The latter is especially important for women, who still tend to do most of the housework; vacuum cleaners spew out all kinds of dust, and cleansers contain irritating chemicals.

Women should also pay close attention to how their symptoms coincide with their menstrual cycle. Researchers from the Medical College of Pennsylvania in Philadelphia reported last year that ER admissions for asthma tended to occur immediately before and during menstruation. Knowing if your symptoms follow a pattern may help you and your doctor develop a strategy to stave off attacks.

For more information Allergy and Asthma Network/Mothers of Asthmatics (800-878-4403; www.podi.com/health/aanma) offers free information packets and access to support groups.

ILLUSTRATIONS BY ALISON SEIFFER

The burden falls most heavily on women, who suffer more than men do from arthritis, asthma, migraine and diabetes, and who feel isolated and frustrated as a result.

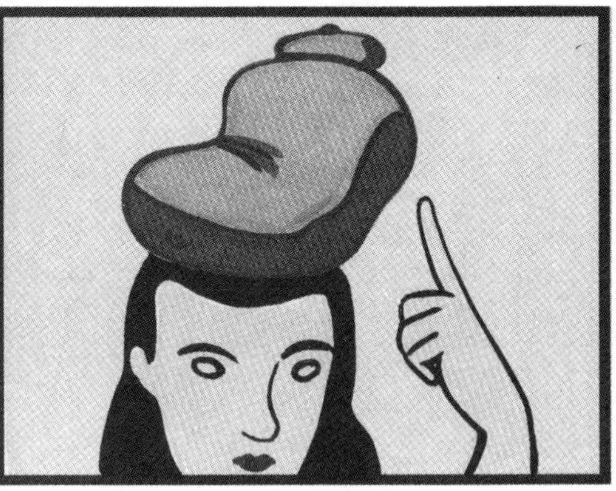

women age, we're likelier than men to suffer from several chronic conditions simultaneously.

In addition to pain and medical complications, the mental health fallout from chronic illness can be severe. Laurinda Poirier, R.N., a program manager at the Joslin Diabetes Center in Boston, sees it every day. "Women with chronic diseases tend to be very isolated," she says. "They think, 'No one really appreciates how I feel.' There's a lot of self-recrimination that feeds their loneliness." Managing their medical care, their family and their career is a challenge. "But they all feel guilty because they can't handle it," she says.

Insurance Inadequacies Doctors and hospitals aren't the only ones feeding the frustrations of women with chronic illness. Many insurance companies don't pay for special services such as assistance with shopping or bathing, or for equipment like ramps and raised toilets. Chronically ill people are often in and out of the hospital or in great pain, making it difficult to hold on to a job, points out Susan K. Golant of Los Angeles, coauthor of *Taking Charge: How to Master the Eight Most Common Fears of Long Term Illness.* "Consequently, they may live in fear they'll lose their jobs and insurance coverage, and rack up high medical bills."

Those who study the problem say these difficulties

The 10 Commandments of Chronic Illness

1. Love yourself *Remember that your illness doesn't define who you are or prevent you from making a valuable contribution.*

2. Love your doctor *Don't settle for feeling rushed and in the dark. Find a physician who listens and who doesn't intimidate.*

3. See a specialist *An M.D. who focuses on your condition can ensure that you're getting state-of-the-art care.*

4. Go to the library or get online *Keep on top of the latest research developments.*

5. Find friends *Hook up with a support group for an emotional outlet and to swap information.*

6. Be vigilant *Study your insurance policy to learn what is and isn't covered. Persist in your efforts to get insurers to pay.*

7. Be patient *Your self-image may change after a diagnosis, so give yourself time to adjust.*

8. Keep your cool *Find ways to let off steam, and schedule them into your daily routine.*

9. Maintain a medical record *Log the dates of office visits, get copies of test results and keep a list of the treatments you've tried and their side effects.*

10. Be selfish *If you care for a chronically ill person, find time to take care of yourself too.*

Migraines: Pain Prevention

Nearly 8 million women between the ages of 18 and 64 experience these recurrent, excruciating headaches.

Symptoms Throbbing, intense headache pain, caused by the tightening and swelling of blood vessels in the brain, is often accompanied by nausea, vomiting and sensitivity to light and sound.

Worst-case scenario Migraine can be very debilitating, leading to lost workdays and greatly restricted lives.

Latest breakthroughs When Imitrex (sumatriptan) debuted in 1993, the injectable medication revolutionized migraine treatment. It was the first drug to mimic the action of serotonin; scientists believe low levels of this brain chemical are the culprit behind migraine.

Imitrex is now sold in pill form, "but it's not a panacea," says J. Keith Campbell, of Rochester, MN, president of the American Association for the Study of Headache. "It doesn't control everybody's headaches or stop an attack from coming on, and some headaches come back within 24 hours."

Consequently, there's been a race among pharmaceutical companies to devise drugs that work better and have fewer harmful side effects than Imitrex, which has the potential of constricting coronary arteries. One of the first out of the starting gate will be DHE [dihydroergotamine]-45, which has been around for years in injectable form but is now awaiting FDA approval as a nasal spray. A faster-acting nasal spray version of Imitrex, which can be taken by people too nauseated to swallow a pill, should be available in the next two years. Also waiting in the wings is a new generation of so-called triptan drugs (Imitrex was the first), including Maxalt (rizatriptan) and Zomig (zolmitriptan).

The next step is figuring out how to prevent migraine. Recent studies have linked the headaches to severe gynecological problems, such as ovarian cysts. This finding may shed light on the relation between hormones and headaches and the reason women in their menstruating years are three times as likely as men to suffer from migraines. The recent discovery of a gene linked to a rare form of migraine may also provide clues to the biological underpinnings of this illness.

Lifestyle Rx Biofeedback, acupuncture, relaxation techniques and avoiding foods that can trigger migraines—cheese, wine, chocolate—may reduce the risk of the headaches.

For more information The National Headache Foundation (www.headaches.org; 800-843-2256) answers general questions, sends information packets, and provides referrals to physicians in your area.

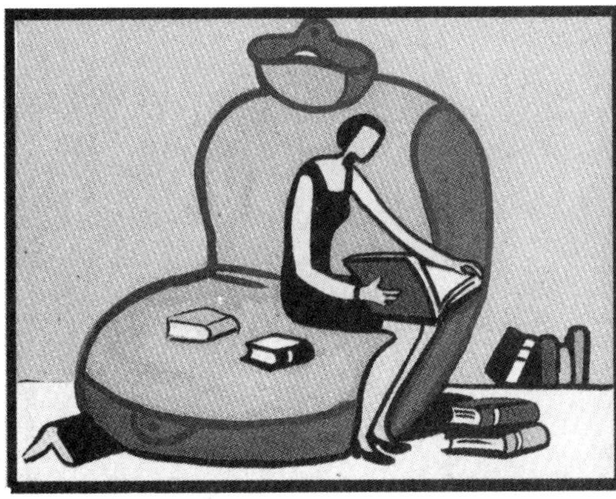

It's up to women to educate themselves and their doctors about their illnesses, to be more aggressive with their insurers and to reach out to others who share their affliction.

Beating High Blood Pressure

More than 8.7 million women under age 64 have hypertension, more commonly known as high blood pressure.

Symptoms Hypertension is often symptomless, though warning signs include dizziness, shortness of breath, tingling and numbness in the arms and legs, blurred vision, bad headaches and angina (a sharp pain or burning sensation in the back, shoulder, neck or arm). The cause of high blood pressure is unknown, but it is linked to obesity, heredity, smoking and a high salt intake.

Worst-case scenario If not properly treated, high blood pressure can lead to heart attack, stroke and kidney failure.

Latest breakthroughs A new class of drugs known as Angiotension 2 receptor blockers, which have fewer side effects than older therapies, were recently added to medicine's arsenal.

Lifestyle Rx Controlling high blood pressure may be easier than you think, according to a new study sponsored by the National Heart, Lung, and Blood Institute. For eight weeks, 459 men and women with mild hypertension consumed a diet rich in fruits, vegetables and lowfat dairy foods, and high in fiber and protein. Participants didn't reduce their salt intake, lose weight, exercise more, take pressure-lowering drugs or use supplements like potassium, calcium, folic acid and magnesium—all of which are known to decrease hypertension. Yet their blood pressure dropped significantly.

The findings reinforce what doctors have been saying all along: Mildly elevated blood pressure levels can often be reduced without popping pills. "The key is to keep your weight down, exercise, watch dietary intake and, since hypertension symptoms aren't obvious, get your blood pressure checked at least once a year," says Norman H. Kaplan, M.D., head of the hypertension division at the University of Texas Southwestern Medical Center in Dallas.

For more information The American Heart Association (800-AHA-USA-1; www.amhrt.org) provides support group resources for people with hypertension.

Arthritis Advances

11.7 million women have osteoarthritis, the most common form of arthritis, a painful and debilitating joint disease.

Symptoms Pain and stiffness result when the cartilage that cushions joints in the fingers, neck, lower back and legs deteriorates.

Worst-case scenario Osteoarthritis isn't fatal, but extreme pain and difficulty moving can prevent some people with the disease from working and leading productive lives.

Latest breakthroughs The phenomenal popularity of *The Arthritis Cure* underscores just how hungry millions of sufferers are for ways to soothe their aching bones. When the book hit stores last winter touting the joint-saving potential of two nonprescription dietary supplements, chondroitin sulfate and glucosamine, it shot to the top of best-seller lists. But the Arthritis Foundation in Atlanta, which funds arthritis research, is dubious about this so-called miracle cure. Though two studies in Europe indicated that the substances eased the pain and discomfort of arthritis, they were preliminary, and the foundation isn't convinced.

One scientifically proven therapy that should be on the market by year-end is Synvisc, a lubricating fluid just approved for use on knees (though it may prove beneficial for other joints as well). The drug is injected once a week in a doctor's office for five weeks. "Some patients don't need any other medication for up to six months," says Roland W. Moskowitz, M.D., a professor of medicine at Case Western Reserve University in Cleveland.

Also expected to be approved is a new class of pain relievers known as cyclooxygenase inhibitors. They're as effective as aspirin, naproxen and ibuprofen but don't cause side effects such as kidney problems, gastric distress and bleeding ulcers. In the research pipeline are drugs known as biological response modifiers that target the mechanisms of disease rather than just treating symptoms.

Lifestyle Rx Keep your weight down to minimize joint overload, and reduce stress through yoga, guided imagery or meditation. Although some people report that avoiding foods of the nightshade family, such as eggplant and tomatoes, minimizes joint pain, there's no scientific proof that this is the case. But it may be wise to up your intake of vitamins C and D: Researchers from Boston University Medical Center reported last year that above-average consumption of these nutrients appears to slow the progression of osteoarthritis. Also exercise regularly, choosing low-impact activities such as swimming. And consult your doctor about strength training: A new study from Indiana University School of Medicine in Indianapolis suggests that strengthening the thigh muscles might forestall the deterioration of the knee joint.

For more information The National Institute of Arthritis, Musculoskeletal and Skin Diseases in Silver Spring, MD (301-495-4484; www.nih.gov/niams/), provides information packages.

There are a few bright spots on the horizon: Women are better able to manage their pain now that doctors are starting to open up to natural, noninvasive therapies.

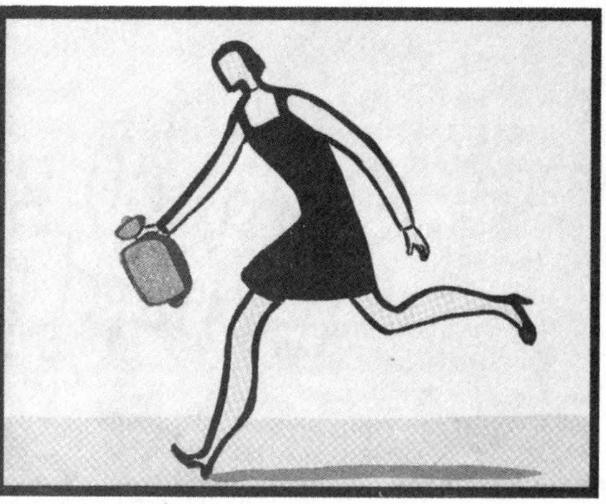

will be exacerbated as more Americans are shifted into managed-care plans. Cost-conscious companies often resist paying for dietitians, physical therapists and social workers who connect patients with community services and teach them how to manage their illness. "There's a tremendous misallocation of resources," says Lewis G. Sandy, M.D., executive vice president of the Robert Wood Johnson Foundation, a nonprofit research group in Princeton, NJ. "We don't blink an eye about spending $40 on a diagnostic test, but we don't pay for outside services like home health aides or long-term physical therapy."

The rush by many patients to embrace alternative medicine is a sign of the times: "Alternative medicine is thriving because we don't have a cure for many of the diseases that plague Americans," says Jane E. Corboy, M.D., an assistant professor of family and community medicine at Baylor College of Medicine in Houston.

Taking the Next Step Fortunately, advances have been made in the treatment of many chronic ailments. Some federal agencies, forward-thinking managed-care companies and academic institutions are formulating standardized treatment guidelines and giving them to patients. They are also developing systems of care that include specialists, physical therapists, dietitians and home health aides. Doctors are starting to open up to natural, noninvasive therapies that help patients manage pain. For instance, a woman might be taught to practice visualization, picturing positive images to prevent the release of stress hormones that might worsen her chronic pain.

Sander's frustrations prompted her to found the Allergy and Asthma Network/Mothers of Asthmatics to help others in similar circumstances find appropriate resources that are not always provided by doctors. Now it's up to women to learn from Sander's lesson: to educate themselves and their doctors about their illnesses, to be more aggressive with their insurers and to reach out to others who share their affliction, so that they can share medical information and be more vocal in their demands as a unified group. "The medical system has to continue to make adjustments," says Karen M. Freund, M.D., clinical director of the women's health group at Boston Medical Center. "Otherwise chronic disease is going to become a giant health care headache as the population gets older. Women will be squeezed the most."

Linda Marsa is the author of Prescription for Profits.

Keeping Diabetes Under Control

About 2.4 million women under 64 have been diagnosed with diabetes. The illness remains undetected in perhaps an equal number.

Symptoms Excessive thirst, frequent urination, extreme hunger, fatigue and sudden weight loss are the hallmarks. Type I diabetes is usually diagnosed in children or young adults, while the more prevalent type II diabetes tends to be diagnosed after age 30.

Worst-case scenario If not diagnosed and treated, diabetes can cause permanent nerve and kidney damage and substantially increase the risk of heart attack.

Latest breakthroughs The talk of last summer's meeting of the American Diabetes Association in Alexandria, VA, was new guidelines calling for testing all adults for diabetes starting at age 45. The ADA also lowered the benchmark for determining whether someone was diabetic from 140 milligrams of glucose per deciliter of blood to 126 milligrams. Officials hope that widespread screening with this new criterion will help identify 2 million of the 8 million Americans believed to have undiagnosed diabetes.

Innovative treatments are also being added to the list of therapeutic options. The FDA has approved the oral medication Rezulin (troglitazone) for use by people with type II diabetes. Humulog, a very fast-acting injectable insulin, was recently approved for type I diabetes. "People can take it right before eating, which gives them more flexibility," says Laurinda Poirier, R.N., a program manager at the Joslin Diabetes Center in Boston. Tests are under way to determine whether low doses of insulin may prevent or delay the onset of type I diabetes in those at moderate risk.

Lifestyle Rx Eat healthy. A 1997 Harvard University study confirmed that a diet low in fiber and high in carbohydrates (white rice, white bread, potatoes, soft drinks) more than doubles a woman's chance of developing diabetes. If you have diabetes, investigate nutritional supplements. Vitamin E may prevent some complications associated with diabetes, but don't add it to your routine without talking to your doctor or a registered dietitian who has experience treating diabetes.

For more information The American Diabetes Association (800-DIABETES; www.diabetes.org) will refer you to your local chapter for information on classes and support groups in your area.

Editor's note: The next article, Part Two of "Conquering Chronic Illness," presents techniques for overcoming the emotional challenges of having a long-term ailment.

PART TWO*

Conquering Chronic Illness

Nurturing Your Emotional Needs

How do some women stay happy and mentally healthy despite a long-term illness like asthma, arthritis or diabetes? Researchers who study these remarkable patients now have a recipe for a beat-the-odds attitude ◆ By Randi Glatzer

The nurse gave her an orange to practice on. She'd always hated needles, and yet here Yvonne Davis was, in a class for people with diabetes, an orange in one hand and a syringe in the other, learning how to give herself an insulin shot. All she could think of was what might go wrong. It was one thing to stick the syringe into the orange's dimpled skin, quite another to plunge the needle into her own flesh. The first tries made her sick to her stomach.

But she knew there was no choice if she wanted to survive. "I made myself do it. I'm the only one who can do it the way it should be done," says Davis, 52, a homemaker in Greentown, IN. Six years later, she gives herself insulin shots twice a day.

For women living with chronic illnesses such as diabetes, asthma and migraine headaches, the unthinkable becomes routine. The disease changes their bodies, and it changes their minds and spirits as well. These psychological changes can be devastating, but often, researchers are increasingly finding, they're positive and profound. This fact has doctors and patient advocates pushing for a new way of caring for the chronically ill—one that takes into account the psychological side of their condition as well as the

*See page 120, *Annual Editions: Women's Health* for part one of this two-part series.

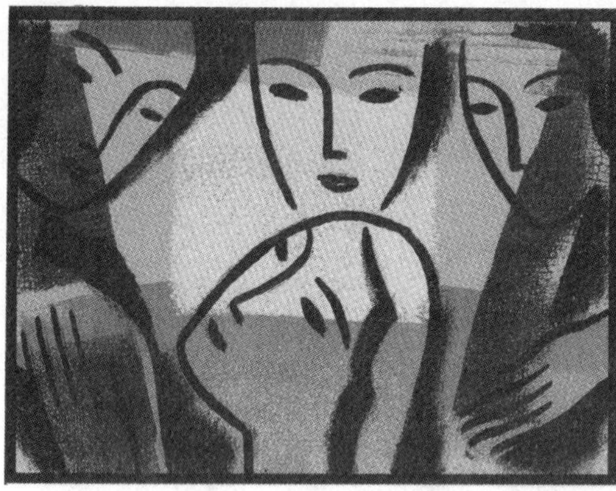

Chronically ill women want to look self-sufficient, yet they still need friends and family to understand that they might need help with shopping or to spend a whole day in bed.

medical, their strengths as well as their weaknesses. The issue is especially important to women, who are likelier than men to have chronic conditions such as arthritis, osteoporosis, lupus, migraine and multiple sclerosis.

AN EMOTIONAL ROLLER COASTER

The mental health repercussions of chronic illness can be far-reaching. It can leave a woman depressed and anxious, place pressure on her family, threaten her relationships, affect her work and leave her in constant contact—and often in a constant struggle—with the medical world.

Chronic pain makes things even worse. Psychiatrist Nelson Hendler, M.D., director of the Mensana Clinic in Stevenson, MD, estimates that 76% of his patients with pain are depressed. He's confident that pain is the reason for their depression, because 89% of them weren't depressed before the pain started.

"Your mental health is always affected by your physical health," says psychologist Royda Crose, Ph.D., associate director of the Fisher Institute for Wellness at Ball State University in Muncie, IN. Dr. Crose gets frustrated with physicians who prescribe antidepressants for chronically ill patients without investigating the reasons for their moods, or who expect them to be relentlessly upbeat in the face of illness. It's better, she believes, to look at what's upsetting the person and see if there are ways to solve those problems.

Dr. Crose collaborated on a study of 40 women who had diseases such as lupus, rheumatoid arthritis, multiple sclerosis and osteoporosis. She found that one of the toughest things for the women to deal with was the unpredictability illness brought to their lives.

"They can't plan anything," says Dr. Crose. "One day they can be feeling pretty good, and the next they're flat on their back." Several women had to retire from their jobs, even though they sometimes felt perfectly capable of working. They had a hard time making plans with friends, knowing they might have to cancel at the last minute if they felt sick. They wanted to look attractive, energetic and self-sufficient ("I don't want a pity party," one woman told Dr. Crose), yet they still needed friends and family to understand that they weren't just like everyone else, that they might need help with the grocery shopping or to spend a whole day in bed. "The women felt like others accused them of being lazy," Dr. Crose says. "But they knew if they pushed themselves they'd be down for days."

Worst of all are the feelings of anger, shock, isolation and despair that come as a woman realizes her life may never be the way she thought it would. Women with chronic illness can hold on to feelings of anger and regret, turning bitter and despondent for years on end. But the likelihood is that they won't. Elizabeth Lindsey, Ph.D., an associate professor at the University of Victoria School of Nursing in Canada, conducted a study of chronically ill people and found that many feel healthy and cheerful despite physical limitations. She determined that these people had gone through a healing "journey," a series of psychological stages not unlike those Elisabeth Kübler-Ross, M.D., describes in the groundbreaking book *On Death and Dying* about the approach to death. But Dr. Lindsey found that her subjects moved through these stages not just toward acceptance, but beyond that to an exploration of new opportunities. Though Dr. Lindsey's stages have different names and time frames, they roughly parallel those that Dr. Crose and Dr. Gordon saw in the interviews they conducted.

In Dr. Lindsey's opinion, the worst part of the healing

Dealing With Doctors: How to Be Heard Without Shouting

Under the best of circumstances, medical professionals sometimes don't take patients—particularly women—seriously. The situation is worse for a woman with a chronic illness, whose disease results in frequent office visits and repeated requests for symptom relief. Even when a woman's complaints are legitimate, some doctors tend to dismiss them. A few words of wisdom: ◆ **Find a physician** who trusts you to know your body and who respects your views. ◆ **Bring a list of questions** to every doctor's appointment. ◆ **To help ensure that you're taken seriously,** write down your symptoms and how often you've been having them before your appointment. Sort through the issues you want to address, so that you can bring them up in an organized fashion. (It will help to get information from the library, the Internet or a nonprofit organization for information beforehand.) ◆ **If your doctor seems rushed,** tell her you have several things you want to discuss and request another appointment. If she won't schedule another visit or call you on the phone when her waiting room clears out, start shopping for another doctor. ◆ **Before you stomp out** of any doctor's office, though, stop for a moment to examine your own attitudes. A 1997 study at the University of Iowa in Iowa City showed that patients with a high level of mistrust and suspicion that physicians don't have their best interests at heart are less likely than the others to follow doctor's orders. The conclusion: Be a skeptic but not a cynic. In return, expect that your concerns will be heard and addressed.

ILLUSTRATIONS BY ANTHONY RUSSO

The recovery process starts when women hit the library or Internet for health information and become more assertive, demanding the most effective, least intrusive care.

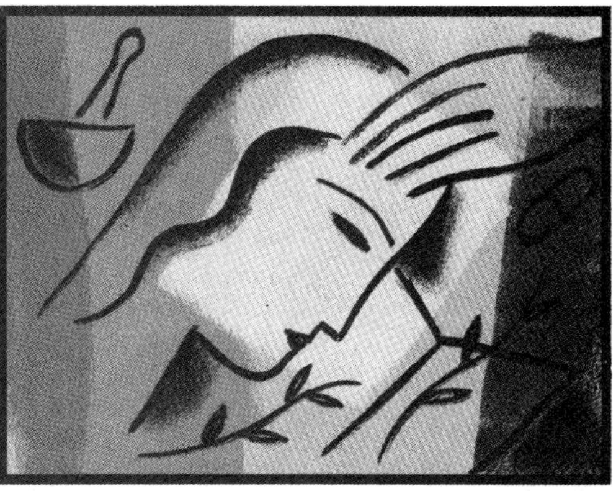

journey occurs shortly after diagnosis, a time she calls "Hitting the Wall," when people bottom out and lose hope. During this period, six of her eight subjects contemplated or attempted suicide. Then they began the next period, which she calls "Turning Around."

CONFRONTING THE CRISIS

The Turning Around process starts when people who are sick begin to take control of their life. For many in Dr. Lindsey's study, that meant becoming their own health advocate. After letting doctors prod and poke at her for a while and feeling there wasn't much to live for, a patient might hit the library or Internet for health information. She might become more assertive with doctors, demanding the most effective, least intrusive care.

Regaining control is a step anyone with chronic illness should take. "Once you've been sick for a while, you know your body better than anyone else," says Dr. Lindsey. It's especially important for women, who are likelier than men to be ignored or not taken seriously by the medical establishment. In a study by the National Multiple Sclerosis Society in Shippensburg, PA, 30% of black women and 11% of white women were initially told that imaginary, emotional or psychological problems were responsible for their symptoms. None of the men were told that; instead they were sent to specialists (see "Dealing With Doctors," page 82).

Another key step is to seek social support, a stage Dr. Lindsey calls "Opening Up." Many women preferred to get help formally, in a hospital support group or an online chat group. "They want to protect their families from some of their feelings," Dr. Lindsey says. "They can't talk about their fear of dying, because their family gets too upset." They also need help with practical things like grocery shopping, running errands around town and cooking meals.

Keeping friendships intact when you're sick can be tough, but the relationships that survive may well be stronger than the ones that existed before. Sandra Cohen, 41, of Washington, saw her way of relating to friends change as her osteoarthritis became more severe. Although she sometimes needed help taking care of errands and had to slow down when she was out with friends, "I kept people at a distance, because I thought, 'Who's going to want to deal with this?'" says Cohen, an occupational therapist. She felt alone at times, afraid to request help from anyone but her parents. Eventually, though, Cohen needed major knee surgery that would keep her in bed for weeks. Once she mustered the courage to let her friends know of her vulnerabilities, they mobilized, taking turns sleeping over, cooking her dinner and stopping by to make sure she did her physical therapy exercises. "People are a lot nicer than we give them credit for being," she says.

Finding techniques that can help you adjust to a new way of life is part of making the healing journey. For example, many of the women Dr. Crose studied dealt with the unpredictability of chronic illness by planning for the unplannable. One woman bought novels and put them aside. When pain and fatigue kicked in and she had to crawl into bed for a few days, she had a good book to take with her.

SEEKING THE SILVER LINING

As unbelievable as it may seem, there's an upside to chronic illness, one that experts are noticing more and more. It takes work to find it, but some women do. In their research, Drs. Crose and Gordon expanded their definition of health to include not just physical aspects, but emotional, intellectual, social, occupational and spiritual dimensions as well. While a woman's body might be withering, her intellectual capabilities, her work, her network of

Illness and Intimacy: The Side Effect No One Talks About

One rarely mentioned side effect of chronic illness is the shadow it can cast over intimacy. Lynn Schlesinger, Ph.D., an assistant professor of sociology at the State University of New York at Plattsburgh, however, has found that many women and their partners are able to keep passion alive. She suggests the following:

Try to figure out what's changed. Are there physical problems? Has the illness resurrected old angers or resentments? Or are you simply tired all the time?

Communicate with your partner—and with your doctor. Try not to criticize your partner or get defensive if he criticizes you. If medication is affecting your sex drive, talk to your physician about whether there's another drug that can help restore libido; the doctor may even recommend skipping doses at carefully scheduled times. If you're uncomfortable with your body, find activities to help you feel more graceful and attractive, such as swimming or yoga.

Don't assume your partner can read your mind. If four nights out of five you're too sick to even kiss, but on the fifth night you're ready to snuggle and see where it leads, you'll have to take the initiative.

Remember that there's a range of options for intimacy. Try showering together, giving foot rubs to each other, or just talking and laughing. The important thing is to stay affectionate during your bad days so you can be more daring on your good ones.

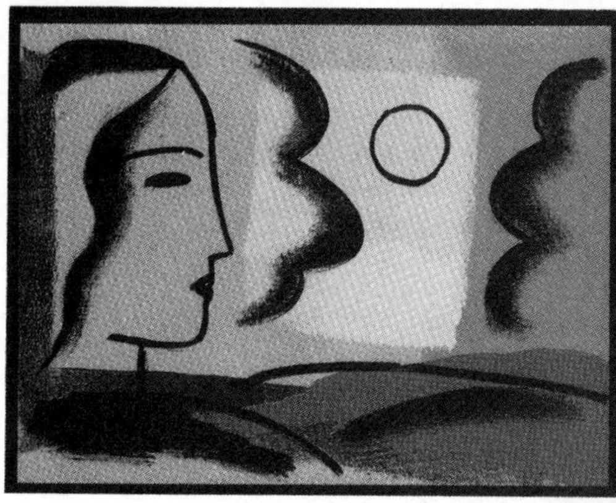

There is an upside. While a woman's body might be withering, her intellectual capabilities, her work, her friendships and her compassion for others might all be growing.

friends, the love between her and her husband or her compassion for others might be growing.

"We went into this thinking we'd find women who'd been abandoned," Dr. Crose says. "We didn't. Most of these women described their relationships with their husbands as improving." The women also tried new things that gave them a healthier, happier sense of self: writing poetry, volunteering or turning to spiritual practices.

Dr. Lindsey's subjects were willing to try a variety of alternative healing practices, including acupuncture, massage, yoga and meditation. "Healing is much more important than curing, because with chronic illness, there is no cure," says Leo Frangipane, M.D., a surgical oncologist formerly with Reading (PA) Hospital and Medical Center. Western medicine, with its emphasis on cures, often doesn't pay enough attention to comfort, something that many alternative treatments address.

It's also important that those who have a long-term disease get involved in some kind of creative activity: painting, writing, photography, singing, gourmet cooking, says psychologist Robert Shuman, Ed.D., of Marblehead, MA, and the author of *The Psychology of Chronic Illness.* It's a way to try to expand their capabilities while the disease is limiting them and to make an effort to find meaning in the suffering. Dr. Shuman speaks from personal experience: He has multiple sclerosis (MS). "People may have an illness, but illness doesn't have to become their identity," he says. "A person can approach illness as a way to understand their place in life's immensity."

Subjects in both Dr. Lindsey's and Dr. Crose's studies did just that. They delved into spiritual practices, from reading the Bible to meditating with a mantra. They had a heightened sense of peace, connection with others and thankfulness. Dr. Lindsey has termed this stage "Acquiring a State of Grace." Drs. Crose and Gordon call it "Transcendence." "They really appreciated their good days, and they didn't let them slip through their fingers," says Dr. Crose. "They'd transcended the disease and become better people."

Illness in the Family

The suffering of a woman with a long-term condition exacerbates the usual emotional and financial problems that can plague marriages. But the effects go deeper than that. "Family members can be up to four times more depressed than the patient," says psychologist Dennis Turk, Ph.D., a professor of anesthesiology and pain research at the University of Washington School of Medicine in Seattle.

In fact, researchers have found that the stronger and healthier a marriage is, the likelier the spouse of a chronic-pain patient is to wince along with him or her, and to experience a spike in heart rate and skin temperature, signs of distress. This means that family members risk developing health problems themselves if they don't care for their own mental and physical health even as they're caring for the patient.

These organizations cater to caregivers:

- **National Caregiving Foundation,** 800-930-1357, provides a free caregiver support kit.
- **Well Spouse Foundation,** 800-838-0879, has support groups for caregivers.
- **Caregiver Survival Resources,** www.caregiver911.com, offers message boards, chats and links to other sites.

Linda Longo-Muth, 49, of Valley Cottage, NY, was diagnosed with multiple sclerosis 30 years ago. At times she's so fatigued she can't get off the couch. Her left leg drags behind her, her eye often wiggles in its socket and her skin burns because of nerve damage. Sometimes she has to hold on to her husband's arm to get around. But in the other hand she carries a carved wooden cane with a brass eagle on the handle ("It's got style," she says). And she forces herself to paint for at least two hours every day. Her works have been displayed in galleries from Washington to Tokyo.

Having multiple sclerosis meant that Longo-Muth had to give up her job as a high school art teacher. "They say that when one door closes, another opens—and it's true," she says. "I can't do many things that other people can do. But they can't do what I can do on canvas. We all have disabilities, and we all have gifts. You have to find out what your gift is and expand on it. MS is part of my life. It's not my entire life."

Randi Glatzer is a New York City writer specializing in health and women's issues.

A H ADDRESS BOOK

Taking Good Care of Yourself

These are resources for women with chronic illness:

- ***Living With Chronic Illness*** by Cheri Register. (Bantam, 1987) This book is out of print; to order, send a check for $12 to Cheri Register, 4226 Washburn Ave. S., Minneapolis, MN 55410.
- ***Taking Charge: How to Master the Eight Most Common Fears of Long-Term Illness*** by Irene Pollin with Susan Golant. (Random House, 1996)
- **American Self-Help Clearinghouse,** Denville, NJ, 201-625-3037. Offers a list of state clearinghouses that assist people who want to find or form support groups.
- **Sapient Health Network,** www.shn.net. Provides information on chronic illnesses, plus access to a message board and medical journals.

The Enemy Within

Millions of women who look perfectly healthy are actually suffering from painful chronic illnesses.

By Randi Hutter Epstein, M.D.

Rosyln Lauterbach had a five-month-old son and a toddler when severe joint pain and fatigue struck her. "Am I not able to handle two kids?" she worried.

Bonnie Granato was finishing high school in Astoria, New York, when she began suffering from frequent high fevers, flulike symptoms and overwhelming tiredness. Granato thought she was losing her mind. Some friends and even a few doctors though so, too.

These women are not chronic complainers. They are chronically ill. They are among the millions of American women suffering from autoimmune diseases, a group of about eighty different illnesses in which a hyperactive immune system turns against the body. No one knows what spurs the body's defense system to run amok. There are treatments, but there is no cure. And some women suffer for years before getting the right diagnosis.

What scares these women is never knowing when or where the disease will strike next. What frustrates them is knowing that they look so completely fine on the outside that friends and family cannot comprehend their pain

For other sufferers of autoimmune diseases, symptoms vary from very mild to extremely severe. These diseases can kill. They include rheumatoid arthritis, which attacks joints; lupus, which assaults random organs; Sjögren's syndrome, which attacks moisture-making glands; scleroderma, which hardens the skin; chronic vasculitis, which inflames and destroys arteries; and multiple sclerosis, which destroys the protective sheaths around nerves, often leading to severely impaired mobility.

"One of the most devastating aspects is that you never know what to expect when you get up in the morning," says Teri Rumpf, Ph.D., a psychologist in Newton, Massachusetts, who has written about this subject. "People often assume you're malingering or depressed. Often these diseases strike women in the age group when they are caregivers, and all of a sudden they must be cared for. This can be a tremendous blow to self-image."

A Female Problem

Women are at least three times as likely to get autoimmune diseases as men—and no one knows why. Not surprisingly, many researchers blame women's hormones.

The hormonal swings of pregnancy, nursing and menopause affect autoimmune diseases, sometimes exacerbating, sometimes calming the symptoms.

"The conventional answer is to blame hormones, but hormones don't explain everything," says Michael Lockshin, M.D., a New York City rheumatologist and former acting director of the National Institute of Arthritis and Musculoskeletal and Skin Disease, in Bethesda, Maryland. "I think hormones determine some expression of the illness, but they don't cause the disease."

Some experts suspect autoimmune diseases may be caused by a genetic defect because the illnesses can run in families—for example, where the mother has rheumatoid arthritis, a daughter has lupus and a cousin has multiple sclerosis.

Reprinted with permission from *Ladies' Home Journal* magazine, February 1998, pp. 78, 82-83, 87, 181.

Other experts wonder whether a virus or bacteria or some other environmental agent wreaks havoc on the immune system. Or, perhaps some women are born with a genetic vulnerability that turns into full-blown disease only after a viral illness. At this point, no one can say with certainty why some women fall to autoimmune ailments and others don't.

A Quiet Epidemic

Since these diseases often go undiagnosed, the statistics on their prevalence are not very reliable. According to the Arthritis Foundation, roughly 2.5 million Americans have rheumatoid arthritis, three quarters of them women, and about 131,000 people have lupus, 80 percent women. Sjögren's syndrome may strike as many as one million Americans, 90 percent of them women.

Even after diagnosis, there is no easy cure. The ultimate goal is to find a treatment that corrects the defective immune system. One possibility: so-called T-cell "vaccines" that would coat the self-destructive immune cells and prevent their next assault. Other scientists are toying with creating fake targets so the body attacks something other than itself.

Paradoxically, despite an overly vigilant immune system, patients are highly susceptible to infections. "The immune system is hyperactive, but it is not normal," says Lockshin. In essence, the body is so preoccupied with self-destruction, it is vulnerable to germ warfare.

But Lauterbach and Granato are fighters. After years of suffering, they have found ways to cope.

Life Redefined

"I was twenty-two and had just given birth to David when the symptoms started," says Roslyn Lauterbach, now thirty-seven, of Flemington, New Jersey. "I had been perfectly healthy, but my hands would lock. And then I had a lump inside my elbow that grew from the size of a cherry to a tomato. I went to three surgeons and they had three different ideas. Sometimes the pain got so bad I couldn't get out of bed."

Lauterbach did not know it at the time, but she had rheumatoid nodules, lumps of tissue under the skin that form in areas exposed to a lot of pressure. These nodules often accompany rheumatoid arthritis.

Rheumatoid arthritis tends to strike the joints in the wrists and hands. It also affects the hips, knees, jaws, ankles and feet—usually in a symmetrical pattern. Without treatment, the disease can destroy tendons, ligaments and bone.

> They look so healthy on the outside that others cannot comprehend their pain

Lauterbach tried to ignore her joint pain. It finally subsided when she became pregnant with her second son, Robbie, now twelve. "Sure enough, when I stopped breast-feeding Robbie, it all came tearing back," says Lauterbach. "I couldn't get out of bed. I couldn't move my arms and shoulders. Finally, I went to a rheumatologist, who told me I had an autoimmune disease, but he wasn't sure which one.

"It wasn't until I was thirty that a rheumatologist at New York University gave me a test for rheumatoid arthritis and told me what I had." The test detects rheumatoid factor antibodies (proteins produced by defense-system cells).

Some autoimmune antibodies can be detected in the blood, such as RF (rheumatoid factor) and ANA (antinuclear antibody, found in people with lupus and other autoimmune diseases). But not everyone who has an autoimmune disease tests positive, and sometimes the test results in a false positive.

"In a way, the diagnosis was a relief. At least I had a path to follow," says Lauterbach. "The worst part has been depending on other people just to get through the day. At one point, I had a nurse helping me. I couldn't bear having my boys see their mother like that. To this day, I'll do anything to get through the pain to see them off in the morning.

"I tried to hide my pain from them, but now I realize they suffered along with me. Just recently, a friend told me that after my divorce, one of my sons, who was five years old at the time, said, 'My daddy's leaving because he's tired of tying my mommy's shoes for her.' "

Lauterbach says the divorce was probably inevitable regardless of her health problems, but she is very thankful that her second husband—they've been married for five years—has been sympathetic during the unpredictable bouts of illness. He understood when she said she did not want to risk another pregnancy.

While medication can sometimes stop the pain and relieve the swelling of rheumatoid arthritis, there can be serious side effects. For example, chronic use of corticosteroids, such as prednisone, can lead to bone thinning, cataracts and weight gain. As with many other patients, Lauterbach's disease attacked the bones in the back of her neck, leaving them dangerously fragile. She needed surgery to fuse them in place.

Severe rheumatoid arthritis sufferers can be helped by joint-fusion surgeries or hip replacements. "I've had five surgeries in the past five years, and I still have a long way to go if I want to be able to roll on the floor with my grandchildren," says Lauterbach.

"Every night I imagine myself getting out of bed in the morning and going for a long walk with nothing hurting," she says. "Positive thinking is my only hope. I have to believe they are going to come up with something that will help me."

A NEW APPROACH TO AUTOIMMUNE DISEASES

Last spring, Michael Lockshin, M.D., a sixty-year-old expert in autoimmune disease, realized a career-long dream. He opened the first multidisciplinary center dedicated to the study and treatment of women with autoimmune diseases. It is located in New York City. The center's staff includes immunologists, rheumatologists, obstetricians and gynecologists.

The name is as complex as the diseases: The Barbara Volcker Center for Women and Rheumatic Diseases at The New York Hospital–Cornell Medical Center. (Sponsor Barbara Volcker, wife of Paul Volcker, former chairman of the Federal Reserve Board, suffers from a rheumatoid disorder.)

Lockshin found his calling when he was a Harvard medical student. "I was in the obstetrics ward, and the first patient I ever saw die was a twenty-two-year-old pregnant woman with lupus," he says. "No one knew why she died."

This tragic episode launched Lockshin's search for solutions. His patients say he is passionate about his work and compassionate about their concerns. "I don't think I'd be alive today if it weren't for him," says Bonnie Granato, whose son, Kevin Michael, is named for the physician.

Says Lockshin, "If you look at things that are particularly destructive to young women, autoimmune diseases rank very high. They strike when women should be in a very healthy, active period of their lives."

He hopes his new center will deal not only with the medical but also the psychological aspects of these diseases. "Anybody who hurts all day, every day and who has to face people who think she is crazy or a chronic complainer would be abnormal if she wasn't depressed," says Lockshin. The disease may also make them prone to depression.

"We want to touch on the very pragmatic things such as daily life, menopause and issues of pregnancy, but a lot of the focus will also be on research," says Lockshin. "We want to solve the biggest problem: What causes these illnesses? Why women?"

For more information, call 212-606-1461.

Shattered Dreams?

Thirty years ago, if someone had told Bonnie Granato that one day she would be happily married with three healthy children, living in Boca Raton, Florida, pain- and drug-free, she would have thought that person was crazy. In those days, she sometimes questioned her own sanity.

Granato's battle with lupus—the complete medical name is systemic lupus erythematosus—began when she was sixteen. "When it really hit me hard," she says, "I couldn't even get out of bed. Everything ached and hurt so badly I just wanted to die. I've suffered a lot of neurologic damage, lots of seizures and many bouts of meningitis [inflammation of the spinal cord]. My skin is so sensitive to the sun, I have to wear tons of sunscreen all the time."

"It wasn't until about a year after these weird symptoms started that my illness was diagnosed. I had a hundred-and-five-degree fever and was transferred from a hospital in Queens to The New York Hospital-Cornell Medical Center, in Manhattan. I remember waking up and Dr. Michael Lockshin telling me I had lupus. I didn't even know what the word meant."

Lupus is Latin for wolf, a name given to the disease because many patients have a butterfly-shaped rash on the nose and cheeks similar to the pattern on the face of a wolf, according to medical lore. But lupus is far more than a skin disease. Attacks by the body's own defense system can strike anywhere at any time. Sometimes the bouts are mild; other times, they are life-threatening. Lupus can attack the kidneys, central nervous system or heart. Patients may also suffer from anemia, low blood counts and chronic joint aches. They are treated with a series of drugs, including anti-inflammatories, antimalarial pills and even anticancer drugs.

"They tried so many different drugs on me, I felt like a legalized junkie with all the IVs, blood transfusions and needles," says Granato. "One drug caused my bones to wither. I've had one hip replacement and need another. Another drug made me go through menopause at the age of twenty-six."

Lupus patients are also prone to early atherosclerosis, or hardening of the arteries, and strokes. Years of steroids can lead to osteoporosis. "And then there is a group who have kidney failure," says Lockshin.

"It takes a big toll on the family and requires a tremendous amount of understanding," says Granato. "But my husband has been with me through it all." The couple even works together—they own a franchise of Mail Boxes Etc.

Pregnancy was another issue. "I never thought I'd be able to have children, so I adopted Lisa, who is now fifteen. Then I was so determined because I didn't want her to be without siblings that I took fertility drugs. At first I didn't tell Dr. Lockshin." (Some experts worry that fertility drugs can trigger a bout of illness and that autoimmune antibodies can cause birth defects.)

"I finally got pregnant with twins when I was forty." On January 20, 1989, Granato gave birth to Kimberly Ann and Kevin Michael. With the twins' birth, Granato's lupus symptoms stopped as mysteriously as they had begun. But she knows the disease can flare up at any time.

"It's a quiet disease eating away at you ever so gradually," she says. "But even though it can't be cured, you can learn to control it and not let the disease control you. If you believe you will feel good, you can lead a normal life."

Randi Hutter Epstein, M.D., is a nonpracticing physician and medical writer.

Heart disease in women: Special symptoms, special risks

Coronary heart disease in women, often overlooked or undertreated, is finally getting its due.

The prevalence of risk factors for coronary heart disease and the death rate from the disease itself have both been dropping steadily in the U.S. for several decades. But those declines have been much less impressive in women than in men. One major reason: Physicians have traditionally regarded coronary disease as mainly a man's disease. So they've diagnosed and treated it less aggressively in women, and they haven't pushed women as hard as men to reduce their risk of the disease by changing their health habits.

Equally important, researchers have traditionally studied coronary disease mainly in men. That has obscured significant differences between the sexes concerning both the symptoms and the causes of the disease—and may have further hindered efforts to prevent or diagnose the disease in women.

The box on the next page focuses on symptoms; here, we tell how the traditional risk factors—and risk-reducing factors—differ in women.

Estrogen may protect the heart in at least four ways.

The differences in risk

The female hormone estrogen, abundant in premenopausal women, may protect the heart in at least four ways: It helps lower the "bad" LDL cholesterol, elevate the "good" HDL cholesterol, increase blood flow to the heart, and distribute body fat favorably. That protection helps explain why heart attack rarely strikes women before age 50, the average age of menopause, while it often strikes men in their forties. After menopause, when estrogen levels fall, the protective benefits generally start to fade, and coronary risk starts to rise; by age 60 or so, coronary disease becomes the leading cause of death in women.

Estrogen's benefits may contribute to at least some of the following differences between women's and men's coronary risk factors:

■ **Low HDL cholesterol.** Average levels of the "good" HDL are significantly higher in women than in men. (For unknown reasons, that gap shrinks only slightly after menopause.) So a low HDL level—less than 35 mg/dl—increases a woman's risk more than a man's, possibly because it represents a greater deviation from the norm in women. Further, a North Carolina study suggests that women may be able to raise their HDL level more than men can. The study found that aerobic exercise increased HDL by 20 percent in female coronary patients but by only 5 percent in male patients. (Other steps that can boost HDL include weight loss, smoking cessation, moderate alcohol consumption, and medications that not only lower LDL but also raise HDL, provided the patient needs both benefits.)

■ **High blood pressure.** Women tend to develop hypertension later in life than men do, so the elevated pressure typically has less time to damage a woman's heart. That difference has led some doctors to treat hypertension less aggressively in all women. But when a woman does develop hypertension, it's just as harmful as in a man of the same age.

In addition, women are more likely than men to develop isolated systolic hypertension, or elevation of just the upper blood-pressure number. While doctors used to consider that condition relatively harmless, research has shown that reducing elevated systolic pressure reduces substantially the risk of both coronary disease and stroke. (To lower blood pressure: Lose weight, exercise regularly, don't drink alcohol excessively, reduce stress, restrict sodium intake, and, if necessary, take medication.)

■ **Diabetes.** Diabetes is more likely to damage the arteries, raise blood pressure, and worsen cholesterol levels in women than in men. Further, it can blunt the protective effects of estrogen. Indeed, diabetes multiplies the chance of developing coronary disease substantially more in women than in men.

So it's particularly important for female diabetics to reduce their alterable risk factors for coronary disease, including the ones listed in this story as well as obesity, inactivity, and high levels of the "bad" LDL cholesterol. In addition, postmenopausal women with diabetes should strongly consider hormone replacement therapy and regular aspirin use to further protect the heart.

Women who have had gestational diabetes—high blood sugar during pregnancy—are at high risk for eventually developing type II diabetes, the most common kind; that, in turn, increases their coronary risk. So they need to take protective steps against both diseases, particularly losing excess weight, exercising regularly, and not smoking.

■ **Body-fat distribution.** Fat tends to accumulate around the hips in women, the belly in men. The male pattern poses greater coronary risk; that's mainly because belly fat breaks down more readily than hip fat, causing metabolic changes that push up the "bad" LDL cholesterol, lower the "good" HDL cholesterol, and increase blood pressure.

Reprinted with permission from *Consumer Reports on Health,* May 1997, pp. 54-56.

But when women do develop that typically male pattern, it may be even more worrisome than when men do, since it often reflects a disorder dubbed "syndrome X." The disorder involves insulin resistance, probably the underlying cause of diabetes; that resistance leads to increased insulin levels, which may contribute to hypertension. Women with syndrome X also tend to have increased male-hormone levels, which reduce the protective benefits of estrogen.

The waist should be considerably smaller than the hips in women; in men, the waist and hips should be about the same size. Fortunately, the instability that helps make belly fat more dangerous also makes it easier to eliminate than hip fat. (Take the same steps you would to lose weight anywhere in your body: Do regular aerobic and strengthening exercise, and follow a low-fat, moderately low-calorie diet.)

■ **Smoking.** Some women incorrectly believe that smoking is less dangerous to a woman's heart than to a man's heart. Smoking not only damages the lining of the arteries but also lowers levels of the protective HDL and can speed the onset of menopause. Smoking may be particularly bad for the heart in women who take birth-control pills.

How the risk reducers differ

Exercising regularly and eating a low-fat diet can provide broad coronary protection by reducing several risk factors at once. Here are three other broadly protective steps that women may want to consider.

■ **Hormone replacement therapy.** Taking female hormones sharply reduces the risk of coronary disease by restoring the protection that women had before menopause. It also eases menopausal symptoms, slashes the risk of osteoporosis, and may decrease the chance of colon cancer, tooth loss, and possibly osteoarthritis and Alzheimer's disease. For most women, those benefits clearly outweigh the treatment's main drawbacks—renewed menstrual bleeding with some regimens, and possibly a slight increase in the risk of breast cancer and blood clots in the legs and lungs. Potential exceptions include women who have a personal or family history of breast cancer; a low risk of coronary disease and osteoporosis; or large uterine fibroids, active liver disease, or a history of blood clots.

■ **Aspirin.** Regular use of low-dose aspirin clearly lowers the risk of heart attack in men by lowering the risk of blood clots. The available evidence suggests that aspirin may have the same effect in women. However, aspirin can also cause gastrointestinal bleeding and may increase the chance of hemorrhagic stroke, the kind caused by bleeding.

So an aspirin regimen is worth considering only by people who are at increased risk of having a heart attack. That includes anyone with coronary disease; postmenopausal women under age 60 or so who have at least two risk factors for the disease; and postmenopausal women over age 60, as well as men, who have at least one risk factor. (Risk factors include the

Diagnosis in women: Why the delay?

Heart attacks are twice as deadly in women as in men. That's partly because the attacks typically strike women when they're older and in poorer health than men. But it's also because doctors often diagnose and treat the underlying coronary disease in women at a later, more advanced stage.

One reason for the later diagnosis is that women's coronary complaints may be harder to interpret than the usually unmistakable symptoms in men. For coronary disease, the hallmark in men is angina, or central-chest pain that comes on with exertion and subsides with rest; for heart attack, it's crushing chest pain, often spreading to the shoulders, neck, jaw, arms, or upper back.

The same symptoms often signal coronary disease or heart attack in women. But female coronary patients tend to be less physically active than male patients, partly due to age and poorer general health. And the disease is often diagnosed at a later, more advanced stage in women. For both reasons, women are more likely than men to develop chest pain when they're resting.

Further, women with coronary disease are more likely to report vague symptoms that can be caused by many other ailments or even medications. Those symptoms include breathlessness, heartburn, nausea, and severe fatigue for coronary disease; and mild chest pain accompanied by breathlessness, dizziness, heartburn, or nausea for heart attack. Researchers theorize that advanced age, diabetes (which is far more prevalent in female than male coronary patients), and unknown causes may all help produce vaguer coronary symptoms in women.

But vaguer symptoms may not be the only reason for the delayed diagnosis: Some evidence suggests that doctors may take coronary disease less seriously in women. For example, a recent study found that when women come to the emergency room with essentially the same coronary symptoms as men do, they're less likely to receive heart medications, and more likely to be handed drugs for an "anxiety attack." Other studies have shown that even when women have *worse* coronary symptoms than men or are actually having a heart attack, they're less likely to undergo angiography, the definitive diagnostic test.

So if you're a woman, you need to know all the symptoms listed above—the classic complaints as well as the vague ones. And you need to take those symptoms seriously, and make sure that your doctor does the same.

items listed in the preceding section, plus high LDL-cholesterol levels, physical inactivity, and a family history of coronary disease before age 60.)

But those guidelines consider only the general risks of aspirin. Many specific conditions and medications can make aspirin excessively dangerous (see *Consumer Reports on Health* March 1997 issue). So it's essential to consult your doctor before starting to take aspirin regularly.

■ **Alcohol.** Moderate drinking may reduce the risk of coronary disease by up to 40 percent, mainly because it boosts HDL cholesterol and fights blood clots. But even moderate drinking has significant risks, such as an increased chance of alcoholism, auto accidents, falls, and breast cancer. In men, the benefits start to outweigh the risks by age 40 or so. In women, that shift doesn't start until after menopause. However, the same precaution about taking aspirin applies even more strongly to drinking alcohol: Talk with your doctor first.

Note that the definition of moderate drinking differs between the sexes, too: no more than two drinks per day for men, one per day for women. That's because women tend to have smaller amounts of a certain stomach enzyme as well as a smaller liver, both of which help break down the alcohol.

Summing up

The following measures are even more important for women than for men—or apply to women only:

■ Try to boost low HDL, stop smoking, and lose abdominal fat.

■ Be particularly diligent about reducing your overall coronary risk if you have diabetes.

■ Make sure your doctor is aware of—and takes seriously—any coronary risk factors you may have, including isolated systolic hypertension.

■ If you're postmenopausal, talk to your doctor about estrogen therapy and possibly moderate drinking. If you're postmenopausal *and* at increased coronary risk, talk about aspirin therapy as well.

Stopping the Deadliest Cancer

Women with lung cancer are the disease's forgotten victims. It's time we cleared the air

BY PATRICIA LYNDEN

See if you know the answer to this one: What's the leading cause of cancer deaths in women? If you said breast cancer, you're wrong. Lung cancer is the biggest killer, and the death rate is soaring, up over 550% since 1950, when the disease was practically unheard of in women. The simple and awful reason is that every day more girls and women become addicted to cigarettes. Still, the extent of lung cancer's threat to our health hasn't sunk in. There are no races for the cure to benefit research, and until last November 14th—the barely noticed first National Lung Cancer Awareness Day—there were no days, weeks or months devoted to the disease.

Women who have lung cancer call it "the hidden disease," even though it now kills just as many of us as it does men. Sandy Eggers, 50, a New York City businesswoman diagnosed last year, recalls lying in her hospital room after having a piece of her lung removed and thinking *I wish I had breast cancer. At least I'd have someone to talk to.*

Unfortunately Eggers has lots of company. There were 80,100 cases of lung cancer among women last year, and it is predicted that by the year 2000 more women than men will die of the disease. Yet because the cancer is 85% preventable, the medical profession and policymakers have paid little attention to finding a cure. (It's worth noting, however, that not all lung cancer patients are smokers; some 8% to 10% have no discernible risk factors.)

Keeping people from getting hooked on cigarettes is important, but it's not enough. All of us must take action in other ways to change society's attitudes about lung cancer, to ensure earlier diagnosis and better treatment and to guarantee cleaner air for everyone.

> 67,000 women died of lung cancer last year, but its threat to our health still hasn't sunk in.

ADVOCACY

No More Blaming the Victim

Those battling lung cancer face a unique problem. "People often say, 'It's their fault, so why should I feel sorry for them?'" says Frank Detterbeck, M.D., director of the multidisciplinary thoracic oncology program at the University of North Carolina in Chapel Hill. And "patients feel guilty because they smoked," adds Paul A. Bunn, Jr., M.D., director of the University of Colorado Cancer Center in Denver.

Even a significant part of the medical community doesn't want to deal with lung cancer. Says Dr. Detterbeck, "A lot of physicians have the attitude that nothing has changed in 25 years, most everyone who has it will die, and there isn't much you can do." Peggy McCarthy, who heads the Alliance for Lung Cancer Advocacy, Support and Education in Vancouver, WA, the only national lung cancer organization, adds that the problem is exacerbated because people with lung cancer often don't get treated at major medical centers that offer sophisticated care. Instead they go to general surgeons in small communities, many of whom share the resignation Dr. Detterbeck complains of, and who don't refer patients to oncologists who could provide radiation and chemotherapy.

A huge, impersonal medical center might be overwhelming for a woman grappling with lung cancer, but it could make the difference between life and death. "We know so much more than we did 30 years ago," and no one doctor can keep on top of all the advances, says Dr. Detterbeck. In his program, every patient's care is discussed by a core group of five specialists, including a medical oncologist and a radiation oncologist. (To learn about comprehensive cancer centers funded by the National Cancer Institute in Bethesda, MD, call 800-4-CANCER.)

SCREENING

Stopping the Shortcomings

Women with lung cancer stand a better chance of survival if the disease is diagnosed in its earliest stages. But in two-thirds of cases, the cancer is not discovered until it is advanced. The scientific community, however, does not recommend screening all women. Because the only widely available test, a chest x-ray (about $125), would detect a relatively small number of lung cancers in a large population, some experts feel periodic x-rays make sense only for high-risk women. This group includes those who smoked 15 years or more, who have been exposed to radon or asbestos or who have a family history of lung cancer, says Chandra P. Belani, M.D., codirector of the lung cancer program at the University of Pittsburgh Cancer Institute. If you know someone with these risk factors, urge her to talk to her doctor about screening. Women heavily exposed to secondary smoke should do the same.

From *American Health for Women,* June 1998, pp. 47-48. © 1998 by Patricia Lynden. Reprinted by permission.

LUNG CANCER: WHAT'S YOUR RISK?

One in nine women who have smoked will get lung cancer, according to Paul Bunn, M.D., director of the University of Colorado Cancer Center in Denver. Symptoms include a persistent or bloody cough; unusual, unexplained tiredness; swelling of the neck and face; shortness of breath; repeated pneumonia or bronchitis; appetite and weight loss; hoarseness; and persistent chest, shoulder or back pain. If you develop any of these symptoms, see a doctor immediately. They don't necessarily mean you have lung cancer, but they shouldn't be ignored.

HOW RISK RISES

Never smoked	**1 in 20**
Smoked 1½ packs a day for 10 years	**1 in 8**
Smoked 2 packs a day for 50 years	**1 in 4**

One new diagnostic tool that finds cancer cells anywhere in the body is the positron-emission tomography scan. Only 60 U.S. centers offer the test, however, and it costs an average of $2,700. R. Edward Coleman, M.D., a radiologist who runs the PET center at Duke University Medical Center in Durham, NC, laments that people aren't better informed about the technique.

PASSIVE SMOKING

Ending Involuntary Exposure

Even if you've never smoked, you could still be at risk for lung cancer. To take action in the fight against the disease, speak out against secondary smoke. The issue has received much attention in the wake of a class action suit brought against the cigarette industry by a group of flight attendants. Norma R. Broin, 43, a flight attendant from Stafford, VA, who led that fight, was diagnosed with lung cancer in 1989, although she had never smoked. She attributes her disease to the carcinogens she breathed before smoking was banned on domestic flights.

While experts and advocates disagree about the extent of secondary smoke's role in lung cancer, there is no question that passive smoking can cause or inflame asthma, chronic bronchitis, emphysema and sinus infections. If you want to get smoking banned in public spaces, take the following advice from Broin and another veteran of the anti-smoking trenches, Joseph Cherner, president of Smokefree Educational Services, who helped ensure that New York City's public spaces are largely smoke free.

Join an advocacy group. Find one in your phone book or on the Internet.

Lobby elected officials. Start with those at the city and state levels. "They live in your community, so they'll vote for what they think their constituents want," says Cherner. Congressmembers may be influenced more by tobacco company money. Use the letter below to contact them; check www.smokescreen.org for letters to other lawmakers.

Complain to the manager. If you stay at a hotel whose lobby is full of smoke, or eat in a smoke-filled restaurant, speak to the manager or write to the company president. Say a smoke-free environment will be a deciding factor when you choose a hotel or eatery in the future.

Use the Americans With Disabilities Act. If your employer won't provide you with a smoke-free work environment, Broin says you have a powerful tool in the ADA. Under the act, sensitivity to cigarette smoke would be considered a disability for which you cannot be discriminated against. Says Broin, "What doctor wouldn't say you're sensitive to the more than 40 known carcinogens and 4,000 toxins in cigarettes if you have repeated sinus problems or bronchitis?"

Patricia Lynden, a writer in New York City, was executive editor of Longevity.

"Breast Cancer Cost Me My Job"

When my boss fired me after my cancer surgery, I was determined to fight back. By Jane Karuschkat, as told to Thomas Clavin

Battling breast cancer was the biggest challenge I have ever faced, but I believed I could beat it. I thought my determination, the love and support of my husband and, yes, even my job as a legal secretary would help. At the office, I had the encouragement of my co-workers, plus the routine of familiar tasks, which offered some stability when everything else in my life was in upheaval.

So it was one of my darkest days when one Friday, in January 1993, I asked my husband, Glenn, to pick me up early at the office.

I told him, "I've just been fired."

For four years, I had been a legal secretary at a law firm in Mineola, New York. A busy office with five attorneys made for very hectic days, but I enjoyed the variety of cases the firm handled. The pay also kept our checkbook balanced while we waited for Glenn's new audiotape production and distribution business to take off.

Then, in October 1992, I was diagnosed with breast cancer. The news left me stunned—I was only forty-one—but I vowed to do whatever was necessary to overcome this illness. I opted for a lumpectomy the following month, but doctors discovered afterward that the cancer had spread beyond the lump, so in December I underwent a mastectomy and was scheduled for a regimen of chemotherapy. The entire experience sorely tested my positive attitude. What helped me hold it together was knowing I had a steady job to rely on.

From the start, I shared the news of my cancer with my employer and my co-workers. I felt it was important for them to know everything, and I wanted their support. To minimize the impact my illness would have on my work, I took less than a week off—a combination of sick and vacation days—to recuperate from the mastectomy. My doctor agreed to schedule my semimonthly chemo treatments Fridays after work so I could have the weekend to recover. At the office, at least, I wanted life to be as close to normal as possible.

People at the firm seemed to be understanding and compassionate—maybe too nice. During that November and December, they stopped giving me work. I would ask the attorneys and secretaries, "Can I help you with that?" or "Let me finish up for you." Not wanting to burden me, they would say everything was okay. But with only trivial tasks to do all day, I no longer felt valued. Still, I hoped that things would go back to normal eventually.

I had my first chemo treatment on a Friday in January 1993, but I still felt rotten on Monday, so I took another of my accumulated sick days and went back to work the next day. Then, early on the following Friday afternoon, my boss, Jessel Rothman, asked me to meet him in the office library. "This is going to be as difficult for me as it is for you," he began after we were seated. "I'm going to have to let you go. I can't afford to keep you any longer."

I knew right away that this decision had nothing to do with money. No other staffers had been laid off recently, and I had more seniority than many of them. And I certainly wouldn't have received my annual Christmas bonus just a few weeks earlier if money had been tight, or if my work had been unsatisfactory.

A part of me suspected what I was really being told was, "You're going to be sick all the time, and we don't want to deal with it. Get out."

Rothman offered a week's severance pay. I asked for two; he refused. That was it. I was out. In a daze, I left the library and put my personal belongings in a box, then I called my husband, and when he arrived, I walked out into the cold.

In the days following my dismissal, I wrestled with many strong emotions. But rising above them all was the feeling that I had to take action. I felt I was being fired for having cancer, and that just wasn't right. And surely I wasn't the only victim of this type of discrimination. I contacted attorneys who were involved in health and employment issues, eventually finding L. Susan Slavin, who was clearly a crusader.

The Americans with Disabilities Act, a federal law that was new at the time, would not apply in my case, because my company employed fewer than fifteen people. Instead, Susan told me, she wanted to file a complaint with the New York State Division of Human Rights, asking them to mandate that the federal law requirements for reasonable accommodation of disabilities be applied to employees with disabilities, including illnesses such as cancer, throughout the state. (The state law applies in companies with more than four employees.) I said, "Okay, let's go for it." Glenn backed me all the way.

It was hard to see my former co-workers testify that I was unable to handle my workload

As anyone who has been involved in a legal procedure knows, it's a lot of hurry-up-and-wait. The law firm chose to fight the complaint, which stretched things out further. Plus, we were asking the State Division of Human Rights to do something that, according to Susan, was unprecedented—rule in favor of a woman in a breast-cancer–related discrimination action, and on top of that, persuade a judge that New York be required to extend its state disability law relating to reasonable accommodation.

The first sign that we had a real shot at success came in March 1994, when the Division of Human Rights ruled that my complaint did have enough merit to take the case to the next level, which was a series of hearings before a judge appointed by the division. Grateful as I was for any progress, the hearings proved to be a painful experience.

It was hard to see my former coworkers—including those who had been my friends—testify against me. I wondered if they were giving this testimony under duress, and I sensed their discomfort as they asserted that I was unable to handle my workload.

In his opening statement, Jessel Rothman said that "no matter how great or competent she was up to October 1992, she lost those skills." He argued that the cancer treatments had affected my time at work. But Susan pointed out that, in fact, I had missed only a few days in the eleven weeks between my diagnosis and dismissal, and

Staying on the job

According to a 1996 survey of five hundred cancer survivors, these patients reported being fired or laid off from their jobs at five times the rate of other workers in the U.S. Of the one hundred supervisors of cancer survivors who were also surveyed, 33 percent believed that the workers could no longer handle their jobs, and 31 percent felt they had to be replaced.

If you have cancer or another serious illness and you've been discriminated against at work, the best course of action is to address the problems early, before they worsen. In a face-to-face meeting with your boss, discuss your diagnosis and treatment program, express your desire and ability to keep working effectively and seek solutions. If the discrimination continues, keep a record of actions taken against you, and if your company has a grievance procedure, pursue it.

These organizations can give you information and assistance: Cancer Care, 800-813-4673; National Alliance of Breast Cancer Organizations, with more than 370 member groups, 888-806-2226 or *http://www.nabco.org*; and the American Cancer Society, 800-227-2345 or *http://www.cancer.org*. The National Coalition for Cancer Survivorship publishes a pamphlet called "Working It Out: Your Employment Rights as a Cancer Survivor." For a copy, call 301-650-8868.

For legal assistance, contact your local Bar Association or send a request for a list of lawyers in your state that deal with employment issues, along with a self-addressed, stamped envelope (with 55¢ postage), to the National Employment Lawyers Association, 600 Harrison Street, Suite 535, San Francisco, CA 94107.

that these fell within my allotted sick and vacation days. It seemed we had made a strong case, but would the judge agree?

We found out in January 1996 that the judge's report to the New York State Division of Human Rights was favorable to us. But now we had to wait for the head of the division, Edward Mercado, to give a final ruling. Around the same time, I was hit with another crisis: My cancer had mestastasized to my hipbone. I needed a more intense series of chemo treatments. (Two years earlier, I had decided to have my other breast removed as a preventive measure.)

That June, Commissioner Mercado's historic ruling was handed down. He said that the firm had illegally discriminated against me because of my illness, that they had not reasonably accommodated my disability and that the New York State Human Rights Law would conform to the Americans with Disabilities Act. He further ruled that as a protection against discrimination, an illness must be equated with a disability, and therefore an employer must make a "reasonable accommodation" (such as flextime, in some situations) for sick workers who are otherwise willing and able to do the essential functions of their jobs.

I've since learned that my case is being used in other states to support the job-discrimination cases of cancer patients. This could have a huge impact, because among the 180,000 new cases of breast cancer diagnosed every year in the U.S., some women are doubtless going to face wrongful discrimination and firing.

The State Division of Human Rights also awarded me close to $70,000—some $20,000 for lost wages, and the rest for "mental anguish." I haven't seen a penny of it and probably never will, because my employer not only appealed the ruling, he also closed his law firm. But my fight was not just about money—it was about informing and empowering myself and others.

Today, though I'm still troubled by hip pain and a cranky digestive system, some of my strength is returning and there is no evidence that the cancer has recurred. I've taken up painting, exhibiting my work and even selling some pieces. Since the ruling, many other women wrongly fired by their employers have contacted me. Many of them were angry; some felt helpless or tossed aside. And I'm sure there are people everywhere who suffer in silence.

What has made the fight rewarding is knowing that my name is attached to a legal decision that is part of the effort to close the door on discrimination and open other doors to opportunity and self-respect.

The battle is far from over. But I won't quit until all cancer patients have the right to do their jobs.

By Peter Jaret

Closing in on Cancer

Treatments now being tested can stop cancer—without the hideous side effects of chemo and radiation. Soon, cancer may be an illness people live with, not die of.

FOR SARAJANE AVIDON, THE WORST PART WAS THE WAITING. "Week after week I'd call the doctor and say, 'Is it here yet?' And week after week he'd tell me, 'Not yet. Soon.' I remember saying to him at one point, 'Hey, come on, what do they have to do to make this stuff?'" Then Avidon, 56, lets loose a husky rollicking laugh—a laugh she's cultivated over 30 years as an actress in Chicago. The stuff in question was an experimental drug code-named IDEC-C2B8. And though Avidon isn't one for melodrama, she knew it might be her last, best hope.

Diagnosed with lymph node cancer in 1993, she'd been through it all: surgery, chemotherapy, radiation. The treatments had beaten back the cancer each time, but the remissions didn't last. "Of course I was worried," says Avidon. "I was worried sick."

Then, in the spring of 1996, her doctor told her about the new drug. "I didn't think twice," she recalls. "I said, 'Let's go for it.'" In November of that year her medical team got the green light to undertake a trial of the therapy, a combination of two drugs. Two shots a week apart—with none of the horrific complications of chemotherapy—and that was it. Within months her tumors began to shrink. More than a year later the disease was still in remission, the longest her cancer had remained quiet since it appeared.

Last November one of the drugs she received, renamed Rituxan, made history when it won FDA approval, becoming the first of a new generation of pioneering cancer therapies to make the leap from experimental to standard therapy. Of 151 patients getting the same drug at cancer centers around the country, half saw their tumors shrink by at least 50 percent. Nine months after treatment almost three-fourths of those were still in remission.

The new therapy, experts say, is likely

the first of many. More promising cancer treatments are moving through the research pipeline today than at any time since the country began its much-vaunted war against the disease in 1971. At least 112 drugs are now in the third and final stage of testing—by pharmaceutical firms where high hopes must toe the bottom line. At the same time the National Cancer Institute is sponsoring some 200 cancer drug trials at respected universities and medical centers.

These ventures offer the first real hope cancer patients have had in a long time. Though the percentage of Americans dying of cancer started to decline slightly in 1991, many experts credit better screening tests rather than advances in treatment. In the *New England Journal of Medicine* last May, a top specialist in the disease put it bluntly: Doctors are no better at curing cancer today than they were 30 years ago.

But that's about to change. "Three decades of basic research is finally beginning to pay off," says Edison Liu, director of clinical research at the National Cancer Institute. "It's a very exciting time. Many of us are confident we're on the verge of taking a giant step forward in the treatment of cancer."

The biggest advance, experts say, is in grasping what they're up against. In the past doctors had to throw everything they had at cancer, scattershot, because they didn't understand the disease. The only options were to "slash, burn, and poison," as some cancer patients grimly labeled the trio of conventional treatments.

True, surgery can eliminate some cancers, but it may be useless if malignant cells have broken loose and infiltrated other parts of the body. Radiation can shrink or destroy localized tumors but often at the risk of injuring nearby tissues.

Likewise, when cancer spreads, or metastasizes, the counterattack is usually chemotherapy—toxic chemicals that poison not only cancer cells but other fast-growing cells, causing hair loss and lowered immunity. And because cancer cells mutate so quickly that they can rapidly grow resistant to drugs, chemotherapies quickly lose their effectiveness.

The latest discoveries will soon change that whole picture. "We're beginning to see what turns a healthy cell cancerous and how that cancer cell manages to grow and spread," says Robert Weinberg, a biology professor at the Massachusetts Institute of Technology. "We're writing the life histories of many human tumors from start to finish. And at every step along the way we're finding points of vulnerability to attack."

Healthy cells don't suddenly turn into killers. At least six separate genetic mutations have to occur, says Weinberg, before a cell begins growing out of control and becomes, in the chilling language of oncology, "immortalized." Genes that tell a cell when to divide must get jammed in the on position. Fail-safe mechanisms that prevent runaway growth must be short-circuited. Systems that check for mutations have to be disabled, and internal clocks that limit the number of times a cell can divide must be shut off.

What allows so much to go so wrong? Some people are born with genetic defects that make certain cells especially vulnerable to mutation. Cigarette smoke, ultraviolet radiation, and toxic chemicals all can damage cells as they divide. Everyday wear and tear on cells takes a huge toll, too—the reason cancer is more common among older people. Eerily, once healthy cells mutate and escape the body's controls, they become unstable, making additional genetic mutations more likely.

The treatments being tested at centers around the country are aimed at stopping virtually all of these dangerous changes. Not every effort will pay off, of course. But, researchers say, four of the new approaches promise to revolutionize cancer treatment. Someday, one of them may save your life.

HEALTHY CELLS DON'T SUDDENLY TURN INTO KILLERS. AT LEAST SIX SEPARATE GENETIC MUTATIONS HAVE TO OCCUR BEFORE A CELL CAN START GROWING OUT OF CONTROL.

1
MONOCLONAL ANTIBODIES
"Guided Missiles" That Seek Out Cancer Cells

"YOU NAME IT, I'VE TRIED IT," says Susan Claymon, 59, as technicians prepare to inject her with one of the latest experimental drugs for breast cancer. It's a Thursday morning at the Mt. Zion Cancer Center in San Francisco, and Claymon settles into an easy chair under a window that frames a sky as blue as one a child might draw.

When she was diagnosed 12 years ago, her cancer had already reached 21 of the 24 lymph nodes tested. "Things looked very bleak," says Claymon. But through two mastectomies, chemotherapy, and radiation, she has battled the odds. Now the cancer has spread to her bones.

Claymon is a woman who belies first impressions. Her gray eyes seem washed out until she fixes her intense gaze on you; her pale skin and thin arms can make her appear frail until you hear the fierce determination in her voice. "You find yourself having to give up a lot with this disease. Like your hair," she says with a grim smile, touching the bright scarf tied around her head. "But one thing I've never given up is hope."

Hope, for now, takes the form of a clear liquid that will drip slowly into her veins for the next half hour. Like the drug that's keeping Sarajane Avidon's lymphoma at bay, Claymon's treatment is made up of monoclonal antibodies: molecules designed to latch onto the surface of harmful cells and bring them to heel. It's a strategy borrowed from the immune system, which produces natural antibodies to seek and destroy invading bacteria and viruses. Researchers can now fashion antibodies that function the same way—as guided missiles that home in on specific targets.

Ground zero, in this case, is a molecular change that shows up when breast cells turn aggressively malignant: the overproduction of a protein called HER2/neu. In a healthy cell, researchers think, the protein signals cells to grow and divide in an orderly manner. "A normal breast cell has about 10,000 of these protein molecules on its surface," says Len Presta, a biochemist at Genentech who helped develop Claymon's treatment. "A cancer cell growing out of control may have 100,000 to a million. So suddenly we have hundreds of thousands of identically shaped targets to zero in on." The idea is that by coating the surface of breast cancer cells, monoclonal antibodies will gum up the works so these cells can't multiply. The antibodies may also alert the immune system, which could target the cells for destruction.

"In lab tests we've seen monoclonal antibodies all but shut down malignant cells," says Susan Hellmann, head of clinical research at Genentech. The results from the first studies in humans look promising, though not miraculous. Five of the first 40 women saw their tumors shrink by at least half during the first year of treatment, according to Debu Tripathy, a cancer specialist at the University of California at San Francisco who directs the research program. "For women with advanced disease, that's encouraging." But several of those who did well initially have recently seen their cancers return.

To increase the killing power of monoclonal antibodies, researchers are devising ways to arm them with destructive payloads. At the National Cancer Institute molecular biologist Ira Pastan has linked antibodies for colon cancer cells with a toxin that enters the cell as soon as the missile reaches its target.

Using a similar approach, NCI researcher Thomas Waldmann has paired monoclonal antibodies that attack leukemia cells with radioactive particles. In one recent test the cancer retreated, at least temporarily, in nine of 16 patients. "Until now, we've been able to deliver radiation only from outside, with large machines," Waldmann says. "Monoclonal antibodies can carry radioactive doses or toxic chemicals into the heart of a cancer cell, offering treatments that promise to be both more effective and far less toxic to patients."

2
GENE THERAPIES

Customized Viruses Sent to Fix Damaged Genes

IF MUTATIONS DEEP INSIDE CELLS trigger cancer, wouldn't it be great to go in and do some repairs? Amazingly, that looks possible. In another strategy designed to zero in on cancer cells, researchers have turned to a surprising ally: viruses. Viruses are really nothing more than strands of genetic material—operating instructions for making new versions of themselves. Once viruses invade a cell, they insert their own genes into its DNA, turning the cell into a virus-producing factory. The high hope of gene therapy is to find ways to tame viruses and then engineer them to carry new or repaired genes into living cells, undoing the genetic mutations that might otherwise add up to cancer.

Luckily, basic research has turned up dozens of targets, from the growth-stimulating genes that get stuck in the on position to genes that normally keep growth in check but become shut down in cancerous cells.

One promising candidate is a gene known as p53, which monitors genetic mutations and orders cells to self-destruct if their inner code becomes too mangled. Usually the system prevents runaway growth. But in half of all cancers the fail-safe system itself becomes disabled, allowing even badly mutated cells to go on proliferating out of control. If p53 can be replaced—or if cells with the defective gene can be destroyed—cells on the way to becoming cancerous might be stopped dead.

At Introgen Corporation in Austin, Texas, researchers have already used a cold virus to ferry p53 genes into cancer cells. Preliminary studies suggest the therapy shrinks tumors. Using another approach, scientists at Onyx Pharmaceuticals in Richmond, Virginia, have tinkered with an otherwise harmless virus so that it targets and kills cells that carry defective p53 genes. If ongoing research pans out, physicians could use the virus to destroy errant cells before they grow into tumors.

At the National Cancer Institute, meanwhile, scientists are

ONE PATIENT WHOSE CANCER HAD SPREAD FOUND DOZENS OF EXPERIMENTAL TREATMENTS TO CONSIDER. "ALL IT TOOK WAS ONE CALL TO A TOLL-FREE NUMBER," SHE SAYS.

What Causes Cancer?

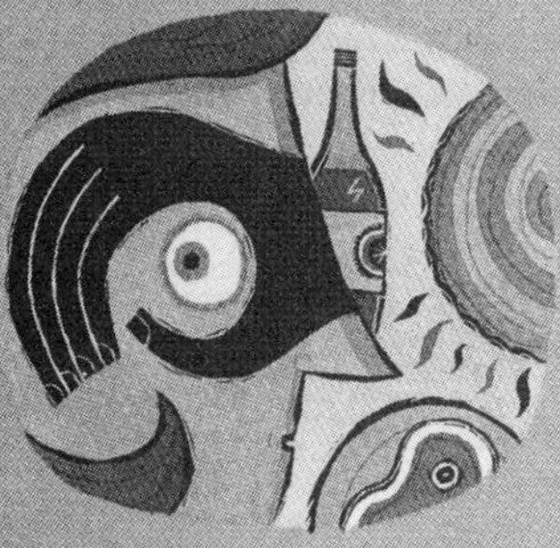

Often it seems to strike with the randomness of a freeway sniper. Yet cancer isn't always mysterious. "We know everything we need to know to cut the cancer rate in this country by about 50 percent flat out," says Graham Colditz, head of the Harvard Center for Cancer Prevention in Boston. That's 600,000 fewer cases a year. Here's what to watch out for.

TOBACCO
Smoking causes one of every three cancer deaths in the United States. While it's to blame for almost all cases of lung cancer, it also doubles the risk of bladder cancer and plays a key role in cancers of the pancreas and esophagus.

RED MEAT
Men in one study who dished up beef, pork, or lamb as a main dish at five or more meals a week were three times more likely to develop colon cancer than were occasional meat eaters. In another study, red meat posed a significant colon cancer risk for women, especially when they ate few vegetables.

JUNK FOOD
Fill up on doughnuts, sodas, and potato chips and you're going to pass up the dozens of cancer-fighting chemicals in fruits and vegetables. People who eat at least five fruit and veggie servings a day are much less likely to develop malignancies.

INACTIVITY
Women who log at least four hours of exercise a week cut their risk of breast cancer by more than a third. As for colon cancer—the third most common form of the disease—active people are about half as liable to get it as inactive ones.

OVEREATING
The more calories you consume, studies suggest, the greater your risk of colon and prostate cancer. Among women, being heavy adds to the danger from breast and endometrial cancer. Weight gain may be one reason breast cancer rates jump among Asians who move to the United States.

TANNING
Malignant melanoma, the deadliest form of skin cancer, kills nearly 7,000 Americans a year; squamous cell carcinoma, more than 2,000. Sunburns raise the risk of both. A study in Israel found that Orthodox Jews, who wear coats and hats or shawls year-round, were much less prone to melanoma than were Israelis who regularly exposed their skin to the sun.

ALCOHOL
Heavy drinking has been clearly linked to cancers of the liver, throat, and esophagus. Women who have just a drink or two a day run a somewhat higher risk of breast cancer. *—P.J.*

already using gene therapy to circumvent cancer's ability to become resistant to chemotherapies. The human body's cells are equipped with tiny pumps that turn on now and then to remove toxins that may find their way inside, explains NCI researcher Ken Cowan. "But when cells become cancerous, they turn the pumps on full-time, so that anything toxic that enters the cell gets churned right out again, including every chemotherapy drug in use."

Scientists recently identified the mutated gene that keeps the pump going in cancer cells, and in a stratagem worthy of their adversary, Cowan and his team are using a harmless virus to insert it into healthy white blood cells. "The hope is that if we can protect healthy cells by giving them resistance to chemotherapy drugs at the outset, we can avoid some of the worst side effects of chemotherapy, like suppression of the immune system," says Cowan. "And we should be able to hit tumors with higher levels of chemotherapy." NCI researchers have succeeded in getting new genes into patients' blood cells. Now they're working to improve the technique so that enough cells receive the gene to confer significant protection.

Another genetic approach to halting cell mutation is using short strands of artificial DNA engineered to lock onto portions of the defective genes and dissolve them. The experimental treatments are called "anti-sense" drugs because they gum up the gene segments that relay operating instructions to the working parts of a cell. They're now being tested against ovarian, lung, brain, rectal, pancreatic, colon, and breast cancers.

3
CANCER VACCINES
Shots That Incite the Immune System to Attack Malignancies

"FROM THE START I knew it was going to be a fight," says Gina Rivera, age 50, a lieutenant commander in the U.S. Public Health Service in Honolulu who found out she had colon cancer in 1994. Since then she's endured a grueling course of chemo and two brutal operations, while the tumors nonetheless spread to her lungs. "Even before the surgery I sat down with my oncologist and said, 'What's next for me? Isn't there something else we should try?'" The answer astonished her.

Dozens of experimental treatments were already being tested on people with colon cancer. "All it took was one call," Rivera says, to a toll-free number maintained by the National Cancer Institute. Three months later she was on her way to its Maryland headquarters to receive her first dose of a new vaccine. Unlike a flu shot, which is designed to *prevent* disease, her vaccine would help fight an illness already raging.

The idea behind all vaccines is simple. The immune system detects invaders like cold or flu viruses by way of telltale molecules on their surfaces—microscopic fingerprints. Once the system spots a foreign print, it attacks and eventually destroys the infectious agent that carries it. Standard vaccines are harmless versions of the same foreign molecules—sometimes in the form of killed or severely weakened viruses—that alert and mobilize the immune system in advance of infection. If the real enemy comes along, the body is ready.

In theory, the same approach could be used to prime the immune system to kill cancer cells. But there's a catch. Unlike viruses and bacteria, tumors aren't foreign invaders; they're our own cells gone awry, and they still look like family to the immune system. That's probably why immune cells seldom disturb tumors. "So the trick is to identify key changes that occur when a normal cell becomes cancerous," says Greg Curt, who directs in-house clinical research at the NCI, "tiny alterations on the surface of the cell that we can wave like a red flag in front of the immune system and say, 'This is a bad guy now. Get him.'"

Rivera's experimental vaccine targets a change that occurs on colon cells when the gene that orders them to divide, called RAS, gets stuck in the on position. It's estimated that up to 20 percent of *all* cancers have defective RAS genes, so the vaccine has promise beyond treatment of colon cancer. NCI researchers are also testing vaccines against mutations of the crucial p53 gene. Researchers hope the shot will alert immune cells to the alteration, prompting them to destroy the tumor.

After three monthly treatments, Rivera held her breath: Only if her tumors had remained the same size or shrunk would she be allowed to go on. "It was a very nervous time," she says. No matter what she'd tried in the past, the cancer had roared back. But tests revealed that the tumors hadn't grown or spread for the first time since her diagnosis. A month later she was back in Maryland to start the next three treatments.

Oncologist Samir Khleif, who's directing the NCI study, is nonetheless cautious. "It's too early to know if the vaccine is making any difference and, if it is, whether it will go on working," he says. Still, many cancer experts are hopeful. Shots against cancers of the skin, breast, ovaries, cervix, colon, pancreas, stomach, and lungs are currently being tested in humans.

At the John Wayne Cancer Institute in Santa Monica, California, researchers have devised a powerful melanoma vaccine called C-VAX. "Not all patients respond," says Donald Morton, who developed the shot. "But among those who do, survival has increased from seven and a half months to 76 months. So we're very excited." The final tests needed to win FDA approval have just begun at 22 cancer centers around the world.

Lifesaving Tests

The surest way to beat cancer is to detect it early. The odds of surviving colon cancer are nine in ten when it's discovered before it spreads but less than one in 14 after.

What's more, a full 97 percent of women diagnosed with localized breast cancer are alive five years later, compared to only 20 percent of those found to have metastasized breast cancer.

While researchers still debate exactly which tests are most important and at what age people should start going in for regular exams, virtually all experts agree that early detection saves lives. Here's what an advance-warning program should include. —*P.J.*

BREAST

Self-examination monthly from age 20. Any new or suspicious lumps should be checked by a doctor.

Breast exam by a doctor every three years from age 20 to 39. Annually from age 40.

Mammogram every year or two from age 40.

CERVIX

Pelvic exam with Pap smear annually from age 18 and for younger women who are sexually active. After three consecutive normal results, some doctors recommend testing less frequently.

SKIN

Self-examination once a month. Look for unusual pearly bumps or red scaly patches. Also check for moles that have changed size or color, or have begun to ooze or bleed easily.

COLON

Fecal occult blood test every year from age 50.

Digital rectal exam, performed as part of a standard physical exam, annually from age 40.

Sigmoidoscopy, a rectal exam using a flexible lighted tube, every three to five years from age 50.

PROSTATE (MEN)

Prostate-specific antigen (PSA) test annually from age 50.

Digital rectal exam, as part of a standard physical exam, annually from age 40.

4

ANTI-ANGIOGENESIS DRUGS

Therapies Designed to Starve Tumors to Death

TO GROW AND SPREAD, cancer cells have to trick the body into creating extra blood vessels to feed their burgeoning masses. Otherwise cancers would exist only as tiny specks, too small to do harm.

Indeed, many cancers lie low for years. A melanoma may appear as a harmless mole on the skin for five or more years; a cluster of breast cancer cells may lurk for years without causing problems. But then trouble hits: Through mutation, some of the malignant cells gain the ability to signal the body to begin producing new blood vessels, a process called angiogenesis.

"It's as dramatic as a switch being thrown," says Judah Folkman, a researcher at Children's Hospital Medical Center in Boston and the world's leading expert on angiogenesis. "It's at that moment that a cancer becomes potentially dangerous." A tumor that was too small to see can swiftly grow to the size of a marble, a golfball, sometimes even bigger—invading organs, nerves, and bones.

To stop the process, Folkman and other researchers have identified nearly a dozen anti-angiogenic factors—compounds that block blood vessel formation, effectively shutting off a tumor's lifeblood. One discovered in 1985, dubbed TNP-470, is being tested at cancer clinics around the country. Researchers are just beginning to evaluate several other powerful blood vessel blockers, including angiostatin and endostatin.

Already there have been surprises—mostly happy ones. Researchers originally assumed anti-angiogenic drugs would stop cancers from growing but not shrink existing tumors; now it's clear they do both. Cancer specialists likewise thought that the drugs would work only against solid tumors like breast and lung cancers. But the latest animal studies suggest they may also fight cancers of the blood, like leukemia.

Better still, they appear to have few side effects. Since adults normally don't produce new blood vessels, blocking the process doesn't cause trouble. Best of all, cancer cells don't become resistant to these drugs, as they do to chemotherapies.

In one astonishing study mice with an aggressive form of lung cancer were given endostatin after their tumors reached 1 percent of their body weight—the equivalent of a one-and-a-half-pound tumor in a human. When the tumors had shrunk to specks, the drug was discontinued. The cancers began to grow again. Researchers allowed them to reach 2 percent of the mice's body weight before they delivered the drug. Again the tumors withered. No matter how many times the scientists repeated the process, endostatin never lost its punch.

Preliminary studies in humans are equally encouraging. At the Dana-Farber Cancer Institute in Boston, half of the brain cancer patients who received an anti-angiogenic drug along with chemotherapy saw their tumors stop growing or shrink. If good results keep coming, says Folkman, the drugs may soon graduate to broader trials.

"One strategy we're looking at," he says, "is using a drug like angiostatin to reduce a tumor down to a tiny speck and then chemotherapy or radiation to kill the remaining cells. Or it may prove more effective to go the other way: Use conventional therapies first to kill most of the cancer cells and then use an anti-angiogenic drug to keep them from growing back into tumors."

Eventually, he says, it may be possible to spot blood vessels forming in patients whose cancer is in the early stages, then deliver the drugs to stop these small tumors from expanding into life-threatening ones. And because blood vessel blockers seem to have few or no side effects, patients could go on taking them for years.

"Every day our lab gets more than a hundred calls from anxious cancer patients or their families—people begging to get into the latest trials," says Folkman. He tries to respond to as many as possible during off hours, but he can't always tell callers what they hope to hear. "Sure, we're very excited about the prospects. But these are just a few drugs, and they're in clinical trials for a very good reason: because we don't really know yet if or how well they'll work."

Consider the news on using monoclonal antibodies to treat breast cancer. Though some women in studies showed remarkable improvement—in a number of cases complete remission—over time many have seen their cancers grow again. So researchers are checking to see how well the drug works when paired with conventional chemotherapy.

The new treatments, in other words, are likely to be cocktails designed to hit cancer cells from many directions—exactly the approach that has scored dramatic successes against AIDS. After surgery doctors may deliver drug-resistance genes to healthy cells before walloping the cancerous ones with chemotherapy. Then, when most of the malignant cells are gone, they may follow up with a blood vessel blocker to stop any surviving ones from mushrooming into tumors.

"In AIDS drug development it took years for researchers to understand the virus well enough to begin to make truly targeted drugs," says MIT's Weinberg. With the latest combined therapies, AIDS death rates have plummeted farther and faster than anyone had predicted. "We may be just about reaching that point in cancer research."

To be sure, no one's promising miracle cures. The single best way to attack the disease remains to stop it before it starts, by eating wisely, getting out for some exercise, and following through on the other day-to-day choices known to markedly lower risk (staying out of the sun at midday, for instance). Furthermore, regular checkups and self-exams can detect tumors early in their growth, so early that they can be completely wiped out with conventional treatments.

"Once cancer has spread, one of the first goals is to turn cancer into a chronic disease—something that people can live with rather than die of," says Edison Liu of the National Cancer Institute. "But I think we're closing in on that. And believe me, that's a lot."

NEW THERAPIES ARE LIKELY TO BE COCKTAILS THAT HIT CANCER CELLS FROM MANY DIRECTIONS—EXACTLY THE APPROACH THAT HAS WORKED AGAINST AIDS.

Peter Jaret is a contributing editor.

"I need everyone on the right to paddle. Now!"

Wendy Rainkin yells from the stern. It's a gray morning, and Rainkin is steering a sharp cut across Oregon's Willamette River in a dragon boat, a large flat-bottomed Oriental canoe whose prow is festooned with a brightly painted carving of the venerated lizard beast. In Portland racing these craft has become all the rage. This morning alone, a half-dozen surge upriver. It takes two rows of ten paddlers pulling with all their might to power one of these boats, in this case a boat containing 21 women recovering from breast cancer.

Rainkin, 50, first felt the lump in her breast in the spring of 1995. A year later, after surgery to remove the tumor and six rounds of chemotherapy to kill off what cancerous cells

HEALING POWER

By Leslie Kaufman

SPECIAL EXERCISES HELPED WENDY RAINKIN BEAT A FRIGHTENING COMPLICATION FROM BREAST CANCER—AND WIN A PRESTIGIOUS SPOT ON A DRAGON BOAT CREWED BY CANCER SURVIVORS LIKE HERSELF.

remained, she was drained but determined to move on. Then she received a letter from the Susan G. Komen Breast Cancer Foundation asking for survivors who wanted to paddle. She knew right away that the boat was just the thing she was looking for to prove to herself she could conquer her illness. The crew's medical adviser, Diane Elliot, an internist at the Human Performance Laboratory in Portland and a leader in the growing movement to treat chronic illness with exercise, met the group in January and told them, "I am talking to you not as patients but as athletes."

Unfortunately, as even Elliot concedes, breast cancer is a lifelong challenge. Chemotherapy leaves many patients perilously weak, and some never fully recover from its effects. Among women who undergo surgery—which is normally accompanied by the removal of lymph nodes at the armpit to see if the cancer has spread—a full quarter suffer lymphedema, an excruciating swelling that occurs when the body can't drain fluids from the arm.

Soon after Rainkin signed up to paddle, she contracted a case of lymphedema so serious she couldn't close her right hand. The pain was bad enough, but even worse was hearing the

From *Health,* October 1997, pp. 75-80. © 1997 by Time Publishing Ventures, Inc. Reprinted by permission.

advice doctors have traditionally given: Avoid unnecessary lifting or gripping. "I went into this depression. Here I thought I had met all the obstacles in front of me, and suddenly there was one more barrier. I was afraid to go to my doctor, because I really needed to join this boat and be with the group of women. I couldn't be told no."

But Rainkin's oncologist surprised her. "You can do this," he said; in recent years doctors have discovered that one of the best remedies for lymphedema is actually exercise. Relieved, she went to a physical therapist who coached her on doing gentle strengthening moves like making a fist or grasping a pulley.

Today Rainkin stands aft on the boat and manages its large awkward tiller. To turn the heavy craft, she grabs the rough handle and throws her entire weight against it. The moves hardly hurt. And Rainkin, tall and broad with cropped brown hair, is the picture of fitness. Of her turnaround she says, "It was like going from the very depths to the heights."

Thirty years ago in America most doctors advised people with chronic diseases to conserve their energy for healing. Heart attack victims were told to take it easy, hypertensives not to exert themselves, people with bad backs to lie down, those with nervous disorders to stay motionless in a dark room, and arthritics to wait for a wheelchair.

What a difference a few decades make. Knowledgeable doctors now prescribe exercise for these ailments and many more. At the Mayo Clinic heart transplant patients get their own stationary bicycles in their rooms. Two days after surgeons open their chests, the organ recipients are pedaling away. (Bypass patients get similar treatment.) At Tufts University elderly women diagnosed with osteoporosis pump plates of iron that often tip the scales at 60 percent of their body weight. Moreover, some 350 U.S. hospitals boast full-service gyms—complete with Olympic-size pools and basketball courts—and the number grows every year.

Why the sea change? Exercise works wonders. It can free diabetics from insulin and hypertensives from blood pressure medication. It allays arthritis pain and lifts depression. When exercise can't halt a disease, it can treat its worst symptoms and delay the need for drugs. It can even reverse the tolls of old age. "No medicine will enable you to do what gets you out of a nursing home, like lifting groceries up the steps," says University of Pittsburgh internist Geoffrey Moore, coeditor of the American College of Sports Medicine's guidelines for patients with chronic disease. "Just exercise."

Put it all together and you see why Steven Blair of the Cooper Institute for Aerobics Research in Dallas—perhaps the nation's most influential exercise scientist—calls physical activity one of medicine's most effective treatments. After all, what other therapy can lengthen and improve the lives of people with everything from asthma and arthritis to chronic fatigue, lupus, and renal failure? Blair's research shows that among people with the same illness, exercisers live the longest. "It doesn't matter how you slice the pie," Blair says. "The fit do best."

IN THIS ERA of health clubs and personal trainers, it's hard to imagine that the exercise prescription was ever anything but common sense. Yet at the turn of the century notions about healing were moving in the opposite direction. Tuberculosis was raging across America. TB patients waste away, so physicians plausibly supposed that hours resting in the sun and a diet of fatty foods were the solution. At the sanatoriums where people with TB and other illnesses were sent, doctors began prescribing this therapy for a widening circle of ailments. By the 1930s patients of every sort, from women who had just given birth to heart attack victims, were urged to lounge about. The advent of the bed rest movement coincided with the invention of the first truly effective drugs, so the genius of the latter hid the folly of the former for decades.

When Elliot and Goldberg proposed **pulling patients off drugs to start them exercising,** other doctors reacted. "You want to do *what?*"

To see how such ideas were finally overthrown, a good place to begin is the Human Performance Laboratory, where Elliot, 46, and fellow internist Linn Goldberg, 50, conduct their research. Neither doctor had entered medical school with the intention of studying exercise, but as gym hounds (both lift weights with a passion) they soon gravitated toward the field. It was the mid-1970s, when fitness therapy was a new proposition and controversial. Several studies indicating that aerobic workouts benefit heart patients had started the ball rolling, yet doctors hardly rushed to embrace the news. In 1975 less than 2 percent of Americans who had heart attacks received any formal exercise rehabilitation. And there wasn't much evidence that working out was effective against other diseases. Of those doctors who wanted to study exercise's curative powers, Blair recalls, "We were lower than nutritionists. We were considered faddists."

The emphasis then was on prevention: to study people at risk for a disease, not already sick with it. Even so, Elliot says, getting approval for studies was difficult. Pulling people off one drug to test another was common practice, but pulling someone off a drug to start an exercise program was unheard of. "They would say, 'You want to do *what?*'" Elliot recalls.

Still, in 1983 Goldberg and Elliot got permission to test out weight lifting on six men and eight women with high cholesterol, a major risk factor for heart disease. After the subjects hoisted progressively heavier weights for 16 weeks, their low-density lipoprotein (bad cholesterol) had dropped nearly 20 percent. The elite *Journal of the American Medical Association* published their findings, winning them a small avalanche of coverage and some latitude for future work. In one study they found that exercisers showing signs of glaucoma (a buildup of fluid and pressure within the iris) could stop the disease in its tracks. In other projects they have investigated exercise's effectiveness for patients with heart disease, fibromyalgia, obesity, hypertension, and Parkinson's disease. By 1994 the two doctors had made enough progress to supervise creation of a bible of sorts, the 344-page *Exercise for Prevention and Treatment of*

Illness. It details how doctors should use exercise against almost every major illness. "There's no longer any doubt," Goldberg says. "Exercise is bona fide medical therapy."

Exercise works its magic in essentially two ways, depending on whether it's building strength or aerobic fitness. With strength training, the body responds directly to the stress of lifting weights by adding bulk to the muscle cells. Larger, better-trained muscles process oxygen more efficiently so the heart doesn't have to pump as hard to keep them supplied, which is why weight lifting is a recommended treatment for cardiovascular disease. And for people with osteoarthritis, whose joints swell painfully because they have lost cartilage between their bones, the best way to compensate is to build up surrounding muscle.

Regular aerobic exercise could potentially **charge up the immune system** enough to stop the spread of existing cancers.

Aerobic exercise's effects are more complicated. By prompting the release of key hormones, it seems to trigger several feedback loops that combat disease. One relatively simple code that scientists think they have cracked relates to hypertension, a condition sometimes brought about by an excess of the hormones adrenaline and noradrenaline. Bodies release the hormones in response to threatening stimuli—an evolutionary development of great use in the Stone Age. But the doses produced day in, day out by an easily agitated modern person cause the heart to race and bring extra sugar into the blood as a kind of fast food for muscles, actions that together raise blood pressure above normal. To treat the disease doctors often prescribe drugs called beta-blockers, which compete with the hormones for position in the cell receptor (called beta) that triggers their effect. The drugs, however, can carry serious baggage: sluggishness and impotence. Thankfully, exercise is a natural beta-blocker. With exertion, muscles become more efficient—practice makes perfect—at processing adrenaline and noradrenaline. The beta cells signal the adrenal gland to slow down, reducing levels of the hormones in the body.

Research confirms that exercising several times a week lowers the average hypertensive's blood pressure by ten points. Some people, Elliot's patients Bill Sugahiro and Bob Earnest, for instance, get more dramatic results. When a person's top number, the systolic pressure, goes above 150, risks for stroke and congestive heart failure double. In 1985 Sugahiro's systolic was measured at 200. Over the next two years Sugahiro, a lawyer, tried half a dozen medications, but all gave him trouble. He recalls feeling so drugged at times that he could barely confer with clients sitting on the other side of his 36-inch-wide desk. "It was like talking to them through a tunnel," he says. Earnest's situation was more dire. Rushed to the hospital in 1987 when his back gave out, he was stunned to learn his systolic pressure was 210. At that rate, a doctor told his wife, she would soon be a widow.

Later that year the two men each responded to an ad that Elliot and Goldberg had placed in the paper seeking subjects for an exercise experiment. Both men worried that they'd be embarrassed. Sugahiro exercised sporadically, an occasional weekend game of golf or tennis. Earnest was totally sedentary. After three months of cycling for 30 minutes five times a week, both showed blood pressure drops large enough that they could greatly lower the dosage of their medications. Having becoming buddies, they decided to keep exercising together. Today their blood pressure is normal: 120 over 80. As long as they keep it up, they are cured.

Aerobic exercise can also charge up the immune system's ability to fight disease. In response to the stress of a brisk walk, run, or bike ride, the body releases two hormones—adrenaline and cortisol—that act to free so-called T cells from the bones and spleen, where they are stored, and flush them into the blood, where they play several important roles in defending the body from invaders. Arthur LaPerriere, an associate professor at the University of Miami's medical school, found that HIV-positive patients who rode stationary bicycles three times a week boosted their T cell count and as a result improved their health. Potentially an exercise-charged immune system might even stop the spread of *cancerous* cells. J. Mark Davis, a professor of exercise science at the University of South Carolina, recently injected mice with tumor cells. After 12 days mice who ran on their version of a treadmill once a day had substantially fewer tumors growing in their lungs.

Even when exercise can't reverse a disease, it can often alter its course. Faith Ottery, a surgical oncologist and nutritionist in Philadelphia, says that 20 to 40 percent of cancer patients die from complications of malnutrition and inactivity. Studies have found that they get caught in a pernicious cycle, she says: Every week of bed rest causes them to lose 4 percent of their muscle mass, the tissue in the body that most demands nutrients. As a result, they take in as little as 500 calories a day. It's no surprise when their lungs collapse or hearts stop. After all, their muscles have no fuel.

Ottery tells of a 49-year-old woman whose weight had dropped from 126 pounds to 84 during her treatment for pancreatic cancer and who, by the time Ottery saw her, couldn't walk across her living room. The tumor had been removed, but she was so weak her life was in danger. As part of a nutrition regimen, the doctor started the woman walking around the house every day, then persuaded her to carry two-pound weights in her hands as she tottered about. Slowly her strength and appetite returned, and she added resistance work with exercise bands. The woman now weighs 115 pounds and is back at her demanding full-time job as a photo assistant; her cancer remains in remission.

EXERCISE IS NO MAGIC BULLET, of course. But Goldberg and Elliot think research has yet to explore its full potential. "No pharmaceutical companies will pay doc-

Your Prescription Is Ready . . .

If exercise were a pill, it would be a medical breakthrough on a par with the invention of penicillin. You can't swallow fitness in gelatin capsules, though. To get the therapeutic benefits, you must find a regimen that's proven to work against your specific illness *and* that supplies enough of a mental and physical lift to keep you coming back for more. Here is the American College of Sports Medicine's get-started advice for the five most common ailments. Ask your doctor for a more specific prescription.

ARTHRITIS (33 million Americans)
WHAT WORKS BEST Daily stretching and low-impact aerobic exercise (walking, swimming), plus two or three weekly sessions of strength training.
WHAT TO EXPECT For people with either rheumatoid arthritis or osteoarthritis, less pain and more freedom of movement. However, be careful to pause when anything hurts, and don't overexert yourself; risks include spinal cord compression and low back pain.

HYPERTENSION (28 million)
WHAT WORKS BEST Moderate aerobic exercise—at a pace that allows for conversation—and weight training. (Before starting a program, people with severe hypertension should lower their blood pressure with medication.)
WHAT TO EXPECT On average, a ten- to 15-point drop in blood pressure after four months. That's often enough to make medication unnecessary. But stay at it: Blood pressure usually rises again if you stop exercising.

OSTEOPOROSIS (25 million)
WHAT WORKS BEST Two or three weekly weight lifting workouts for arms and legs.
WHAT TO EXPECT A halt of bone loss; some women actually rebuild bone.

DEPRESSION (17 million)
WHAT WORKS BEST Group aerobic and weight workouts. Among women, weight lifting in particular seems to improve self-image.
WHAT TO EXPECT Regular exercise relieves symptoms in many, though not all, sufferers.

DIABETES (8 million)
WHAT WORKS BEST Daily walking, running, biking, or other aerobic exercise—the more vigorous, the better.
WHAT TO EXPECT For insulin-dependent diabetics, greater control of blood sugar (though exercise needs to be coordinated with insulin shots and meals.) For Type 2 diabetics, weight loss and a reduction in medication dosage; some eliminate the need to take insulin altogether. *—L.K.*

tors to have patients exercise and not take drugs," Goldberg says. Without large controlled studies pushing exercise to the forefront, many doctors find it easier to write prescriptions than to urge patients to put their muscles to work.

An even more formidable limit is what Goldberg calls the compliance problem. Less than 20 percent of healthy Americans exercise regularly. For the tens of millions with a chronic illness, the challenge is all the more daunting. Studies show that among heart attack victims who know that their lives depend on their getting up and moving, fewer than half stick to a program of moderate activity. People with less threatening ailments—arthritis, say, or chronic fatigue—are even less inclined to work out. Only with repeated prodding, says Elliot, does she manage to overcome such resistance among her own patients at the Oregon Health Science's outpatient clinic. "Most doctors just give up," she says. "I have faith in gentle persistence."

Gentle persistence made the difference for Wendy Rainkin. By the time she started going to practices with her boat last winter, the special exercises were helping her lymphedema, but it was obvious that as a paddler she couldn't keep up with the team's pace—nearly 72 strokes a minute. Still, she couldn't bear to give up. Keeping her doubts to herself, she volunteered to take the tiller. Other women had rotated through the position, but Rainkin, who has a background in sailing, understood intuitively how to maneuver the rudder. Of course, the job required a strong grip—just the thing her ailment might have made impossible. But Rainkin wanted it badly. Off the boat she and her therapist kept exercising her hand and arm; on the boat she just winced when she felt pain.

The homestretch of a dragon boat outing is the real test of a helmsman's skill, especially on a day like this, when all the boats head for the dock at the same time. To get there, they have to pass through a narrow opening into a harbor and make several tight turns. Six boats jostle for a space 20 feet wide. The voices of paddlers mix noisily with the pounding of the drummers that several teams employ to keep rhythm. But Rainkin stands calmly in the back, clasping the tiller and pushing hard against the weight of the river. Her teammates know this is her moment and cheer her on. "Go, Wendy!" "You're doing a great job." "Keep it up, Wendy!"

Sure enough, the boat slips through the bustle and slides smoothly alongside the dock. It is a moment of the will's triumph over the body. Her lymphedema is behind her along with her cancer, and what makes it sweet for Rainkin is that, unlike all the treatments that came before, this wasn't bestowed upon her by a hospital. "You know," she says, "I feel I've earned it."

Leslie Kaufman is a staff writer at Newsweek.

Unit 6

Unit Selections

Key Points to Consider

❖ Based on the readings, why do you think the experience of addiction is different for women than for men?

❖ What issues would be of special concern to women seeking treatment for addiction?

❖ Of the substances discussed in this section, which do you consider to be the most harmful and why?

❖ Why is noncompliance such a costly problem for our society?

❖ What precautions would you take to ensure your safety if you had to take medication?

DUSHKIN ONLINE Links

www.dushkin.com/online/

22. **National Clearinghouse for Alcohol and Drug Information**
http://www.health.org/women.htm
23. **National Institute on Drug Abuse (NIDA)**
http://www.nida.nih.gov/WHGD/WHGDHome.html

These sites are annotated on pages 4 and 5.

Substance Abuse: New Trends for Women

The title of this unit reflects the necessity of discussing drug-related issues beyond the realm of drug abuse or addiction. Conversely, issues of addiction often encompass substances and behaviors that have little to do with drugs or alcohol.

The discussions begins with "What Does Being Female Have to Do with It?" In this article the author makes the distinction between men and women clear in terms of both the diagnosis and treatment of addiction. Unless and until these distinctions are addressed, women will remain reluctant to enter treatment, and they will experience a lesser degree of success in treatment. "Why Women Drink" helps to support this distinction by discussing the specific effects of alcohol on the female body. "An Alcoholic in the Family" puts a human face on the concept of addiction. In this selection, the author describes the history of alcohol addiction in her own family and its meaning for her own life and the lives of her children. Along the same lines, "Prescription for Addiction: Confessions of a Pill Popper" tells the story of a normal girl from a normal family as she battles both depression and addiction.

Continuing the examination of addictive substances, "Stop Smoking" illustrates the power of nicotine on the human brain. Of the 16 million Americans who want to quit, only about 15 percent of them will be able to. "Kickin' Butt" addresses the same issue but profiles the problem in a younger audience. To complete the discussion of addictive substances and women, "Way Out West and Under the Influence" acquaints the reader with the growing problem of methamphetamine abuse.

Turning attention to problems involving nonaddictive substances, "Legal Drugs' Lethal Side Effects" alerts the reader to a little-known fact. More people die as a result of side effects from legal drugs than do from street drugs. This selection points out the disturbing flaws in the system that is meant to protect the public from harmful drug effects. Finally, "Prescription for Disaster" deals with another deadly serious yet frequently overlooked drug-related problem: noncompliance. Noncompliance means the failure to use medication properly. Failure to do so costs this country dearly both in terms of money spent and human suffering.

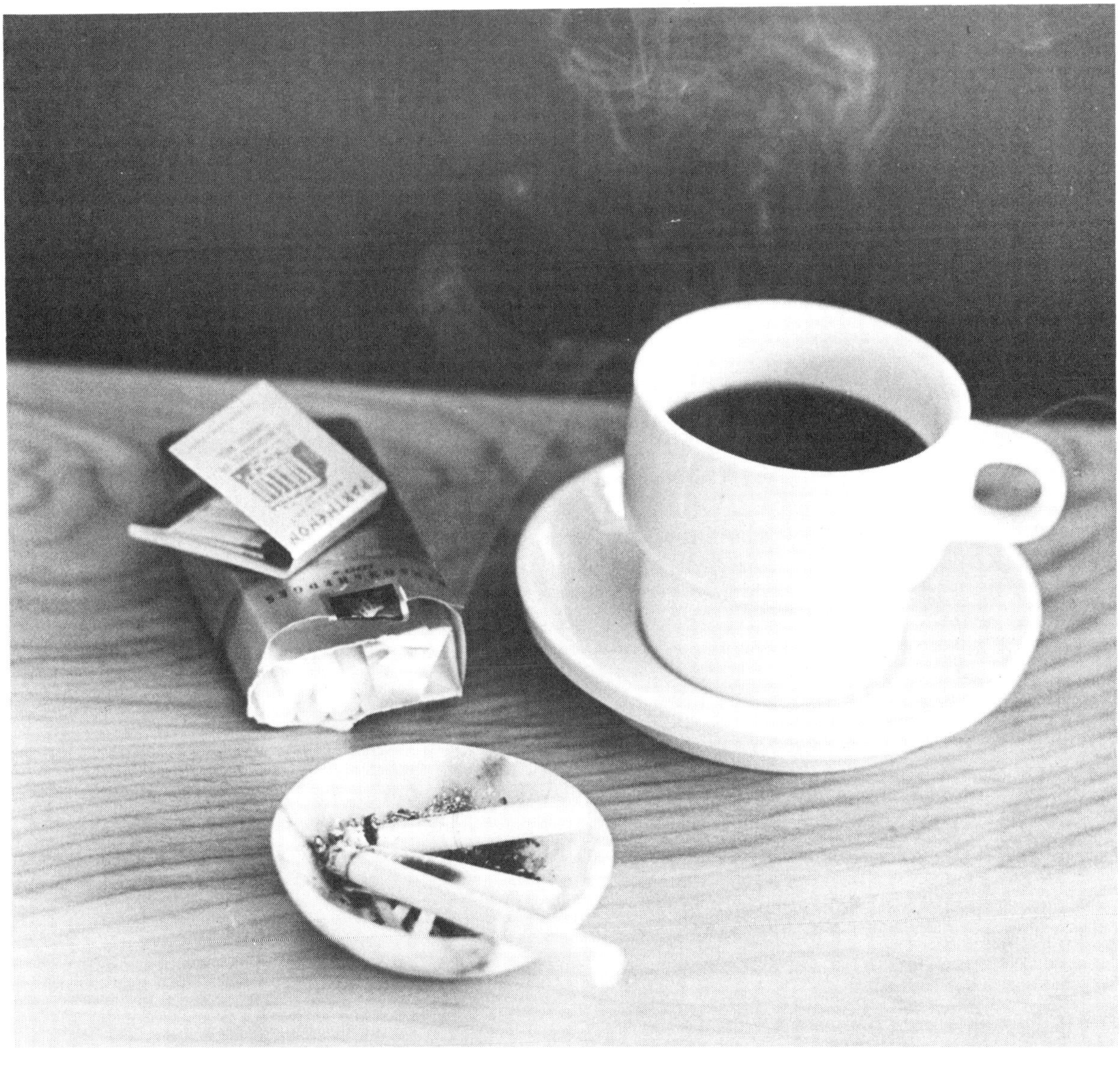

What Does Being Female Have to Do With It?

ROKELLE LERNER

Rokelle Lerner is an international consultant, lecturer and author on addictions and family systems, and clinical advisor to Marworth Treatment Center and Sierra Tucson.

The developmental and psychological pathways that lead women to drug use are different than those followed by men. Female addicts and alcoholics exhibit more depression and more suicidal tendencies than males, and report a far greater incidence of physical or sexual abuse as well as a greater incidence of family substance abuse.

Women also tend to get to treatment at much later stages of the disease than men, due in part to our society's reluctance to acknowledge female alcoholics and addicts.

It starts early. One study revealed that the average age of a child when she or he learns of Dad's alcoholism is approximately 12.6 years. The average age of the child who recognizes that Mom is an alcoholic is 18.3 years. The fact that women hold many more menial positions in the workplace — or do their work in the confines of their home — helps them to more easily "hide."

We also have to acknowledge that culturally women have lower self-esteem than men. The shame of being a woman goes way back, as is evidenced by the quote of Thomas Aquinas: "A woman is a man gone wrong"; or the Orthodox Jewish prayer: "Dear God, thank you for not making me a woman."

Women who are addicted carry not only the cultural shame of being a woman, but also being a woman who is alcoholic or addicted. If a man drinks he may be considered to be funny, just acting foolish or simply having a good time. When a woman drinks she is called a lush, a "floozy," sometimes a whore.

Because of their sensitivity to relationships, women will often take care of others before they care for themselves. Recent studies on women's development reveal that this is not necessarily pathological. Men are trained to develop an ethic of "justice" while women are trained to develop an ethic of "care." Nevertheless, women are as often called codependent and, again, shamed because of their caring.

Many woman have medicated themselves with drugs or alcohol to avoid dealing with the pain of childhood sexual abuse. In fact, the *majority* of addicted women have a history of incest, sexual abuse and physical abuse. In these cases, women have used alcohol or drugs to self-induce a dissociative state. Once sober, these painful memories may recur.

Counselors who deal with women need to be aware of women's inherent shame and low self-esteem. Because of these feelings, it is possible that once a woman is sober, rather than feeling better many recovering women find that they need help for depression, obsessive compulsive disorders or eating disorders — all powerful triggers for relapse.

While delving into these issues may not be totally appropriate in early sobriety, women need to learn how to soothe themselves when flashbacks and anxiety occur. If a woman brings these issues forward in treatment, then it will be crucial for her to know she can get help.

Communication is the key to success. I suggest to women in recovery that if they find that during or after treatment they suffer from depression, anxiety, eating disorders or other problems, they should communicate this to their loved ones. It will not only help them to understand why the woman may be having a difficult time, but it will also provide the woman with the support she needs and deserves.

It is of utmost importance for women inpatients to talk about their relationships with their spouse and their children before returning home. One aspect of the homecoming that recovering women fear most is their ability to be intimate and sexual with their partners. Many women feel that they can only be romantic or sexual when they are using. We need to remind women to be gentle and patient with themselves while they discover their sober, recovering lives.

If a recovering woman is reluctant to return home, we cannot assume that her reluctance is simply a normal response to returning to family life; it may be violence or battering she fears.

If we ask a woman if she is being beaten at home, she will probably say no. However, if we ask specifically, "Have you been shoved, slapped, bruised or threatened?" we may get a very different response. If a woman is returning to a home where she is battered, then her sobriety and, quite possibly, her life are at risk. We must provide her with resources for help.

With most of the addictions research based on men, it is no surprise why many women have difficulty in the treatment and recovery process of addiction. Carol Gilligan, author of *In A Different Voice*, puts it eloquently: "It all goes back to Adam and Eve, a story which shows, of course, that if you make a woman out of a man, you're bound to get into trouble!"

Recovery means finding a way of living that works for us: spiritually, emotionally and physically. We need to attend to the special needs of women to help them find ways of making their lives more joyful, peaceful and loving.

Why Women Drink

For millions of women, being the life of the party has become a dangerous addiction.

By Bob Trebilcock

New research shows that alcohol abuse has become a very serious problem for American women. In this special report, we'll tell you why more and more women are driven to drink. Plus, one woman's journey from the bottom of the bottle to recovery.

Kim Stapleton's car spun out of control on a dark Connecticut highway, then smashed into a guardrail. Shaken but unharmed, Kim stumbled out onto the road. She was drunk, just as she'd been almost every night for the last few weeks. A friend's words rang in her ears: "If only you could see what I see right now, you would stop drinking."

This wasn't the first time someone had urged Kim to give up alcohol. At twenty-four, she had been drinking for nearly half her life. But it was the first time the words made an impact.

"Alcohol was making me crazy," Kim says now from her home near New Haven, Connecticut. "I knew that if I didn't get sober, I'd be dead. I could not go on."

That was thirteen years ago, and Kim has not had a drink since. Today, at thirty-seven, she is a personnel consultant for an employment agency. She and her husband of eight years have a five-year-old daughter and an eleven-month-old son. "Each thing that I have achieved is a miracle," says Kim—a miracle she attributes to sobriety.

Kim's journey into alcoholism is a familiar story, according to a comprehensive two-year study of the impact of alcohol and substance abuse on women by The National Center on Addiction and Substance Abuse (CASA) at Columbia University, in New York City. Today, 4.5 million women are alcoholics or alcohol abusers. While more men than women have traditionally drunk to excess, the gender gap has been closing since World War II, especially among women under thirty-five. Adolescent girls are now equally as likely to drink as adolescent boys.

THE FACTS ABOUT WOMEN AND DRINKING

- Number of Americans with a drinking problem: **13.8 million**
- Number of women with a drinking problem: **4.5 million**
- Number of women who consume at least sixty drinks per month: **2.5 million**
- Alcoholic beverage women drink most often: **wine**
- Age at which most female alcoholics start drinking: **thirteen**
- Estimated number of children who live in households with at least one alcoholic parent: **6.6 million**
- Percentage of Alcoholics Anonymous (AA) members who are women: **35**
- Percentage of AA members aged thirty and under who are women: **43**
- Most frequently reported barrier to treatment for alcoholic women: **lack of child care**

—B.T.

SOURCES: THE GALLUP ORGANIZATION, THE NATIONAL INSTITUTE OF ALCOHOL ABUSE AND ALCOHOLISM, AND THE NATIONAL COUNCIL ON ALCOHOLISM AND DRUG DEPENDENCE

None of these findings comes as a surprise to Kim. "I know there are other women experiencing the shame and loneliness that I experienced as an alcoholic," she says. "As women, we're supposed to carry the emotional strength of the family and be in control. When you're drinking, you're not in control. You feel worthless."

All in the family

For Kim, alcoholism was a family tradition. Her maternal grandmother died of alcohol-related diseases. Kim's mother, Sue, began drinking at age fourteen; by the time she was thirty, she was a functioning alcoholic, divorced and raising three young daughters.

A shy and lonely child, Kim felt estranged from both her parents after their divorce. Although her father often visited, he was preoccupied with his restaurant business. Her mother was completely unpredictable. Sober, she was attentive and nurturing; returning home drunk from a night out, Sue was loud and belligerent.

Late one night when Kim was ten, she heard her mother arguing with a boyfriend, then knocking over furniture after he left. When Sue came upstairs, Kim accused her of being drunk. Sue lost control, screaming and yelling. Kim locked herself in her bedroom.

The next morning, when Kim and her sisters crept out of their rooms, Sue was passed out on the sofa. When she finally came to, "all three of the kids were just looking at me, terrified," recalls Sue, who is now an addictions counselor in Florida. "That was my bottom. For the first time in my life, I connected with my mother's alcoholism. It was devastating."

That was 1971. Once Sue decided to get sober, she threw herself into Alcoholics Anonymous (AA) with the same zeal she used to have for parties with her friends.

But despite the fact that Kim had seen what drinking had done to her mother and grandmother, she didn't shy away from alcohol. In fact, she had her first beer at a beach party when she was just fourteen years old.

At first, says Kim, drinking was like donning Wonder Woman's costume. Normally shy and reserved, she found alcohol made her inhibitions fall away. "Drinking allowed me to open up, become more social and spontaneous," Kim remembers. "I used alcohol as a way to get what I thought I couldn't get sober."

Gradually, Kim graduated from beer to wine to scotch. She blacked out for the first time at age fifteen. "I woke up the next morning extremely hungover and scared because I didn't know where I'd been or what I'd done," remembers Kim. "It was the first time I said to myself, I'll never drink again." Six hours later, she had a beer in her hands.

At sixteen, she had her first drunk-driving accident, killing a neighbor's German shepherd. But no one realized she'd been drinking. The neighbors attributed Kim's hysterics to her shock at having run over the dog.

Kim also managed to hide the extent of her alcohol abuse from her mother. "There were times when I could tell she had been drinking," admits Sue. "I confronted her on occasion. But I didn't realize how frequently she was doing it."

Drinking: A passion

Kim's slide into uncontrolled alcoholism began at college. Drinking or planning to drink consumed her. By the end of the first year, she was asked to leave school. Kim moved to Florida to work as a cocktail waitress in one of her father's restaurants—the perfect job for an alcoholic.

Four months later, she flew home to be the maid of honor in her best friend's wedding. The night before the ceremony, she spent the evening in a bar with her high-school pals. The next morning, Kim didn't wake until eleven A.M., an hour before the ceremony. Reeking of alcohol, she arrived at the church with just enough time to remove the curlers from her hair before the wedding march sounded.

"I was humiliated, and my friend was extremely hurt, disappointed and angry," says Kim. "We're still friends, but it's one of those incidents that will never be forgotten, and that I'll never get over."

Over the next few years, her drinking increased, and she was fired from her restaurant job. Sue realized that her daughter had a serious problem, but she also knew she couldn't prevent her from drinking. "Recovery in AA is about learning to let go of the control of other people," says Sue. As a mother, she adds, "that's the hardest thing that I've ever learned."

In late 1984, Kim, who was now working in another one of her father's restaurants in Connecticut, did try to get sober. "I was screwing up at work, and my relationships with my family were horrendous," she remem-

Why Drinking Is **Worse** For Women

When it comes to alcoholism, the sexes weren't created equal. Women become intoxicated more easily, and suffer more quickly from the long-term effects of drinking. Female alcoholics are twice as likely to die as male alcoholics in the same age group.

The differences begin as soon as an alcoholic beverage passes a woman's lips. Because women have a smaller quantity of body water than men, liquor is concentrated in their blood at a higher level. And due to differences in stomach enzymes, women metabolize alcohol less efficiently. The result: A woman becomes just as drunk as a man after drinking roughly half as much as he did.

Heavy drinking is associated with women's increased risk of hepatitis, pancreatitis and heart disease, and is related to menstrual disorders, infertility and an increased risk of early menopause. Some studies have also linked two or more drinks a day to an increased risk of breast cancer.

bers. She attended AA meetings and stayed sober for a month. Then, one night, she decided to have a drink. She was going to prove to herself that she wasn't an alcoholic.

She failed miserably. Soon, she was drinking every night. Her binge culminated several weeks later in mid-January 1985. She had been drinking at work since eight o'clock that night. After the restaurant closed, she went out to breakfast with a co-worker with whom she had fallen in love. As he tried to explain to Kim that he didn't want a relationship with her, she became angry.

"If only you could see what I see right now, you would stop drinking," he told her. Then he left.

"It was a moment of humiliation and despair," Kim recalls. "I was a drunk."

She got in her car, and a few minutes later, smashed into the guardrail. The next morning, she called her mother for help. "I'm willing to do anything," Kim told her.

Sue told Kim about Arms Acres, a substance-abuse treatment center in Carmel, New York. "It's a place for alcoholics," Sue said.

"I'm not an alcoholic," Kim insisted. "I'm having a breakdown."

"Honey," Sue said, "they'll address all of your problems, but I really think this is the place for you."

Kim hesitated, then said, "I'll go."

The road to recovery

Sue was thrilled that Kim was finally willing to ask for help. "I was feeling such relief," she says. "I saw her as really beaten down, and this was something that could save her."

Kim spent a month and a half at Arms Acres. After an initial forty-eight hours in detox, every minute of her day was scheduled around meetings and therapy. "They break you down," explains Kim. "In treatment, you're forced to face up to your drinking, and that leaves you feeling very vulnerable."

A large part of it, she adds, was

Treatment That Works

In 1976, Jean Kirkpatrick, Ph.D., founded Women For Sobriety (WFS), a self-help group exclusively for women alcoholics, when AA couldn't help her overcome her drinking problem. Today, the group, which is based in Quakertown, Pennsylvania, has more than three hundred fifty chapters. "I believed that women require a different approach," says Kirkpatrick.

The difference between WFS and AA, says Kirkpatrick, is in the underlying philosophy. "AA believes the key to sobriety is your humility and turning your life over to a higher power," she explains. "But alcoholic women need to get their lives back. To maintain sobriety, a woman needs more self-esteem, self-value and self-confidence."

Today, there is a growing awareness that women's needs could be better met in single-sex treatment programs. While the protocol is the same for both female-only and coeducational programs, single-sex groups provide an environment where women can face issues that are unique to them, such as eating disorders and physical or sexual abuse. "Those are significant issues that are unlikely to be addressed or receive the same level of attention in a coed group," says Nancy Waite-O'Brien, Ph.D., director of psychological services at the Betty Ford Center, in Rancho Mirage, California.

At Betty Ford and the Hazelden Foundation, the two best-known centers in the country that offer women-only programs, the average stay is twenty-six to twenty-eight days. The first few days are spent in detoxification, followed by three to four weeks of intensive group therapy. The average cost of treatment at both institutions is about $13,000.

Health insurance no longer routinely covers the total cost of a rehabilitation stay, but "both Betty Ford and Hazelden have assistance programs, as do many other institutions," says Waite-O'Brien. For more information on treatment programs and women-only support groups in your area, contact your local or state social-service agencies, or the United Way, which is often an umbrella group for a number of local programs. Information is also available from:

- **Betty Ford Center at Eisenhower Hospital, 39000 Bob Hope Drive, Rancho Mirage, CA 92270; 760-773-4100**
- **Hazelden Foundation, Box 11, Center City, MN 55012-0011; 800-257-7800**
- **Women For Sobriety, Box 618, Quakertown, PA 18951-0618; 215-536-0826; *www.mediapulse.com/wfs/***
- **National Council On Alcoholism And Drug Dependence, Inc., 12 West 21st St., New York, NY 10010; 800-622-2255.**

What Drives Women To Drink

There is no one reason that women drink, just as there is no simple explanation why men drink. Here are some of the many factors involved:

- **GENETICS AND ENVIRONMENT Female alcoholics are more likely than male alcoholics to have a family history of the disease.**
- **EMPLOYMENT Women who work in male-dominated occupations tend to drink more heavily than those in other occupations. According to the study by CASA, women who work outside the home are 67 percent more likely to drink heavily than homemakers.**
- **MARRIAGE Women who have never been married are 50 percent more likely to drink heavily than married women.**
- **CHILD ABUSE Alcoholic women are twice as likely as nonalcoholic women to have been beaten or sexually abused as a child.**
- **SEXUAL DYSFUNCTION Women alcoholics are likely to suffer sexual dysfunction because alcohol depresses their sexual response. They may then drink to try to "treat" the problem, but alcohol only makes it worse. —B.T.**

learning to understand the things that were the catalysts for her to drink. "Once you acknowledge that you're an alcoholic, you need to connect with people who are going to support and understand that," she explains. "When I got a taste of what my life could be like sober, it was amazing. I felt great. Things looked brighter. The obsession to drink was removed."

After she left the treatment center, Kim stayed at a halfway house, an added measure of support before reentering the real world. She also went into therapy.

A few months later, Kim enrolled in business school, and after graduation in 1986, she walked into an employment agency looking for work. They offered her a job as a recruiter. She has been in the employment industry ever since.

That same year, Kim met Mark Stapleton, a doctoral student in clinical psychology. Kim told him her entire story. "He was incredibly accepting," Kim says. Three years later, they were married.

Occasionally, Kim still craves a drink, especially at the holidays. "In AA, they teach you to think the drink through," she says. "The first sip is wonderful. Then I ask myself, Is the first sip worth what happens five hours later? The answer is no every time for me."

Kim is well aware that her children are predisposed to become alcoholics. "When they are old enough, I'll tell them about my drinking. I want to create an environment where they will feel safe to say anything to me, an environment of open communication."

What does she tell other women who have drinking problems? "That they're not alone, and that there is another way of living," says Kim. "The road to recovery is challenging and difficult, but what's on the other side is truly beyond your wildest dreams."

Bob Trebilcock writes for Reader's Digest and other publications.

MY MOTHER LIKED TO DRINK AND EVENTUALLY BECAME AN ALCOHOLIC. I LIKE TO DRINK, TOO. SO WHAT DOES THAT MAKE ME?

an alcoholic in the family

By **Dorothy Foltz-Gray**

My mother was an early riser who buttered my toast and poured orange juice while I was getting ready for school. But for herself she set out a different breakfast: a cup of creamy, sugared coffee; a tall, iced Coca-Cola; and a pack of cigarettes. At night she curled up on the sofa, watching old movies and beating the gloss off a ribbon of homemade fudge or scooping up handfuls of fresh popcorn.

My mother was drawn to pleasure like a cat. Her indulgences, when I think of them now, seem dangerously childlike, unrestrained by shoulds or shouldn'ts. If she wanted to butter her doughnuts, she did—with gusto. And she schooled me in her enthusiasms, teaching me to roll peppermint creams in salted spanish peanuts. To grill peanut butter sandwiches. To keep candy in my bedside drawer. She was no more embarrassed by these excesses than she was by her big feet.

Except for one: She loved to drink.

I'm not sure I knew how much until I hit drinking age myself, although there were signs—the flow of alcohol at my parents' parties, the array of scotch and ice left behind after cocktails with friends (my sister and I would taste the contents of each glass), the liquored kiss my mother gave me when she returned home from an evening out.

But my mother also associated drinking with a bagful of things nice ladies didn't do, and if Mrs. Smith down the road had a drinking problem, then Mrs. Smith was a no-account, lurching around her house in bare feet, opening the door only to toss out empties. The message I got was this: It is okay to drink but not to talk about it; not to indicate a love for it; and never, ever to get drunk.

My mother had a good reason to keep her love of drinking secret. Her father had been a traveling salesman who drank on the road, an alcoholic who sometimes vanished for days. For my mother, his addiction carried shame and sadness but no warning signal.

Instead, she let my disciplined father curb her impulses. He had drinking rules: only on the weekends, and never alone. Those rules probably held my mother's tendencies in check for years. But I suspect she began drinking alone after my brother, sister, and I left home, occasionally adding a nip of Crown Royal to her late afternoon cola.

Even so, when my father called me years later to say she was drinking too much, I didn't believe him. I thought his need for discipline was spilling over, her pleasures finally getting on his nerves.

And yet I also knew it was true. We were all recovering then from the death of my sister, and my mother remained despondent. But who could blame her? My sister, a psychologist, had been shot by one of her patients, and my mother's grief, so physical, unnerved my father. In that first year of mourning she sat alone in the house, on the sofa where she had once beaten fudge, and let vodka numb the death she carried inside her.

My mother denied her problem for months, despite urgings from my father and aunt to enter a treatment program. When I was home visiting she sometimes asked me to bring her a drink. If I refused, she would respond with fury and a cold shoulder. Eventually my father took her to a nearby treatment center, and within weeks she became one of the lucky ones who quit and actually stick with it.

But her addiction scared me. My adulthood had always been a rumba between my father's restraint and my mother's self-gratification, and it was unclear which side would win. If I let go of my father's stern work ethic, would I sink into my mother's hedonism?

It's easy to think so as I act out the rumba, moving from discipline to pleasure and back again. In fact, the two drives sometimes seem fed by the same source: fear, compulsion, a taste for oblivion. From nine to five I work so hard I beat back anxiety and ego and self-defeat. And then, blessedly, it is dinnertime. I set some peppers and onions simmering and pour a glass of wine. I put my feet up and read the paper. I put out a plate of cheese and crackers or a bowl of peanuts. My husband comes home. He pours a beer. Our two sons join us for hors d'oeuvres. The wine relaxes me, my back stops aching, my work seems far away. I seem far away.

On nights when I drink too much wine, I turn sleepy. I go to bed, and hours later I wake up. My heart is pounding, and my mouth is dry. I am scared. I am my mother.

This is a ritual I love. It lifts me from my kitchen to a remote French bistro. But on nights when I drink two or three glasses of wine, I turn sleepy or grouchy. I go to bed, and hours later I wake up. My heart is pounding, and my mouth is dry. I am scared. I am my mother.

Still, it's not the occasional nights of too much wine that scare me most. It's the fear that one day I could slip over some invisible line into my destiny. Or worse, that Matthew and Jacob, my 11- and 13-year-old sons, could slip as well. They have grown up in a household where drinking is what my husband and I do to relax, to celebrate, to entertain friends. And through me they, too, share my mother's genes.

My mother's turn into alcoholism caught me by surprise—and her as well, I think. Suddenly, it seemed, she had crossed from sobriety to alcoholism. I had always loved the life-embracing enthusiasms I inherited from her, but now I wonder if that trait will one day kill me—or one of my sons.

On most days I'm rational about this. I'm not a heavy drinker. But I have also read Caroline Knapp's memoir, *Drinking: A Love Story,* and seen the ways alcoholics can cloak their addiction in normalcy and denial. And I saw plainly the inheritance that Knapp hid from herself for years: her father's alcoholism. So my questions swirl. How far can genetics propel me and my boys toward addiction? Why do people like my mother and me seem so much more attached to pleasure and its routines than other people? Are these attachments predictors of addiction?

Scientists have known for many years that children of alcoholics face an increased risk for alcoholism. But Marc A. Schuckit, a psychiatrist at the University of California at San Diego and director of the Alcohol Research Center for the Veterans Affairs Medical Center in San Diego, wanted to know precisely what they inherit that increases their risk. For ten years he tracked 450 men, sons of both alcoholics and nonalcoholics.

"What I found is that being able to hold liquor well is a strong predictor of alcoholism," says Schuckit. "What seems to be inherited is a low level of response to alcohol." In other words, sons of alcoholics can drink more than most people before feeling the effects. Schuckit was not surprised by this. "People have a varying level of response to most drugs," he says, "and those responses are usually genetically influenced.

"I don't necessarily think there's a gene for alcoholism," he adds. "But I think there are genes, probably a bunch, that make it more likely you'll drink a lot in a society like ours where drinking is encouraged. You can take any organism, from rat to dog to person, and give it high enough doses of alcohol for a long enough period of time, and it will become physically dependent. What I'm studying is why some people voluntarily take high enough doses over a long enough period to develop dependence."

Indeed, as Schuckit describes in his

research, what struck me was not that my mother and I could easily drink our peers under the table, but that we chose to drink despite our family history. And among the adult children of alcoholics that I know, most drink, worry about it, and still drink. Why?

On the surface, drinking moderately is fun. It's a leavening for the soul, a little buzz-on, as a friend calls it. But for some, liquor's pleasure is more complicated. In my case, drink musters powers against a formidable foe: me. With my oversensitivity, my occasional melancholy, my harsh self-assessment and demanding ego, I can be a drag to inhabit. I sometimes want out of my skin, and liquor takes me there—or at least I believe it does.

This belief, that liquor will tranquilize what's normally inconsolable, may be as dangerous for me as my history is. In studying college binge-drinkers, G. Alan Marlatt, a clinical psychologist and director of the Addictive Behaviors Research Center at the University of Washington in Seattle, found a link between addiction and a belief in alcohol's powers. Drinkers who tended to become dependent gave alcohol what Marlatt calls the magic elixir profile.

"They think, Drinking's the only way I can sleep or be comfortable dating or keep from being depressed," Marlatt says. "They believe that if they don't drink, they will feel worse." To Marlatt's surprise, students who thought they were drinking alcohol but were actually given placebos began to feel as they expected to feel: more relaxed, more comfortable, less depressed.

I don't usually attribute magical powers to liquor. But last year, after writing an article about the dangers of alcohol, I was shaken and decided not to drink for a week. The first evening I began pacing nervously, divorced from my nightly routine. I was anxious and brooding. Where was my bistro? Finally, I took down my wineglass and filled it with bitter tonic water, put my feet up, and read the newspaper. Away went my anxiety, and my body relaxed.

But at the week's end I went back to drinking wine with dinner. I had no desire to eliminate that pleasure. Still, the experience made me realize I had built for myself a life in which alcohol and its trappings played a part. As I paced my kitchen I was responding to cues—the dinner hour, the newspaper, the wine goblet, the cheese plate—that automatically made me reach for a glass of wine.

This type of response has been an important part of the work of Edythe D. London, director of the Brain-Imaging Center at the National Institute on Drug Abuse in Baltimore. To study cocaine addiction, London showed addicts a video of other addicts, crack houses, white powder, and ten-dollar bills, while measuring their brain responses. Two areas of the brain lit up: the amygdala, associated with the recall of pleasant or painful consequences of experiences; and the hippocampus, associated with learning and short-term memory. That research has convinced London that addiction involves the creation of memories and that those memories alone can stir up powerful cravings.

I believe her, for certainly memory, ritual, and routine play parts in all my pleasures, not just alcohol. Would I love pâté as much without my French hors d'oeuvre plates, or my nightly chocolate without a good book and plump comforter? But after acknowledging the power of rituals and their associated cues, I'm still puzzled. Not everyone seems as captive to pleasure and its routines as I am. How come?

None of the experts I spoke with acknowledged an addictive personality per se. But they do believe that certain personality characteristics seem to place people at risk—thrill-seekers, for instance, who expect to like alcohol, or whatever substance they become addicted to, from the start. And as Schuckit shows in his research, these types tend to tolerate substances like alcohol better than most. People who have never learned to funnel stress into a hard bang on the piano may also be at risk.

My mother could have used a dozen pianos. She was anxious about almost everything: what friends thought about her, what her clothes looked like, whether she was gracious enough. And despite her flair for taking pleasure, she was congenitally sad.

"Some people have constitutionally high levels of anxiety or depression, and they haven't been taught to deal with that," says Barbara Wood, a psychologist in Bethesda, Maryland, and author of *Raising Healthy Children in an Alcoholic Home*. "That's a powerful combination that could move someone along the path to addiction."

This explanation helps. When I think of my mother's addiction, it's not genetics that leaps to mind. It's a picture of my salesman grandfather moving from one yard goods store to another in rural Arkansas during the Great Depression. It's my mother growing up at the knee of his darkness, watching her mother, a former elementary school principal who pinned naughty schoolboys to the wall by the neck, scold her self-deprecating father. It's me watching my own mother disappear on the sofa, chiseled away by sadness and a marriage to a man as critical as her mother was. It's the palpable, physical haunt of shame and anxiety that hard work, and wine, and chocolate will anesthetize.

I can say I'm at risk for alcoholism. I can also say I won't stop drinking any more than I'll stop living. But I will think about alcohol's threat like I think about the night after my sister died, when I took a huge goblet from the shelf and filled it to the rim with wine. I was going to drink it all, because I believed that glass could carry me elsewhere. Of course all it did was give me a terrible headache.

I haven't used that goblet since. It sits there on the shelf, a reminder of oblivion and unresolved choices. For now it remains available, empty as air.

Being able to hold your liquor is a strong predictor of alcoholism. And most children of alcoholics can drink their peers under the table.

Dorothy Foltz-Gray is a contributing editor.

prescription FOR ADDICTION

Confessions of a pill popper

by Malina Sarah Saval

There's not much to do in a mental hospital. Mostly we sit around drugged out of our skulls or stand in line at the pill dispensary to get even more drugged out. If we talk too loudly or say something too intelligent, they call us "agitated" and shove tranquilizers down our throats. I am on Tegretol, a mood stabilizer prescribed to manic-depressives and sufferers of epilepsy. The doctors prescribed it to me within 10 minutes of my entering the hospital. All the cool kids on my unit are on Tegretol. Lithium is passé. It makes you shake.

They wake you up early in a mental hospital. The phlebotomist comes every other day at 5 a.m. to draw blood. He runs some tests to make sure the "bad" drugs are out of my body and the "good" drugs are in. Good drugs, bad drugs—it makes no difference to me. As long as I'm not left alone with my mind.

By breakfast time I'm weak and tired, and fall asleep in my plate of wet eggs. A nurse yanks me by the neck, force feeds me a spoonful of runny yellow yoke and tells me I'd better eat. I've lost 10 pounds since I got here. Rumor has it I'm anorexic. Anorexic? I don't want to be skinny. I just want to be stupid.

I explain all this to Dr. Strong*, a detox specialist. We meet every morning for six minutes. And every morning he asks me to explain why I tried to kill myself.

"It was an accident," I say.

"An accident?" he asks.

"An accident. I never tried to kill myself."

"You took five Ativan pills, six Valium tablets and 10 milligrams of Xanax, and you didn't think it would kill you?"

"That's how much I took every morning," I say.

"Tell me why."

"To numb the pain. To stop my brain."

"So you didn't want to die?"

"Of course not! I just wanted to be blank. I wanted to stop the noise in my head. It races all the time. It won't shut up. I never meant to end my life. I only meant to stop the noise so I could get some sleep."

The doctor grunts. It's what doctors do when they don't understand.

"Let me ask you a question," he says. "[Grunt.] How long have you felt this way?"

I shrug, "I don't remember *not* feeling this way."

"Let me ask you another question. [Grunt.] Where on earth did you get all these drugs?"

• • •

Flashback to 1986 . . . I'm in my pediatrician's office, practically screaming, "Give me something to sleep!" My heart is racing. My mind is wired. I'm tired, pale and cranky. I haven't slept in three nights. My pediatrician writes out a prescription for Valium. I'm only 13 years old.

What is that last line in *Casablanca*? Something like . . . This could be the start of a beautiful friendship?

Friendship?

Love affair is more like it.

The Valium works. I sleep. Ah, how I love my little white pills! But then the Valium runs out. My insomnia starts again. I want more Valium. Now!

The pediatrician won't give me a refill. So I find someone who will. I get pills from the allergist, the gynecologist, the ophthalmologist—any doctor ending with an –ist.

At 16, I get my wisdom teeth pulled and leave with a lollipop and a prescription for codeine. It's not Valium, but it helps.

At 17, I contract mononucleosis and have to be put in a hospital. I get Demerol to calm me down, Percodan to dull the pain, Dalmane to make me sleep. It's like a vacation. But the mono clears up and the pills are gone. And back home, I lay awake all night—my mind racing.

By the time I enter college, I've probably lost 1,000 nights of sleep, a fact that frightens me as I sit in my Psych. 101 class listening to my professor lecture about the detrimental effects of sleep deprivation. He says for every hour of sleep lost, that's five minutes off of your life. I must be dying!

I scurry to the health center and beg one of the attending physicians for something, anything to save my life. And, depending on the physician, I get every prescription from Valium to Xanax to a suggestion to take up yoga.

One time I get a referral to a psychologist who doesn't believe in medicine at all. He diagnoses me with "hyperideation." He says I think too much. Duh! He suggests I stay off medicine and start keeping a daily journal of all my thoughts. As silly as his advice seems at the time, it's probably been the best I've gotten.

But even this advice grows quickly out of hand. I don't need a journal. I need many journals. And notebooks and napkins and the backs of menus in restaurants. My thoughts amount to novels. And I still don't feel any better. I am sick.

That's when I hook up with a shrink who diagnoses me with atypical depression (which basically means I'm bummed out

I just **wanted to be blank**. . . to **stop the noise** in my head.

all the time) and starts me on Paxil, an antidepressant. When Paxil doesn't work, he puts me on Ativan, then Klonopin, then Librium. We basically work our way through the entire benzodiazepine family. Maybe I *am* depressed. I don't know. I do know these pills are all downers, and eventually I sleep.

But I wake up feeling awful. Woozy, nauseous, like I have a head-splitting hangover. Even so, I am willing to make the sacrifice to sleep and be blank. Blank feels so good. In fact, I want to be blank all the time, not just when I'm asleep but when I'm awake as well. In order to do this, my doctor has to constantly up my doses of medication. When my body becomes tolerant to two milligrams, he ups my daily intake to three, then four, then five . . . until I'm taking 20 milligrams of Valium. A normal dosage might be five. When my body becomes tolerant of one pill altogether, I switch to another, then another. Before I know it, I'm a college senior juggling five classes, applications to graduate school and a smorgasbord of sedatives.

I alienate all my friends. I lock myself in my room listening to the depressing lyrics of depressed songwriters. I lie in my bed, curl up in a ball and pray for death. And then I get to graduate school. . . .

I spend most of my first semester at the University of Southern California film school slicing my forehead with razor blades, crashing my car and swallowing more pills. I try Ritalin (by this point, I'm so scattered my current psychiatrist thinks I suffer from attention deficit disorder) and Zoloft, an antidepressant in the same family as Paxil. When in doubt, doctors often just prescribe a different drug. It's easier than figuring out what's wrong. But no pill can curb the racing thoughts, the desire to die and the delight in endless sleep. The pills continue to make me nauseous. Yet I take them, hopeful that one day they will work.

And then one morning, something changes.

I don't wake up nauseous. I wake up sick. My hands are clammy and the room is spinning. When I stand up my knees buckle. My throat is red and raw. I can barely talk. I look like Ewan McGregor in *Trainspotting*.

I go from doctor to doctor to find out what's wrong with me now. And doctor after doctor comes up with a different diagnosis, from a relapse of mono to chronic fatigue syndrome. Finally, a specialist in infectious diseases takes one look at my chart and says, "You're a drug addict."

"Drug addict?" All I was ever trying to do was to get some sleep and calm the thoughts and voices playing over and over in my mind. Okay, so I took a few too many pills. And, yeah, the pharmacists at Longs Drugs do know me by face. But a drug addict? Come on. My problem has to do with depression and insomnia, not with drugs. Anyway, none of the other doctors I've seen ever even mentioned drug addiction.

But then the blood test results come back. They confirm that over all these years, the various medications—Valium, Xanax, Ativan, Librium, Klonopin—have wreaked havoc on my central nervous system. The tremors, the sweating and the fevers are the result of spending the last decade using my body as a chemistry lab. I *am* Ewan McGregor in *Trainspotting*.

Two days later, I'm admitted to Thalians Mental Health Center at Cedars-Sinai Medical Center in Los Angeles.

• • •

There's not much to do in a mental hospital, but there is a tight schedule. They map out our entire day, from morning 'til night. Wake up. Breakfast. Exercise. It's like camp. Minus the fun.

Recreation time is the worst. In occupational therapy we make rawhide moccasins—very expensive moccasins when you consider the cost of all the doctor's visits, tests, psychiatric sessions and meals. One day in our spare time, we figured out that a night at the Ritz Hotel is cheaper than a night in a private hospital.

What's really crazy is that, even though I'm supposed to be a drug addict, the doctors are pumping me with even *more* pills. I get a pill to calm me down, a pill to even out my moods, a pill to make me less depressed and a pill to make me sleep. But maybe it's not that crazy after all, because this time, for the first time since I was 13, the drugs actually seem to be working.

I sleep.

After all these years, I finally sleep and have dreams. Dreams about not needing medicine. Dreams about getting released. Dreams about never leaving. And when I awake, I don't feel sick. I feel calm. I feel refreshed. I feel . . . normal.

• • •

It's been eight months since I left Thalians. No one ever did really figure out what's wrong with me. In my 15 days there, I received several diagnoses from several psychiatrists—manic-depression (high highs and low lows, with periods of normalcy in between), bipolar rapid cycling disorder (high highs and low lows, with no normal breaks) and atypical depression. I do know that insomnia is often a symptom of depression, which has plagued me in some form or another throughout my life.

What the doctors finally succeeded at was finding a combination of drugs—Tegretol and Zoloft—that made me feel "normal."

Now I sleep. The racing thoughts have disappeared. I even recently sold my first screenplay. And I certainly don't spend my days curled up in a ball, crying, wishing someone somewhere would "fix" whatever is wrong with me. I, for the most part, am fixed. And it only took 11 years.

**Name has been changed.*

Stop Smoking

BY STEPHANIE WOOD

The Best Ways To Do It For Good

Only 15% of smokers who try to quit actually succeed. We screened dozens of **products and programs** to boost the odds that you or someone you love remain smoke free

"FOR MOST OF MY LIFE, I WOULD HAVE SMOKED THAN EATEN," admits 37-year-old Carla Sarver, an artist in Columbus, IN. Sarver got hooked on cigarettes at 19 and maintained her pack-a-day habit through her diagnosis of diabetes at 34. She thought she'd smoke forever. Then her diabetes worsened to the point where she needed a daily insulin injection.

On her doctor's advice, she tried to quit with the help of nicotine gum. It worked. "The first few weeks were hard," she says, "but then I was motivated by the improvement in my health. Four months after my last cigarette, I no longer needed the insulin. Now when I want a cigarette, I imagine a syringe, and it kills my craving."

More than 16 million Americans try to kick the habit each year, many of them because of failing health. Besides the obvious connection to lung cancer and emphysema, smoking also doubles the chance of a heart attack. Diabetics who smoke, like Sarver, are six to 10 times likelier to have heart disease. In fact, regular exposure to secondhand smoke increases a nonsmoker's risk of developing heart disease, according to a recent study of 32,000 women.

The first challenge is figuring out how to quit. Americans spend $1.2 billion on over-the-counter and prescription nicotine replacement products (about 300,000 boxes of nicotine patches and gum are sold each week), yet only 10% to 15% of those who pledge never to light up again actually remain smoke free for at least six months, according to the Centers for Disease Control and Prevention in Atlanta. To increase your chances of being a successful quitter, most doctors suggest researching what type of smoking-cessation therapy would work best based on your personality type, gender and smoking frequency. Then run your decision by your doctor to make sure it doesn't interfere with any medical conditions you have.

To save you time, we pored over the latest research and examined studies on effectiveness. Our expert guide covers a dozen methods with one goal in mind: Quit smoking for good.

Percentages on the following pages indicate success rates.

CARDIOSTAT

About 24 hours after your last cigarette, your heart attack risk drops, and in a year it's half that of a smoker.

PHOTOGRAPHS BY DAVID COOK

From *American Health for Women,* September 1997, pp. 78-82. © 1997 by Stephanie Wood. Reprinted by permission.

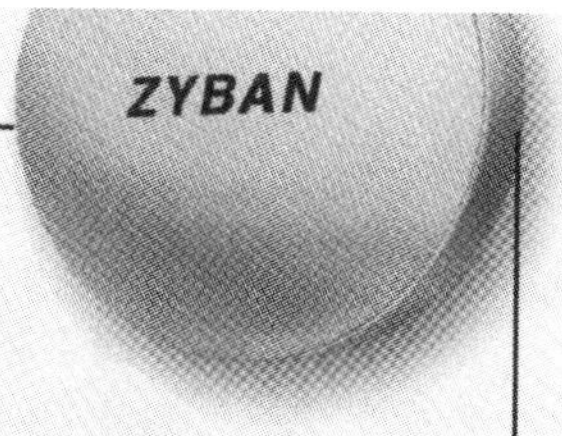

35-50%

Antidepressant

Best for: People who smoke more than a pack daily and have been smoking for at least a year. Those with a history of seizures and eating disorders should avoid the drug.

The lowdown: *Last May the FDA approved Wellbutrin, a prescription drug used to treat depression since 1987, to be marketed for smoking cessation under the name Zyban. It stimulates the production of brain chemicals that have been found to create the same pleasurable sensation as nicotine. Doctors generally prescribe one 150-milligram tablet for the first three days, and then two daily for seven to 12 weeks, depending on your response.*
Cost: $80 to $100 for a month's supply
Biggest hassle: It takes two to six weeks to feel the effect of the drugs.
Insurance coverage: At press time Zyban's manufacturer, Glaxo Wellcome, was meeting with insurers to request that the drug be covered for this purpose.

Hypnosis

20%

Best for: People who smoke mainly in social situations and those with an ability to work well with imagery or suggestion. Heavy smokers should use it in conjunction with a nicotine patch, gum or spray, because it doesn't address the physiological addiction to nicotine; two out of three patients quit smoking when hypnosis is used in conjunction with other therapies such as the patch.

The lowdown: *Upon entering an unconscious state, a patient may reveal her emotional reasons for smoking. The practitioner then helps her develop alternative behaviors to replace the need for cigarettes in her life. Although a hypnotized patient seems to be in a deep sleep, her mind is alert and focused, and she generally remembers what went on during the entire session.*
Cost: Prices usually range from $100 to $200 per session. Plan for five sessions.
Biggest hassle: Finding a trustworthy practitioner. Your best bet is to go to an M.D., such as a psychiatrist, who has experience with hypnotherapy.
Insurance coverage: Likely if it's performed by an M.D.
Resource: For information on how to find an experienced hypnotist, call the Institute for Clinical Hypnosis in Great Neck, NY, at 516-482-1220.

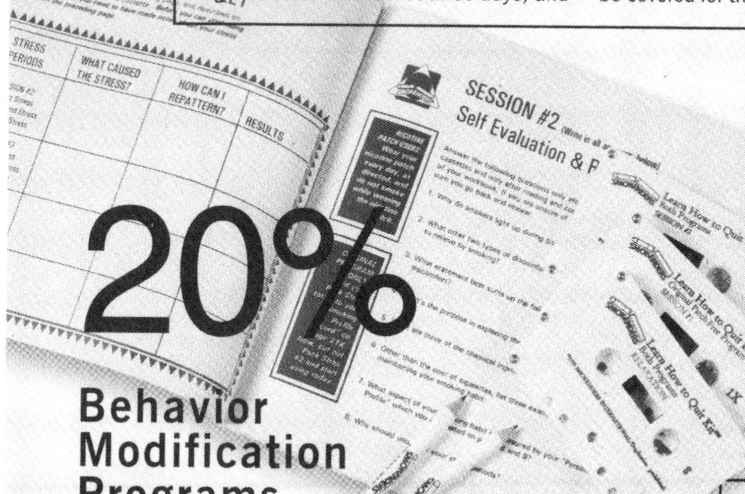

20%

Behavior Modification Programs

Best for: Light smokers. Heavy smokers (two or more packs daily) need to use a nicotine patch, gum or nasal spray too.

The lowdown: *Smoking cessation groups (such as Smoke Stoppers and Smokenders), one-on-one counseling and self-help kits are designed to give smokers the emotional support to quit.*
Cost: When offered by employers, many programs are free. Smoke Stoppers charges $160 for eight meetings. One-on-one counseling ranges from $60 to $95 per session. Kits from Smoke Stoppers or Smokenders cost $75 and $129 respectively.
Biggest hassle: It's time intensive.
Insurance coverage: About half of managed-care plans offer smoking-cessation programs, and the majority of them cover the cost.
Resources: For more information, call the American Lung Association at 800-LUNG-USA, Smoke Stoppers at 800-243-0876, x384, or Smokenders at 800-828-4357.

Ear Acupuncture

(AURICULAR THERAPY)

Best for: Heavy smokers (two packs or more daily), because they have the greatest need to reduce nicotine craving. One caveat: There are no large-scale scientific studies to support the effectiveness of acupuncture in smoking cessation, though anecdotal evidence is strong.

The lowdown: *By tapping into the points on the ear that release endorphins, experts in this Chinese medical procedure can combat nicotine cravings.*
Cost: Per-session fees vary from $20 to $75. Plan on taking five sessions.
Biggest hassle: Time consuming.
Insurance coverage: Unlikely
Resource: To find an acupuncturist in your area, contact the Center for Better Health in Baltimore at 800-396-8525.

SMOKE SCREEN

To see which method will work best for you, take this quiz developed by Elliot Wineburg, M.D., director of the Stop Smoking Medical Center in New York City. **Instructions:** *Rate how often you're likely to smoke at each of the following times. Give yourself four points for "always," three for "sometimes," two for "seldom" and one for "never." Add up your points and check your score.*

I like to smoke:
1. In bed before I get up
2. In the bathroom in the morning
3. With my breakfast or first cup of coffee
4. On my way to work
5. At work, on the phone, on the computer
6. During my morning break
7. With or instead of lunch
8. During my midafternoon break
9. On the way home from work
10. Before supper
11. At supper
12. While listening to music or watching TV
13. In a bar while drinking
14. With others at parties or in couples
15. Before bed or in bed
16. When I'm awake in the middle of the night
17. During a break at a movie or play
18. In the car
19. Before stressful situations
20. After stressful or emotionally draining situations

TOTAL ________ **SCORING** *(see next page)*

20%

Nicotine Gum
(NICORETTE)

Best for: People who get lots of intense urges, as they can tailor their dosage to match their cravings. If you have heart disease, an irregular heartbeat, high blood pressure or severe gum disease or take medication for depression or asthma, consult your doctor before buying the gum.

The lowdown: *This peppery-tasting over-the-counter chewing gum helps relieve withdrawal symptoms by releasing nicotine into the system without the harmful effects of tars and carbon monoxide. Most smokers should start by using a two-milligram piece every one to two hours. Those who smoke more than 25 cigarettes daily should begin with the 4-mg dose and use it as part of Nicorette's free "Committed Quitters" behavior modification or independent therapy.*

Cost: $50 for a two-week supply. You'll need about three months' worth.

Biggest hassle: You can't constantly chew the gum, because you'll get too much nicotine and feel sick, so you'll have to "park" it between your cheek and gum to chew every 30 minutes. You also can't drink fluids when you have the gum in your mouth.

Insurance coverage: Unlikely now that it's available over the counter.

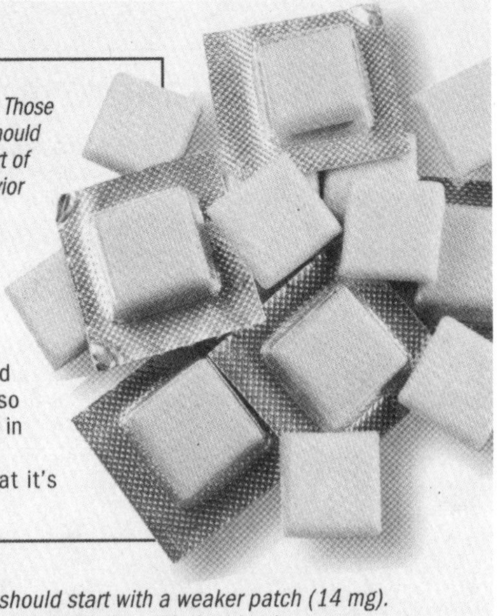

Patch (NICODERM CQ, NICOTROL, HABITROL)

35%

Best for: People who smoke more than a pack a day. Those who smoke less may not do as well on the patch, most likely because their addiction is psychological rather than physiological. Women are more apt to be successful than men. People with heart disease, an irregular heartbeat, high blood pressure or a skin disorder, or who take medication for depression or asthma should consult their doctor.

The lowdown: *Worn on the arm for 16 to 24 hours a day, this small adhesive cloth patch releases nicotine into your body. If you smoke more than 10 cigarettes daily, use a full-strength patch (21 mg of nicotine daily). Lighter smokers should start with a weaker patch (14 mg). Using the patch in combination with the blood pressure medication mecamylamine is eight times more effective than using the patch alone, says Eric C. Westman, M.D., medical director of the nicotine research program at Duke & Durham V.A. Medical Center in Durham, NC. Dr. Westman reports that Sano Corporation in Miramar, FL, is close to requesting FDA approval for a patch that contains mecamylamine. In the meantime, talk with your doctor about using the two together. Since it was only tested on smokers with normal blood pressure, Dr. Westman advises those with high or low pressure to avoid using the combo until more research is done.*

Cost: $50 for a two-week supply of patches. You'll need about two months' worth.

Biggest hassle: Your skin may become irritated, and you'll need to change patch sites frequently.

Insurance coverage: Unlikely.

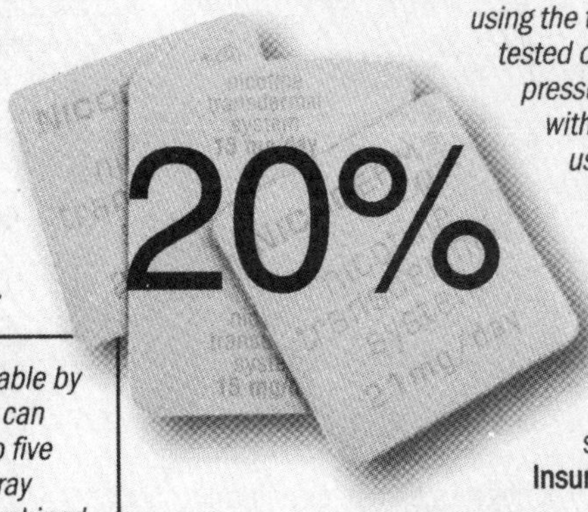

20%

Nasal Spray
(NICOTROL NS)

Best for: Heavy smokers who haven't succeeded with other products. People who suffer from allergies, asthma or other chronic nasal disorders should avoid it unless their doctor gives them the green light.

The lowdown: *A form of nicotine-replacement therapy is sprayed into the nose and absorbed through the nasal membranes. It's available by prescription only. You can use it as needed up to five times an hour. The spray doesn't have to be combined with other treatments.*

Cost: About $35 to $40 per week initially; $20 to $30 as you require less of it.

Biggest hassle: The nasal irritation experienced by virtually all users in the first week or two.

Insurance coverage: Fewer than half of managed-care plans cover it. Be sure to ask.

SCORING

70 to 80 points: Nasal spray or 24-hour maximum-strength patch
60 to 70 points: 16- or 24-hour patch in moderate strength, or nasal spray
50 to 60 points: Moderate-strength patch plus nicotine gum
40 to 50 points: Low-dose patch plus nicotine gum
30 to 40 points: Nicotine gum and hypnosis, acupuncture or behavior modification
20 to 30 points: Hypnosis or behavior modification
If these therapies fail, ask your doctor about Zyban *(see previous page)*.

WEATHERING THE WITHDRAWAL

Popping a pill or putting on a patch is no guarantee of success. Follow these guidelines for getting through the critical first two weeks, when withdrawal symptoms and cravings are strongest.

- **Devise alternative behavior patterns.** For example, if you normally sit down and have coffee with a cigarette, stand up instead.
- **Avoid alcohol.** Drinking can decrease your willpower.
- **Don't try to diet at the same time.** Most people will gain four to five pounds when they quit smoking, partly because smoking increases your metabolism and partly because some smokers were substituting a cigarette for food. Munch on low-cal, lowfat snacks like fruits and vegetables when you crave a cigarette, but don't diet; it may divert you from your important focus: kicking the habit.
- **Start exercising.** Working out will get your mind off smoking and help build your motivation as you begin to feel the energy-producing effects of clear lungs. Plus you'll be less likely to gain weight.

For a copy of *American Health for Women*'s recent article on teen smoking, send a large SASE to *American Health for Women*, Attn: Reader Service, 28 W. 23rd St., New York, NY 10010.

While it's no secret that smoking is bad for your health, 6,000 of you will light your first cigarette today. Oh sure, it can seem kind of glam and almost harmless when you're only taking a couple puffs at a party. But before you strike that match, you might want to check out this report. It could save your lungs (and your life).

kickin' butt

Of all the young people in the United States who are currently younger than 18, more than 5 million will die prematurely from a smoking-related disease

By Dana Silbiger

"I KNOW I'M NOT GOING TO BE A SMOKER when I get older," says one Bethesda, MD, high school student. "It's just a phase. I smoke socially."

That's exactly what 90 percent of adult nicotine addicts told themselves once upon a time. Ask any chronic smoker, and nearly every one of them will admit that he or she started out as a teenage "social smoker." No one, however—not even that pruny old lady who constantly sucks on cancer sticks—wakes up one morning and decides, "Hmmm. Today think I'm going to become a chain smoker."

Often, the habit kicks in long before your brain realizes you're hooked. In fact, your very first cigarette triggers the addiction process, says Jack Henningfield, Ph.D., an associate professor of behavioral biology at Johns Hopkins Medical School and an expert on addiction. While your head says things like, "I'm different. I'm not really a smoker," the nicotine is fast at work,

From *Jump,* May 1998, pp. 68-72. © 1998 by Welder Publications. Reprinted by permission.

Calling it Quits

By Christy Turlington

I started smoking at about age 13. My father smoked all of my life and I remember hating it when he would smoke in the car on long drives with the windows rolled up. I don't quite know why or when my feelings about smoking when from disgust to interest, but I do recall that it was around the time my older sister and some of her friends began to smoke. We had horses and spent much of our spare time at the stables. A lot of the people at those stables smoked. By the time I started high school, I was smoking in other social circles as well, along with most of my friends.

In the meantime, I started modeling. My mother often accompanied me to work. I really wanted to be seen as sophisticated, which was difficult with her in tow. When she wasn't around, however, I could smoke freely without any questions asked or judgments made. There are many smokers in the fashion industry.

My father had had a heart attack when I was 14. He was a commercial airline pilot, and because he had endured angioplasty surgery, the FAA prohibited him from doing what he loved to do most. He quit smoking briefly, but wasn't able to stick to it.

I, like many people, couldn't see myself in my father's position. I thought I could stop any time. I did quit the first time at age 19. I had heard that hypnosis would work best, and I didn't smoke for two years. But at some point, I became interested again. I felt that I was stronger and could handle it in moderation. No such luck—I was hooked and went back to smoking the same amount as I had before. I attempted quitting once again about a year later with the patch, which was only temporarily successful. Then I went through a series of other attempts such as acupuncture, and I had another go at hypnosis. Nothing worked. Along the way I encouraged my dad to quit too.

Finally, at the age of 26, three years ago almost to the day, I gave up—cold turkey. I couldn't stand not having control. I'd broken so many promises to myself and others who cared about me, and I was fed up, embarrassed.

I decided one night not to smoke ever again, and I haven't once looked back.

I know that I will never smoke again.

I tried to help my dad quit after I did, explaining that I was proof he could do it. It was mind over matter. He went into a week-long cessation program in December 1996 and finally quit. He had been coughing up blood prior to quitting and had been feeling achy and tired for a few months.

Sadly, my dad was diagnosed with lung cancer two months after quitting smoking, and he died in June 1997. He was 64 and had smoked for more than 50 years.

I was so thankful that I wasn't still smoking during my dad's illness, though I'm certain that if I were, I would have stopped.

My father was the quintessential outdoorsman—a skier, runner, hiker—tall and great looking. He was my greatest role model. But he just didn't believe in himself enough to kick this habit.

I want to share my story in hope that I can prevent young people from smoking. And for those who have already started, I am proof that quitting is difficult but possible. I feel that I have experienced this issue on every level and can speak from my heart, but also with the facts. I want people to understand the ramifications of this drug—there is no excuse for ignorance any longer.

As told to The National Field Hearing for the U.S. Senate Democratic Taskforce on Tobacco.

stimulating chemical responses in your body that mimic the feel-good responses you get naturally from doing things like chowing down or making out. When you smoke, your body creates extra receptors to try to protect itself from the sensory overload. The result? "Once they start, it's difficult for people to function and feel right unless they keep the nicotine coming in," says Henningfield. In another word: addiction. And there's plenty of research to prove it.

Of teen smokers who said they wouldn't be smoking in five years, 73 percent were still puffing away. Worse, two-thirds of teen smokers say they want to quit already (that's how fun it is!), and 70 percent say if they could do it all over again, they would never start smoking in the first place. Even so, in recent years, the number of teens smoking has climbed steadily, and puffing among high school seniors has reached a 19-year high of 36.9 percent. Each and every day, 6,000 teens light up for the first time. They think it's temporary. But more than half of smokers puff away up until the year before their (premature) death. Kind of takes your breath away, doesn't it?

YOU DECIDE No one's gullible enough to get suckered by tobacco companies, right? Then explain why the three most highly advertised brands—Marlboro, Camel and Newport—are smoked by 85 percent of adolescent smokers (and only 35 percent of adults).

TOBACCO: *the truth and consequences*

Most teen smokers think they haven't been smoking long enough to do any harm. Here's the head-to-foot fiasco that starts with the first drag.

HAIR
You'll have nice, smelly locks.

NOSE
Weekends will be spent with a thermometer. Smokers get more respiratory tract infections, like bronchitis and pneumonia. Oh, and when you *do* feel good? You'll probably have to skip sleepovers with friends. Smokers snore—a lot!

HANDS
No guy will hold your hand because your fingers will stink and your nails will have yellow-brown discoloration.

LUNGS
Two words: LUNG CANCER!

OVARIES
When you're ready to have kids, you'll have a higher chance of being infertile.

Taking the pill and smoking dramatically increases your risk of having cardiovascular problems, especially blood clots.

WALLET
Your automobile insurance may go up. Smokers crash cars more often than non-smokers.

If you're a typical smoker, studies show you fork out $700 per year on cigs. That's a lot of missed concerts, movies and, well, fun!

You'll spend lots of cash on Kleenex and/or therapy. Smokers are more likely to be depressed, to engage in high-risk sexual behavior and to get into fights. They also have a higher rate of suicide.

YOUR ENTIRE BOD
With each puff, you inhale 4,000 chemicals including cyanide, carbon monoxide and formaldehyde.

LIPS
You'll ruin your makeup. When you suck on cigarettes, wrinkles develop around your lips and, tahdah, your lipstick bleeds.

You won't get many kisses because your breath stinks. (Kissing a smoker is like licking an ashtray.) Besides, in a survey, 49 percent of guys said smoking makes a girl look insecure, and 78 percent of boys said they don't want to date someone who smokes.

Forget flashing your pearly whites—you'll have discolored teeth.

HEART
The resting heart rate of teen smokers is two to three beats per minute faster than that of nonsmokers. So in competition, your body wastes a lot of heartbeats just to keep up.

BACK
Teenage girls who smoke have a lower bone mineral density, which can cause all kinds of yucky stuff, including osteoporosis, later on.

SKIN
You'll speed the aging and, therefore, wrinkling process. Wanna look like the freak à la *Scream?* Smokers get hollow cheeks from the repeated muscular motion of inhaling.

Way Out West and Under the Influence

CAREY GOLDBERG

SPOKANE, Wash.

It was like the buzz of 1,000 cups of coffee, Joy said. It kept her up for days at a time, and set her to cleaning the house like the old white tornado commercials for Ajax. It whisked away her postpartum depression and made staying slim a breeze.

The only problem, said Joy, who asked that her last name not be used, was that it wrecked her life, costing her custody of her 3-year old son Conor (she is now fighting to get him back) and it proved so hard to kick that she went through four in-patient programs to get to the point where she is now, with six drug-free months behind her.

"I was a garbage pit," she said.

The illegal drug that seduced and almost destroyed Joy is methamphetamine—also known as crank, speed or meth.

Its growing popularity, almost entirely in the West and Midwest, has brought warnings from Federal officials that it could become the 1990's version of crack cocaine. It is easy to make, cheap, powerfully addictive and so long-lasting that $25 can buy a four-day high.

From Crack to Crank

The biggest difference between crack and crank, experts say, is the constituency: Crank users are mainly white and come from rural or suburban areas.

And crank appears to be popular among women in unheard-of proportions.

At a recent regional conference on methamphetamine held in San Francisco, researchers from the National Institute of Justice, a Federal research center, reported that crank users in their 20's were likelier to be women than men. In eight Western cities, they said, methamphetamine was found more often in bloodstreams of women than in men who had been arrested, and women were likelier to use it than any other drug.

The statistics are still preliminary, researchers say, and it's not yet established why women are especially drawn to it. Popularized by bikers and truckers as long ago as the 1950's and nicknamed crank because it was often hidden in their crankcases, it was also once known as "blue-collar cocaine." Later it became popular among gay men.

But now, said Gen. Barry McCaffrey, director of drug policy for the Clinton Administration, "women are testing positive at a higher rate than men, and that's the first time we've seen that on any drug.

"There may be a piece of it related to weight loss," he said, and "a piece of it related to enabling prostitution—it's a drug that allows you to deal with your feelings of remorse."

The spread of methamphetamines also fits into a broader picture of rising drug use among women, he said. Last summer the National Center on Addiction and Substance Abuse at Columbia University issued a report showing that 3.1 million American women regularly used illegal drugs, that 40 percent of crack addicts were women and that among teen-agers, girls and boys were equally likely to have used drugs.

Mr. McCaffrey said he found the spread of methamphetamines among women especially scary because crank users, like crack users, are prone to violence and child abuse. It is, he said, one of the few things "powerful enough to shatter a mother's love for her child."

Speaking at the San Francisco conference, Senator Dianne Feinstein of California noted that in one Sacramento hospital, there are now more babies addicted to methamphetamines than to crack.

Spokane, a regional center of 400,000 on the sparsely settled eastern edge of Washington state, typifies the kind of territory where methamphetamine use is increasing rapidly. Barb Richey, an outreach worker who helps mainly pregnant women on drugs, said that many women have gotten hooked on crank—which can be smoked, injected or snorted—as a weight-loss drug. Of the 335 pregnant women she has helped get into drug treatment since November of 1995, she said, about 40 percent of them were on crank.

"Eight years ago I thought injectable cocaine was the worst drug in the world," said Lynn Everson, who staffs a needle exchange program in Spokane. "Six years ago I thought crack was the worst and now I think it's crank."

Joy said the drug is readily available at bars or through small groups of casual friends. Users don't often have to deal with violent gangs to get it, because small-time manufacturers and distributors abound.

That is part of its appeal to women and other users, said Thomas Constantine, head of the Federal Drug Enforcement Agency, in an interview at the San Francisco conference. "It can be bought in rural and suburban areas, without venturing into a high-crime area," he said.

The prevalence of women on crank also seems to hark back to old patterns. Women, who suffer disproportionately from anxiety and depression, have long been prone to abusing prescription tranquilizers, anti-depressants and weight loss pills, researchers say. The only difference is that crank, which delivers a much more potent and long-lasting high, is illegal.

Mother's Little Helper

Crank "is kind of a drug of the times in that it's a drug for people who don't have enough time," said Michael Gorman, a University of Washington researcher running a study of methamphetamine use in Seattle. "You have the sense that it's moms trying to juggle jobs and three kids and day care, and women working as waitresses on their feet for 12 hours a day. And it's truck drivers, carpet layers, people who work long hours doing tedious, repetitive tasks."

Dr. Gorman's research has focused mainly on crank's prevalence among gay men who sometimes use it to enhance sex. But he said it was clear that among women, the weight-loss component of crank was also very strong. In Hawaii, where "ice"—a smokeable form of methamphetamine—has been in wide use since the late 1980's, doctors and the police have become much more familiar than their mainland colleagues with its effects on users, and have noticed a peculiar difference between the sexes.

Dr. Tom Leland, a psychiatrist at Queens Hospital in Honolulu, said one can often tell where ice is being smoked, because the woman in the house will be a compulsive cleaner, and the place will be spick-and-span. The man, meanwhile, will have become what police officers call a "tweaker," overcome with a manic urge to take things apart, and so car and machine parts will often be scattered on an immaculate lawn.

That urge to clean is what Joy, a 36-year-old janitorial supervisor, experienced in her Spokane home, where she tended her tiny garden and cleaned compulsively.

"Things got done," she said. "It's not like cocaine where you use it and automatically you're out looking for more."

For days at a time, she said, she would be gloriously numb, able to forget all her troubles. But whenever she would stop using it, she would be forced to face "the wreckage of the last 15 or 17 days."

Joy, who weighed 130 pounds on crank, is now at 200 pounds and struggling toward recovery, thankful she was never arrested and trying to win custody of her son from her mother.

But she knows she is fighting the odds: "They say that with crank, there's such a high rate of recidivism they just about write you off," she said.

Legal Drugs' Lethal Side Effects

Ordinary medicines can be extraordinarily hazardous. We'll tell you how to stay safe

BY STEPHEN FRIED

My wife, Diane, took a single dose of an antibiotic she was given for a minor urinary tract infection and ended up disoriented and hallucinating in the emergency room. While waiting for Diane's condition to improve—a wait we expected to be hours, but which turned out to be months—I learned a lot about the system that should have prevented her severe adverse drug reaction (ADR) or at least ensured that she and her doctor were sufficiently warned of the risks. It's a safety net that nobody likes to look down at too often, because the holes in it are terrifyingly large. And unfortunately women fall through more often than men.

Side Effect Surprise: They're More Common Than You Think

Most people are amazed (as I was) to learn that far more Americans die each year from adverse reactions to prescription and over-the-counter medications than succumb to illegal drug use. Up to 11% of hospital admissions are the result of "drug-induced sufferings," as they're referred to in Japan. And more than a quarter of U.S. inpatients have adverse reactions to the drugs they're given in the hospital.

Why does this happen? Sometimes it's bad luck—every drug is going to harm a small percentage of patients—but just as often it's bad science. Drugs are approved for sale on the basis of what the FDA calls "adequate and well-controlled studies" of some 3,000 to 4,000 test subjects. After approval, a drug's safety profile in the real world is supposed to be continually assessed and studied. That process goes by the European term "pharmacovigilance." It's an elegant name for what has been so far an appallingly inelegant system—an inadequate, out-of-control study that we unwittingly volunteer for every time we swallow a pill.

The problem is especially acute for women because many of the drugs they take were developed while pharmaceutical companies were all but prohibited from testing new medicines on women of childbearing age. Even today many test subjects are men, and as a result adverse reactions tend to show up in women after a new medication reaches the market.

How the System Works—And Doesn't Work

After a drug is approved by the FDA, there is generally no mandatory postapproval research to ensure that the drug continues to do what it did in the initial studies or produces the same side effects. Instead there's a voluntary monitoring system. Doctors and patients can submit confidential reports to manufacturers and the FDA about drug side effects, but there's no requirement that they do so. Consequently, the FDA and its sister regulatory agencies around the globe estimate that 90% of all ADRs, and perhaps as many as 99% of the most serious ones, are never reported. Patients at least have a decent excuse: Most of us have no idea we're supposed to report drug reactions to our doctors, let alone to the FDA. Doctors have no excuse. But privately they'll offer some explanations: They're pressed for time; they don't have to do it; and it pains them to admit that a drug they prescribed could have hurt a patient (guilt and fear of lawsuits are a potent combination). But mostly doctors just don't want to get involved. They know that bad news about a drug is never welcome news—except to the manufacturer of the drug's competitor.

ADR reports are supposed to be forwarded to MedWatch, the FDA's drug-monitoring program, even if a doctor merely suspects a drug created a problem. That way someone with more specific expertise in that particular medication can stop a disaster such as the fen-phen diet drug debacle in its earliest stages. (For an idea of how the fen-phen story unfolded, see "How a Drug Is Pulled Off the Shelves.") Yet the reports aren't always made, even if the link is patently obvious. And when doctors do send in reports, they often don't bother to fill out the paperwork fully. As a result, the records are so incomplete that they're nearly useless to the FDA, and early signs of problems get missed. Furthermore, drug companies can almost always claim the spotty reports represent a skewed sampling and don't give an accurate picture of a drug's safety.

It doesn't help that the FDA has a shoestring budget for pharmacovigilance. American drug sales topped $90 billion last year, yet the budget for MedWatch is still a mere $140,000 annually. Although MedWatch statistics are ultimately analyzed by some 50 FDA employees, the frontline monitoring for the entire nation is handled by four people. Until recently the staff worked with low-tech systems that were still run "pretty much like a library card catalog," according to Murray M. Lumpkin, M.D., deputy director of the FDA Center for Drug Evaluation and Research in Rockville, MD. A new $3.5 million computer system was put in place last November, but shortly before the installation, Dr. Lumpkin's boss, Janet Woodcock, M.D., director of the CDER, admitted to the Associated Press that she was "real unhappy" with the system.

Since the FDA Reform Act passed

From *American Health for Women,* May 1998, pp. 44-48.

GETTING SMART ABOUT SIDE EFFECTS

When you fill a new prescription, ask your pharmacist for a copy of the package insert, or look up the drug in the *Physicians' Desk Reference* at your library (the *PDR* is updated yearly, so make sure you're looking at the current version). Keep a medical dictionary handy; the fine print and medical jargon contain crucial safety information. Once you have a package insert in hand, examine these sections:

INDICATIONS This section lists the conditions the FDA has approved the drug to treat. "Most of the time the pharmacist isn't aware of what the drug was prescribed for, so you should look to see whether the condition you have is on the list," says Nancy Best Mabie, a registered pharmacist and manager of member services at the U.S. Pharmacopeia in Rockville, MD. If your diagnosis isn't on the list, ask your doctor why she chose this particular medication. (Many so-called off label uses are fine, but it would be a good idea to hear your doctor's explanation.)

CONTRAINDICATIONS This section lists people who should not take the drug.

WARNINGS The louder they scream at you from the page, the more important they are, says Mabie. Pay close attention to information that appears in capital letters or bold-faced type or is enclosed in a black box.

PRECAUTIONS These are milder cautions. This is also the section of the label where you'll find advice about tests you may need while taking the drug long-term.

ADVERSE REACTIONS This list of side effects associated with a drug can be a little scary. Remember that some of the side effects are rare, while others are more common. Pay special heed to symptoms such as sleepiness or dizziness that might impair your ability to drive, work or think clearly.

DOSAGE Check to see that the dosage your doctor has prescribed falls into the recommended range. If it's lower or higher, ask your doctor or pharmacist why.

last year largely ignores the specific drug safety problems of women, *you* should be real unhappy too, because the best chance of finding out about a gender-specific problem is if it comes up on MedWatch's blurry radar.

Protect Yourself: Read Labels, Write to the FDA

What can you do about all this? Make sure you and all your doctors are pharmacovigilantes. If you have an adverse drug reaction, tell the doctor who prescribed the drug about it right away. There are certain classes of drugs—such as fluoroquinolone antibiotics, which include Floxin (the medication my wife took)—that patients should stop taking the moment certain reactions begin to occur. (My wife was lucky that her doctor took her symptoms seriously and sent her straight to the ER; she was unlucky that some of her complications are permanent and controllable only by medication she'll be on for the rest of her life.)

After your acute symptoms have passed, make sure your reaction gets reported to both the FDA and the company that manufactures the drug. Reports are to be made regardless of whether the doctor is certain the drug caused the problem. If your doctor is reluctant to file a report, you can do it yourself. Call 800-FDA-1088 for the form you'll need, or print a copy from the MedWatch Website, www.fda.gov/medwatch.

MedWatch specifically asks doctors to report reactions that are *serious,* but this is a pretty loaded word, especially for women, who often have trouble getting their complaints taken seriously by physicians. The FDA considers an event serious when it's fatal (obviously) or life-threatening, or when it causes or prolongs hospitalization, results in a disability that is "significant, persistent or permanent" or requires "intervention to prevent permanent impairment or damage."

There's a lot of wiggle room in that list. FDA epidemiologists have determined that the drug my wife took can cause insomnia that may become permanent, as well as other neurological and psychiatric changes. Would your doctor consider such symptoms serious? Would the physician check a year later to find out whether such problems persist and then bother to do a follow-up report?

There is one other aspect of personal pharmacovigilance: You can try to compensate for the flaws in the system by becoming a hyperinformed consumer. The best way to do this is to assume that the most up-to-date information about a drug has *not* reached your physician. It's wise to spend a few minutes looking into any drug prescribed for you—especially if it has been approved only recently. When your doctor hands you a prescription, ask what she knows about the drug, starting with how long it has been in use. A medication that has been on the market for only a few months may not have been used by enough patients, and particularly by enough women, for side effects to show up in any significant number.

Technically, your physician should share the warnings in the "Information for Patients" section on the drug package insert with you, but many doctors do not. So you'll also want to read up on the drug at your pharmacy or library. (For more advice on how to decipher a package insert, see "Getting Smart About Side Effects.)

It's also a good idea to make sure you know the generic names of all the drugs you take, because the label warnings never list interactions by brand name. Also learn the drug's class, or "family"—not just "antibiotic," for example, but penicillin (Amoxil, Polycillin), cephalosporin (Keflex, Ceclor) or macrolide (erythromycin). Once you have that information, make sure all your doctors have it too; any physician who treats you should be aware of all the medications you're taking—prescription or over-the-counter—so possible interactions can be averted.

Tell your doctor about an adverse reaction **right away**. There are some drugs you should **stop taking** the moment side effects begin to occur.

HOW A DRUG IS PULLED OFF THE SHELVES

When enough people report suspected side effects, a drug can be removed from the market. Nevertheless, the fen-phen fiasco is a reminder that just because a drug is FDA approved doesn't mean it's free of side effects.

1973 The FDA approves fenfluramine for weight control.

1992 Michael Weintraub, M.D., an associate professor of community and preventive medicine at the University of Rochester Medical Center in Rochester, NY, reports that combining fenfluramine with another drug, phentermine, produces significant weight loss. Word of fen-phen's success seeps out to patients and doctors.

1993 French investigators report a cluster of cases of primary pulmonary hypertension (PPH), a rare lung disorder, in patients using derivatives of fenfluramine.

June 1996 Dexfenfluramine (Redux), a cousin of fenfluramine, enters the market and becomes the newest prescription weight loss drug in more than two decades.

July 1996 Fen-phen is practically a household word and is being prescribed by national weight loss chains such as Jenny Craig and Nutri/System.

August 1996 A study in the *New England Journal of Medicine* links dexfenfluramine to PPH.

July 1997 Doctors at the Mayo Clinic in Rochester, MN, report that 24 women who had taken fen-phen developed a rare but serious heart valve abnormality.

August 1997 The *New England Journal of Medicine* reports that a woman died of PPH after taking fen-phen for 23 days. The FDA receives 82 MedWatch reports on the drug combo.

September 1997 At the FDA's request, manufacturers withdraw fenfluramine and dexfenfluramine from the market after doctors submit new information showing the drugs might cause heart valve defects in a third of users.

—Julie Christie

After complaints from doctors and from patients like my wife, the FDA investigated central nervous system side effects from fluoroquinolone antibiotics such as Floxin. As a result, the drugs' labels now include a slightly stronger caution of the risk of these side effects. But many doctors still aren't aware of the risk, and I'm sure some patients will continue to slip through the cracks and suffer side effects. All drugs cause adverse reactions in some people, and no individual patient can compensate entirely for the failures of pharmacovigilance. But as my wife and I learned in the aftermath of her drug reaction, it's best to learn everything you can before swallowing.

Stephen Fried is the author of Bitter Pills: Inside the Hazardous World of Legal Drugs. *His investigative articles on drug safety, written for* Philadelphia *magazine, won a 1994 National Magazine Award.*

Prescription For Disaster

Patients' refusal to take their medicine causes 2.5 million emergencies each year. Will your family pay a high price for playing doctor?

By GLORIA HOCHMAN

Kay Redfield Jamison, of all people, should have known better. After all, a critical part of her job as a clinical professor of psychiatry at Johns Hopkins University School of Medicine in Baltimore is to encourage people with manic-depressive illness to take their lithium. "Manic depression is a destructive disease," she would tell them. "Untreated, you can expect to experience at least 10 major episodes of depression or mania in your lifetime, and you are at high risk for suicide."

Nonetheless, Dr. Jamison turned her back on her own advice, even though her moods ricocheted from euphoric highs to paralyzing lows. "I knew the inevitable, bleak consequences of not taking lithium," says Dr. Jamison. She describes them in her best-selling memoir, *An Unquiet Mind:* "When you're high it's tremendous. The ideas and feelings are fast and frequent. But somewhere this changes. The fast ideas are far too fast, and there are far too many; overwhelming confusion replaces clarity you are irritable, angry, frightened, uncontrollable and enmeshed totally in the blackest caves of the mind."

At one point, Dr. Jamison became convinced that if her mind did not start working normally again, she would kill herself by jumping from a nearby 12-story building. Yet, despite her suicidal thoughts, she took lithium for only a few months, until her initial mania and subsequent depression were gone. Then, against medical advice, she stopped cold. That decision, she acknowledges, was a "devastating lack of judgment for which I and my family paid an exceedingly high price."

The Medication Mess Dr. Jamison's recalcitrance, known in health care lingo as "medication noncompliance," is common. Whether it's lithium to regulate mood swings, antibiotics to zap an infection or diuretics to control high blood pressure, there is a 30% to 50% chance that people will not take prescription drugs as directed by their physicians, according to the National Council on Patient Information and Education in Washington.

At least 7% of patients never fill their prescriptions in the first place. Others stop taking a drug as soon as they begin to feel better. Thirty-two percent fail to purchase refills. Many skip doses or down one pill when they should really take two; others take too much medication, reasoning that if one pill is good, two must be better. Even people with serious conditions such as high blood pressure or diabetes neglect to take the medicine that may save their lives. Some simply forget; others don't feel motivated to swallow a pill when they're feeling no immediate discomfort.

Doctors and pharmacists call noncompliance an unheralded but insidious medical problem that affects not only patients but also their families. In 1993 a task force made up of government and industry representatives estimated that it costs the U.S. $100 billion annually in reduced productivity, absence from work, hospital admissions and added treatment costs. According to Jon C. Schommer, Ph.D., an assistant professor at Ohio State University College of Pharmacy in Columbus, noncompliance results in as many as 2.5 million medical emergencies and 125,000 deaths every year.

Patients in Denial The reasons consumers give for ignoring physicians' prescriptions are as varied and complex as the colors in a Cézanne landscape. For many people, including Dr. Jamison, the resistance has psychological roots: Taking medication would

From *American Health for Women,* July/August 1997, pp. 66-67, 106, 108.

Good to the Last Dose

"An infection is like a campfire," says Paul L. Doering, a professor at the University of Florida College of Pharmacy in Gainesville. "On the first day, the 'fire' is raging and you need antibiotics to put it out. But unless you keep pouring on pills, the smoldering bacteria can roar back to life." His timeline shows why it takes 10 days' worth of penicillin to douse strep throat.

Day 1	Days 2 and 3	Days 4 to 6	Days 7 to 9	Day 10
Start medication. Your symptoms are at peak intensity, reminding you constantly to take your medicine. You can't wait for it to work.	You begin to feel better, but symptoms are still present.	You're feeling much better—so good that you're tempted to skip the drugs altogether. But though the bacteria count is down, the infection hasn't been eradicated.	If you stopped taking your medication around Day 4, the infection rebounds and comes back with a vengeance. In the following weeks, you could find yourself fighting rheumatic fever, a complication of strep throat.	Finish medication. The infection should be vanquished.

force them to admit they have an illness. These people often associate drug therapy with weakness, a shameful willingness to let medicine do what they should be able to handle on their own. "Their stubborn mindset makes them believe that they should be able to tough it out without medication," explains Gertrude Copperman, M.D., a family physician in Bala Cynwyd, PA.

Other patients are philosophically opposed. "My mom always told me, 'You're the captain of your soul and master of your fate,' " says Joan Lester*, a 54-year-old Philadelphia communications consultant. "I was influenced by her belief that you are in control of your life. For me, that means healing your mind, body and spirit in a natural way."

Lester takes Prozac for her depression only as a last resort. "When nothing I try on my own—yoga or meditation or better nutrition—works," she says, I reluctantly turn to the Prozac I keep in my dresser drawer. But even then, I skip doses and stop taking the pills the minute I feel some relief."

Tori Hudson, N.D., a professor of gynecology and oncology at the National College of Naturopathic Medicine in Portland, OR, says Lester probably isn't getting any therapeutic benefit from taking Prozac erratically. Only when the drug is taken consistently are blood levels adequate to relieve depression. "There are excellent, natural therapies for depression," says Dr. Hudson, "but if they don't help, I urge patients to try conventional therapy."

The Fear Factor Every day, it seems, newspapers report on the long-term side effects of drugs once considered safe. "Women especially are afraid, and rightly so," says Dr. Copperman. "A lot of medicines have not been adequately studied, and many were tested only on male subjects." Women's smaller bodies and fluctuating estrogen levels also put them at higher risk for side effects from some drugs.

Cost is also a problem. Prices can be high enough to deter those whose insurance plans don't cover prescription drugs or those who have only partial coverage. Some people fill a prescription but deliberately cut the drug regimen short to keep a few precious pills in reserve for the next time.

The smorgasbord of side effects that accompanies many drugs also leads many people to stop taking medication sooner than they should, or to take it erratically. When Sandra Fusco-Walker's daughter, Morgan, 15, refused to take her asthma medication because of its side effects, Fusco-Walker had to alter her work schedule so she could go to Morgan's school to administer the drug. "I couldn't count on her to do it on her own," says Fusco-Walker, who lives in Kinnelon, NJ, and is a director of outreach services for the Allergy and Asthma Network, a nonprofit patient education group based in Washington. "I worried every minute." Morgan says she stopped taking the medication because "it makes me spacey and gives me the jitters, like I've just had 20 cups of coffee." Besides, the inhaler she has to use to deliver the drug is inconvenient and embarrassing. She isn't eager to appear "different" to her classmates, so she skips doses even though she knows she may pay for it later.

The High Price of Noncompliance

Family members often suffer as much as the noncompliant patient, and disrupted work and school schedules are the least of the problem. Dr. Jamison's refusal to use lithium took a wrenching toll. "In my blind manic rages, I was physically assaultive, screaming insanely at the top of my lungs or impulsively trying to leap from cars,"

**Name has been changed.*

she says. "I destroyed things I cherished, pushed to the utter edge people I loved and survived to think I could never recover from the shame."

The health fallout from noncompliance varies according to the medication and the condition for which it was prescribed. For example, not taking high blood pressure drugs may produce no short-term problems but could lead to heart damage or stroke later in life, notes Eileen Hoffman, M.D., associate director for education at Mount Sinai Women's Health Program in New York City. Likewise, stopping antibiotics too soon may result in a return of the original infection, warns James R. Allen, M.D., vice president of science, technology and public health standards for the American Medical Association in Chicago. "In some cases, if you don't finish the full course of therapy, some of the hardiest bacteria may hang on and cause a new infection," he explains. "And because these bacteria may have become resistant to the original medication, the infection will require a more potent antibiotic. Do this enough times and you start running out of antibiotics."

Such antibiotic abuse can cause problems on a national, even global scale. The mid-1980s surge in cases of tuberculosis came about in part because people didn't take antibiotics as directed. "TB is prevalent among homeless people who start and stop medications inappropriately," says John Stern, M.D., who runs the infection control program at Pennsylvania Hospital in Philadelphia. "Over time their noncompliance affects the rest of the population." Several drugs are needed to rid the body of the infection. "If patients take only one or two or don't take the medicine in the first place," says Dr. Stern, "they permit the organism to flourish, and this highly contagious disease spreads." The problem is so serious that medical centers in many cities require people being treated for tuberculosis to report twice a week to take medication under observation.

Six Questions to Ask Before Filling Any Prescription

Medication noncompliance is a family health issue that frequently falls into the laps of women, who end up monitoring not only their own compliance but their children's as well. When a drug is prescribed, take a few minutes to ask the doctor these questions:

◆ **Why are you prescribing this particular medication?** Often, several drugs can relieve a certain medical problem. But their potential side effects may help you and your doctor determine which one is best for you.

◆ **What are the instructions for taking the medication?** Listen carefully and write them down.

◆ **What are the consequences of not finishing the medication or not taking it at all?**

◆ **What are the short-term side effects, and how long should they last?** Expecting certain side effects may make them more tolerable and tip you off to medication-related symptoms that are out of the ordinary.

◆ **If the side effects are intolerable, is it safe to stop taking this drug without first calling my doctor?**

◆ **If this drug is new, what is known about its risks, long-term effects and interactions with other medications and foods?** If after the doctor answers these questions you aren't willing to give the drug a try, ask her to recommend alternatives with better-known side effects.

Getting Back on Track Steps are being taken to chip away at the noncompliance problem, and pharmacists have been front-runners in bringing about change. With computers they can track medication usage and notify people who don't pick up prescriptions or order refills on time. In addition, drug manufacturers are preparing more medications in convenient, less forgettable one-a-day doses, and services have sprung up that will remind consumers, via computer or telephone, that it's time to take their medicine.

Ultimately, though, the responsibility for taking medication rests with the patient. When you fill a prescription, take a few minutes to note in your calendar the day you should finish the medication; make it a point to refill prescriptions on time. Whether the prescription is for yourself or a family member, you can monitor compliance by keeping the medication in an accessible place that's easily visible to you, so you can check its usage. If you have trouble remembering to take medication, set a timer as a reminder, jot a note on your calendar or take the drug with meals, if possible. To remind a child to take medication attach a note to her lunch box or school notebook; also alert the teacher, school nurse or camp counselor.

The key to compliance is education. "Doctors have the responsibility of informing and educating patients," says Dr. Hudson. "We need to make sure that people understand why a medication is being prescribed, how it should be used, what side effects are possible and what the consequences of not taking the drug could be. If patients hesitate when handed a prescription, doctors should encourage them to ask questions and present them with other treatment options." You should never leave the doctor's office feeling uncertain about what medication you'll be taking or why.

"Many doctors believe their responsibility ends with writing a prescription," says Dr. Hoffman. "But women need to have a trusting relationship with doctors before they feel comfortable acting on the advice. We don't like to be told what to do, especially by male authority figures. We don't want to hear 'Just take the pills, honey.' Those days are over."

Gloria Hochman is coauthor, with actress Patty Duke, of A Brilliant Madness: Living With Manic-Depressive Illness.

Unit 7

Unit Selections

Key Points to Consider

- Female genital mutilation is justified by its practitioners as a cultural tradition. How do tradition and health collide when people immigrate to a new country?
- What can be done to make the issue of violence against women more easily discussed?
- Victims of rape are often told that they brought it upon themselves through their dress or behavior. Do you think this is ever true? Why or why not?
- Many cultural images show violence against women. Do you think that these images promote or cause actual violence?
- A group's history helps to form its views on issues such as violence. How does the history of African Americans in the United States shape their view on aggression against African American women?
- What is the role of health care providers in responding to and preventing violence against women?

DUSHKINONLINE Links

www.dushkin.com/online/

24. **Crisis Resources**
    http://www.access.digex.net/~nova/resource.htm
25. **Domestic Violence**
    http://www.s-t.com/projects/DomVio/domviohome.HTML
26. **Sexual Assault Information Page**
    http://www.cs.utk.edu/~bartley/saInfoPage.html

These sites are annotated on pages 4 and 5.

Violence in Women's Lives

Violence in women's lives can take many forms. It can be images of violence in the media; it can be the fear of being out late at night; or it can be fear at home because of a violent partner. Violence can also take the form of culturally accepted rituals that involve violence. Whatever the form, most women report some experience with violence and take the need to deal with it as a necessary part of life.

In this section we have tried to highlight some of the most pressing issues facing women today. It is important to recognize that there are other forms of violence we have not been able to touch on, particularly the issue of violence in relationships between teenagers.

As the world is made smaller, through travel and technology, we become aware of cultural practices that are violent and yet are clung to. One of these is female genital mutilation or clitoridectomy. In "Female Genital Mutilation: Balancing Intolerance of the Practice with Tolerance of Culture," Layli Bashir discusses how health care providers should respond when encountering patients who have been mutilated or who practice mutilation. How are tolerance and respect for cultural differences balanced with our concept of the ethical practice of medicine? Can a violent practice ever be justified by cultural norms?

Violence within a relationship does not begin overnight. Violence can be seen at all stages of a relationship and can take many forms. In "A Woman's Killer Is Likely to Be Her Partner, a New study in New York finds," Pam Belluck examines the data on who kills women. Most of these murders are the culmination of repeated instances of violence, and health care providers need to recognize the signs and be prepared to assist women in need of help.

In "Domestic Violence Can Be Cured," the response of one community to domestic violence is examined. Here is how one community responded to the concerns of its residents and instituted a multifaceted response system that includes health care providers, the police, and the therapeutic community.

The article "I Was Raped," by Lori Robinson, addresses the role of power and aggression in relationships. In her examination of a rape that divided two colleges and revived her own memories of a rape, the author touches upon all the issues of acquaintance rape. According to the Centers for Disease Control and Prevention, 15 to 25 percent of male college students admit to involvement is some form of sexual aggression and 80 percent of rapes on college campuses are committed by someone known to the victim. By addressing the issues of responsibility, alcohol use, racism, and institutional attitudes, the author raises as many issues as she resolves.

Lastly, the cycle of violence and its legacies are looked at in "The Consequnces of Violence against Women." These include physical and psychological damage. This damage may have an impact on individuals, families, neighbors, friends, and the larger community.

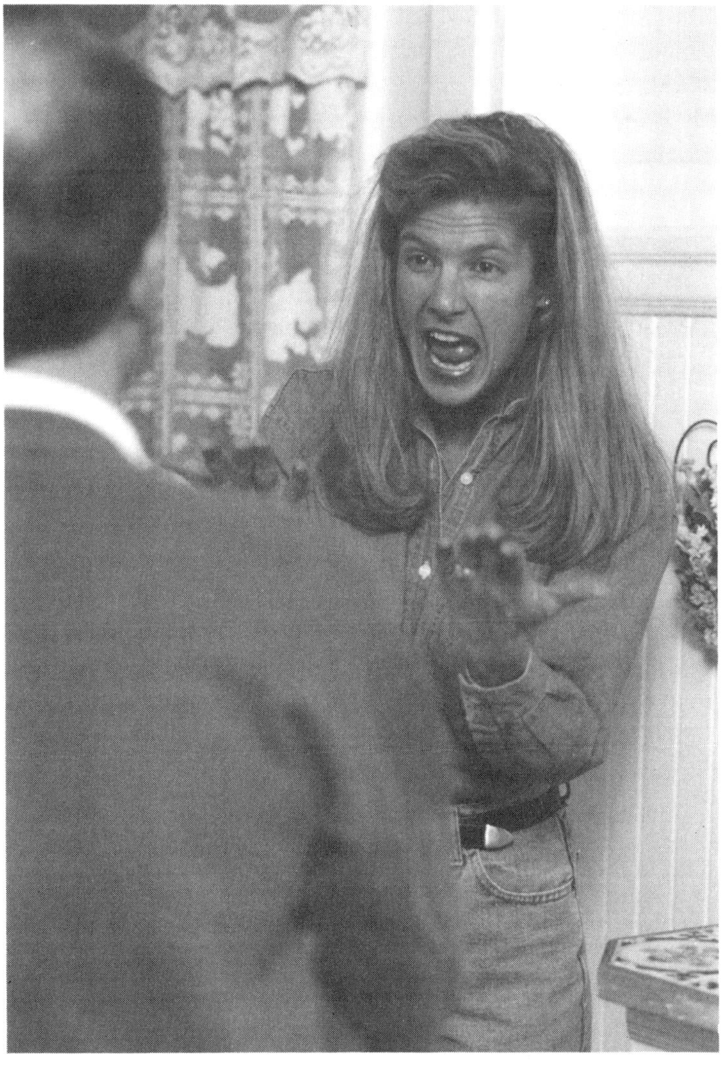

Lex et Feminae

Female Genital Mutilation: Balancing Intolerance of the Practice with Tolerance of Culture

LAYLI MILLER BASHIR, J.D., M.A.*

Female genital mutilation (FGM)** is a cultural rite of passage performed in many African and some Asian countries[1] on an estimated 114 million girls and women. Typically performed under unclean ritual circumstances and without anesthetic, FGM often causes serious medical complications, pain, and sometimes death.

Recently, the influx of immigrants from countries where FGM is performed has caused the practice to gain increased attention in the United States. This is reflected in the recent media spotlight given to women requesting asylum in the United States in order to avoid the ritual and women requesting that FGM be performed on their daughters at American hospitals.[2] The World Health Organization (WHO) declared in 1994 that, because of recent immigration patterns, FGM has become a public health issue in the United States.[3] In addition, the Centers for Disease Control and Prevention estimated that in 1996 more than 150,000 women and girls in the United States were at risk of genital mutilation.[4]

The growing presence of FGM has placed the medical community—particularly women's health practitioners—in the middle of this cultural, ethical, and now, legal dilemma. Last fall, Congress passed a law making FGM a felony,[5] following similar action in several states. In addition, medical associations recently have spoken out against the practice. Practitioners should be aware of their legal liabilities and ethical responsibilities in this area, as well as the cultural circumstances that surround this practice.

WHAT IS FGM?

FGM has several forms, which may vary in severity but always result in permanent damage to the clitoris. Nahid Toubia, M.D., a Sudanese physician at the Columbia University School of Public Health, advanced a system of classification that groups the most common forms of FGM into two broad categories: clitoridectomies and infibulations.[6] Type I clitoridectomy (Sunna circumcision) is the least severe form of FGM and involves the partial or complete removal of the clitoris. Type II clitoridectomy (excision) involves the excision of

*Ms. Bashir received her Juris Doctor from the Washington College of Law at American University and her Masters degree in International Relations from American University in 1996. She currently works at the United States Department of Justice, Board of Immigration Appeals. The opinions expressed in this column are solely those of the author and are not intended to represent those of her employer.

**There is a controversy over the terms used to refer to this practice. Some feel that the description of the ritual as mutilation is offensive and insulting, while others argue that the use of the term "female circumcision" evokes improper comparison to male circumcision. I follow the usage of the Inter-African Committee, which voted that "female circumcision" did not accurately reflect the ritual practice and decided that it should be referred to as "female genital mutilation" (Marilyn Milos, NOCIRC Newsletter, Fall 1993 at 2). I must note, however, that I feel that no suitable term for this ritual practice has been identified.

From *Journal of Women's Health*, February 1997, pp. 11-14. © 1997 by Mary Ann Liebert, Inc. Reprinted by permission.

the clitoris and part of the labia minora. In a type III infibulation (modified infibulation), the clitoris, labia minora, and parts of the labia majora are removed, and the anterior two-thirds of the labia majora are sutured together, leaving a posterior opening. Type IV infibulation (total infibulation), the most severe form of FGM, involves the same amount of cutting as a type III, but the labia majora are sutured together to cover the urethra and the vagina, leaving a very small opening for the passage of urine and menstrual blood.

FGM frequently causes serious and prolonged physical complications. In a 1993 Kenyan study, more than 80% of women reported at least one medical complication after undergoing FGM.[7] Other reports estimate that between 15% and 30% of all girls and women who endure FGM die from bleeding or infection.[8] Serious early adverse effects include severe pain and vaginal hemorrhage, which sometimes may lead to shock and death. Other effects include wound infections, abscesses, ulcers, septicemia, tetanus, and gangrene. A serious long-term consequence of FGM is hematocolpos, which may lead to chronic pelvic infections, back pain, dysmenorrhea, infertility, and urinary tract infections. The most common long-term complication is the formation of painful dermoid cysts and keloid scarring. Childbirth creates additional risks, particularly among immigrants in the United States, as most American obstetricians have not been trained to deal with infibulated women.[9] If an infibulated woman is not properly cared for during childbirth, complications, including perineal tears, vesicovaginal fistula, and even fetal death, may result.

The rationale behind FGM is a matrix of superstitions, perceptions of gender roles, beliefs regarding health, and religious customs. The most frequently cited reason for the continuation of FGM, however, is that it is perceived to preserve virginity, prevent promiscuity, and, consequently, preserve family honor. Parents who insist on this ritual for their daughters frequently state that if the ritual was not performed, their daughters would be perceived as immoral, would be unable to find a husband, and would be ostracized by the community.

LEGAL AND ETHICAL OBLIGATIONS

In September 1996, Congress passed a law that makes FGM a felony punishable by up to 5 years in prison.[5] The bill authorizes the prosecution of anyone who "circumcises, excises, or infibulates the whole or any part of the labia majora or labia minora or clitoris of another person who has not attained the age of 18." The law punishes both the parents who arrange for their daughters to be cut and those who perform the procedure.

Th[e] new federal law also seeks to prevent FGM through a process of education and cultural sensitivity. It requires the Secretary of the Department of Health and Human Services to identify ethnic communities in the United States that practice FGM and to engage in outreach activities to educate these communities on the physical and psychologic effects of FGM. These activities must be "designed and implemented in collaboration with representatives of the ethnic groups practicing such mutilation." The law also requires the Secretary to develop recommendations for the education of medical students regarding FGM. The federal law will go into effect on March 30, 1997.

In the past 2 years, numerous states have passed laws that criminalize FGM. Such states include California, Minnesota, Tennessee, Rhode Island, and North Dakota. South Carolina and Colorado are currently considering similar laws.

In addition to criminal penalties for performing FGM, medical practitioners also must be cognizant of ethical statements on the practice, recently developed by national and international medical organizations. The WHO has declared it unethical for a physician to perform FGM.[9] In 1994, the International Federation of Gynecology and Obstetrics passed a resolution that calls on all doctors to refuse to perform FGM.[10] In addition, the American Medical Association (AMA), in Policy 525.987(A-91), pronounced that it "opposes all forms of medically unnecessary surgical modification of female genitalia."[11] The AMA recommends that "[p]hy-sicians who are requested to perform female genital mutilation on a patient provide culturally sensitive counseling to educate the patient and her family members about the negative health consequences of the procedure, trying to discourage them from proceeding. If possible, physicians should refer the patient to social support groups that can help them cope with changing societal mores."

THE REAL SOLUTION

Criminalization of FGM is one step toward its eradication and may assist in fostering an environment in the United States that is clearly intolerant to FGM. The example of other Western nations that have criminalized FGM, however, demonstrates the inadequacy of merely making it illegal.[12] In Britain, for example, FGM has been a crime for more than 11 years, and despite this, there have been no convictions, and the rate of the mutilation of immigrant girls is reportedly on the rise.

While criminalization will assist in deterring the practice, the medical community can play a prominent role in protecting young girls and women from FGM by educating its members about the anatomic and psychological effects of FGM. The psychological and emotional side effects of FGM are particularly important to understand. A failure to appreciate the loss of dignity an FGM victim often feels when going to the doctor, let alone undergoing a pelvic examination, may contribute to poor patient attendance at prenatal care obstetrics services, or for routine physical exams.

When faced with a request to perform FGM, the practitioner must balance the legal and ethical obligation to emphatically refuse to perform the ritual with a sensitivity for the family's perspective. A reaction of anger or disgust will likely embarrass or alienate the patient and her family, and jeopardize the physician/patient relationship. The health care professional, in this situation, should explain to the patient and her family the serious dangers to the life, health, and well-being of a victim of FGM. Also, the practitioner should inform the patient and family that the practice is a crime in the United States.

Health care professionals should understand that many immigrants are surprised by what they perceive to be the flagrant sexual behavior of American youth and an apparent moral decay of our society. They are genuinely and seriously concerned that having moved into a culture where their values of virginity and chastity are in the minority, their children may fall victim to American immorality. To some families, FGM may be seen as even more important once in the United States in order to safeguard their family honor and culture against the contrasting tendencies of American society.

Although the criminalization of FGM may intimidate those who want to have the ritual performed on their daughters, health care professionals can have the greatest impact by understanding the root causes of FGM and, through culturally sensitive education and counseling, communicating its dangers to patients and their families. Health care professionals can help convey to a family requesting that their daughter undergo the ritual that, although the family's values are legitimate and their concerns are understandable, a girl or a woman has the ability to make rational decisions regarding sexuality and, if she shares her family's values, will be able to remain chaste and uphold her family's honor with her clitoris intact.

ACKNOWLEDGMENT

I am grateful for the invaluable assistance of R. Martin Bashir, M.D., in the preparation of this column.

REFERENCES

1. According to the World Health Organization, over 30 African countries and Muslim populations in Indonesia, Malaysia, India, Pakistan, Oman, South Yemen, and the United Arab Emirates practice FGM.
2. See, e.g., Ostrom CM. Doctors at Seattle hospitals consider circumcising Muslim girls. Seattle Times, September 29, 1996 (describing the dilemma of Seattle doctors at Harborview Medical Center faced with requests to perform FGM on Somali girls); Dugger C. Women's plea for asylum puts tribal ritual on trial, New York Times, April 15, 1996 (discussing the case of Fauziya Kasinga who fled from Togo to escape FGM and requested asylum in the United States).

3. UN calls for end to female genital mutilation. Chicago Tribune, May 5, 1994.
4. Dugger CV. Tug of taboos: African genital rite vs. American law. New York Times, December 28, 1996.
5. Federal prohibition of female genital mutilation act of 1996, Pub. L. 104-140, 110 Stat 1327 (1996).
6. Toubia N. Female circumcision as a public health issue. N Engl J Med 1994;331:712.
7. Okie S. Female circumcision persists: Tribal rite worries Kenyan health officials. Washington Post, April 13, 1993.
8. H. Lightfoot-Klein H. Pharaonic circumcision of females in the Sudan. Med Law 1983;2:353. (estimating that one-third of all Sudanese FGM victims die); Mann J. Torturing girls is not a cultural right. Washington Post, February 23, 1994 (quoting Rosemary Mburu, a Kenyan gynecologist, who estimates that 15% of all circumcised females die of bleeding or infections).
9. Female circumcision: state of World Health Organization position and activities. Submitted to the UN sub-commission on the prevention of discrimination and protection of minorities (Press Release WHO/10, June 1982).
10. Adolph C. Doctors must become advocates for women, conference is told. The Gazette (Montreal), October 1, 1994.
11. Report of the Council on Scientific Affairs. CSA Report 5-I-94, 1994.
12. For a broader discussion of European legislation against FGM and its effectiveness, see Bashir LM. Female genital mutilation in the United States: an examination of criminal and asylum law. Am UJ Gender L. 1996;4:415, 433.

Address correspondence to:
Lynn Sargent Berner, J.D., M.P.H.
Editor of Lex et Feminae
The Cleveland Clinic Foundation
9500 Euclid Avenue-KK53
Cleveland, OH 44195

A Woman's Killer Is Likely to Be Her Partner, a New Study in New York Finds

PAM BELLUCK

More women in New York City are killed by their husbands or boyfriends than in robberies, disputes, sexual assaults, drug violence, random attacks or any other crime in cases where the relationship between the murderer and victim is known.

That conclusion, long suspected by family violence and criminal justice experts, has been confirmed by a study of every woman killed in New York City over five years, one of the first studies of its kind in the country.

To piece together a portrait of these women, researchers from the New York City Department of Health spent nine months teasing clues out of the documents that are the residue of murder: autopsy findings, crime scene reports, witness statements, toxicological and sexual assault tests, ballistics reports, and descriptions of stab wounds and strangulation marks.

For a study that has yet to be released, researchers looked at files on each of the 1,156 women age 16 and over killed in New York City from 1990 through 1994. In only 484 murders could investigators determine the killer's relationship to the victim—friend, stranger, acquaintance or relative. From that narrower pool, researchers learned that nearly half of the women were killed by current or former husbands or boyfriends, a much higher proportion than expected. Nationally, the figure is 40 percent, compared with 6 percent of men who were killed by wives or girlfriends.

The portrait derived from the homicide files is telling in its details of how the women lived and graphic in the specifics of how they died.

More than half the women killed in the city during those years died in private homes, usually their own. In the majority of the cases in which the killer was identified, the murderers were people they knew.

When they were killed by their husbands, one-third of the time the women appeared to be trying to end the relationships. In one-quarter of the cases where husbands or boyfriends were the killers, children were also killed or injured, or they watched the murders or found their mothers' bodies.

And, unlike men, who are killed most often by guns, women "are very likely to be punched and hit and burned and thrown out of windows," said the leader of the study, Dr. Susan A. Wilt, the director of epidemiology and surveillance for the Health Department's injury and prevention program. "We were surprised by the degree to which some of these murders just spoke of enormous rage. Some women were stabbed and also strangled," she said.

"What's very clear is that female homicides are so different from male homicides," Dr. Wilt added, noting that her research staff attended monthly support group sessions and deliberately avoided looking at gruesome autopsy photographs.

Understanding the women's deaths, city health officials say, will help map a plan for hospitals, law enforcement officials, clinics and community organizations to identify and protect women at risk.

The study also provides concrete information at a time when domestic violence policy is a heated issue, with victims' advocates pressuring city and state officials for more help for battered women and more serious penalties for their batterers.

Dr. Margaret A. Hamburg, the New York City Health Commissioner, said the study showed a need for different strategies to protect women. "On-the-street police strength is not effective when the majority of women are killed in an individual's home," Dr. Hamburg said. "Health care providers should be trying to identify women who are at risk for domestic violence because often women do have early contact with the medical system. And we need to reexamine laws that apply to domestic violence."

Two-thirds of the domestic violence killings were in the poorest boroughs, the Bronx and Brooklyn, and three-quarters of the women killed by husbands and boyfriends were black or Hispanic. These findings run counter to the public impression that "domestic violence knows no class and color boundaries," said Dr. Jeff Fagan, director of the Center for Violence, Research and Prevention at Columbia University's School of Public Health.

"The myth of classlessness of domestic violence is one that has persisted since the 1960's," Dr. Fagan said. "The truth is, it is a problem of poverty, associated with other characteristics like low marriage rates, high unemployment and social problems. Whatever we've done to prevent domestic violence has been more effective for white women and we have to figure out how to make it apply to poor women in poor areas."

Also surprising was that in nearly one-third of the cases where husbands and boyfriends killed women, the men also tried to kill themselves.

"Now, when a man comes into a psych clinic and acts like he's suicidal, we should know to screen him to see if he has a family and what kind of relationship it is," Dr. Wilt said. "And women who come into an emergency room because they get hurt by their intimate partners should be aware of the risk to children in the house."

The fact that one-third of the women killed by their husbands were not living with them suggested to Dr. Wilt that these women were trying to leave the relationships.

Overall, many fewer women are killed than men—during the five years in the study, the proportion was nearly seven to one. As total crime decreased in those years, murders of women decreased also, but not as sharply as those of men. At the same time, the number of domestic violence murders increased slightly.

Public health officials worry that the incidence of domestic violence has not dropped as precipitously as the overall crime rate in the past few years. And they are finding that domestic violence rates are not responding to the most common types of crime fighting techniques.

Vivid stories sprang out of the files and forms and documents used in the study.

A 35-year-old woman in Brooklyn was stabbed 12 times with a hunting knife and bludgeoned with a baseball bat by her boyfriend in a case described as "very typical" by Dr. Wilt, who said confidentiality concerns kept her from proving names or identifying details of the victims. The Brooklyn woman's boyfriend killed her on a night he had come home drinking and accused her of having an affair. He also stabbed the woman's sister, who survived.

In another typical domestic violence case, Dr. Wilt said, a 28-year-old woman in the Bronx was killed by her live-in boyfriend after they argued about her leaving him. Neighbors said the boyfriend had abused the woman before and that there was a protection order barring him from seeing her. The boyfriend hit the woman in the face, shot her with a .38 caliber handgun and then shot himself in the head. When the police arrived, they found two children, 5 and 7, in the home with the bodies.

The researchers also looked, of course, at the highly publicized murder cases of those five years, but said that many of them were not typical. Those included the deaths of 87 clubgoers (31 women, 56 men) in the Happy Land Social Club in the Bronx in 1990, which was set on fire by the ex-boyfriend of an employee. And the 1993 murder of Danielle Almonor, a Federal probation officer shot in the back of her head by her estranged husband at the Brooklyn Family Courthouse while she was waiting for their case to be called.

Other unusual cases were the deaths of a woman whose doctor was accused of malpractice and a 16-year-old girl who died of AIDS after being infected through childhood sexual abuse.

Of the 1,156 women killed in New York over the five-year period, more than half were black, even though only one-quarter of the city's female population is black. Sixteen percent of the victims were white, although they make up nearly half the city's female population. And 29 percent of the victims were Hispanic, about the same as their proportion of all women in the city.

Black women were likely to be younger, in their 20's or 30's, and to live in poorer neighborhoods. White women were likely to be older (nearly half were over 50).

Almost one-third of all the murders of women were in the Bronx, even though only 16 percent of the city's women live in there.

Sixty-eight women were killed by their children, grandchildren or other family members who were not husbands or boyfriends. Those murders tended to be more brutal than "intimate partner" murders and other killings because women were more likely to be stabbed—and stabbed more than 10 times.

Domestic violence victims were much less likely to be using cocaine, marijuana or other illegal drugs than other women who were killed. But they were just as likely to be drinking. Dr. Gelles said if a woman in a troubled relationship used alcohol to help her cope, she would be "less able to perceive a threat, more vulnerable to a lethal assault."

Still to be studied, Dr. Wilt said, was whether these victims had sought help from hospitals, the police or other places.

"We're very interested to know," she said, "if women didn't avail themselves of the system, or if the system doesn't work, or if the system can't save them at all."

THE TALLY

A Demographic Portrait

Of 8,932 victims of homicide in New York City from 1990 to 1994, 1,156, or 13 percent, were female. Some predominant characteristics:

Most female victims were black . . .

Black	**52%**
Hispanic	29
White	16
Other	3

. . . and 21 to 40 years old.

21–40	**58%**
Other	42

Nearly half were killed by an "intimate partner"* . . .

An intimate partner was almost always a current or former husband or boyfriend.

Intimate partner	**49%**
Stranger	17
Acquaintance	15
Relative	14
Other	6

*For the 484 homicides for which the relationship between the victim and the assailant could be identified.

. . . and in their homes.

Home	**50%**
Public place	37
Other home	10
Unknown	3

Percentages may not add up to 100 because of rounding.

Source: City Department of Health

"I Was Raped"

A survivor explores an accusation that has divided the Spelman and Morehouse family

LORI S. ROBINSON

A BRISK NOVEMBER WIND GREETED ME when I returned to Spelman College last year. Fall in Atlanta was cooler than what I remembered as a freshman at the historically Black, all-women's school. But that was a decade ago, and much more than the weather had changed. A three-story parking deck sat on what was an asphalt lot in my day. The tiny Guest House near the entrance of the small, fenced campus was gone, replaced by the year-old Camille Olivia Hanks Cosby Academic Center, an elegant five-story building with a museum and auditorium. Even Johnnetta Cole, affectionately known as Sister President, had announced her resignation after 10 years.

Still, as I strolled past the new guard booth, I easily slipped back into the campus' comforting energy. College anywhere is a special time. I was blessed that my time was spent at Spelman, where people didn't assume they were smarter or better than me because of the color of my skin. All around me that November day, young women raced in and out of red brick buildings and cut across lush green grass with confident strides. Spelman strides. I was home again.

And my heart was crumbling because of what had brought me back. I was home to write about rape.

For nearly a month, Spelman and its brother school, Morehouse College, had been in an uproar over a freshman student's accusation that four Morehouse men had sexually assaulted her in a Morehouse dorm late one Friday night. The two schools are educational meccas for the Black middle class and share a special relationship. They are next to each other, and Morehouse men and Spelman women often marry. But in the weeks before my return, the schools had been rocked as rape allegations garnered newspaper headlines and were reported on local television newscasts, packed courtrooms and seriously strained their bond.

There was irony in my returning for the case. In May of 1995, I was supposed to attend my five-year reunion at Spelman. I didn't make it. That was the week that I was raped. In my Washington, D.C., apartment. On my bed. By two men with a gun who accosted me on my doorstep. I was 26 and forever changed.

More than a year later, when I suggested during an *Emerge* staff meeting that we write about rape, I had no idea that in a matter of weeks I would be back in Atlanta. I had mentioned the Spelman–Morehouse case as another example of how serious and complicated the issue is for African-American communities. When senior editors called me back for a private meeting to ask if I would return to Spelman to write the story, I hesitated. They knew about my rape, but there were many issues to consider. Could I write fairly? Could I handle it emotionally? Would it be safe for me? After all, my attackers had never been caught, and *Emerge*'s offices are not far from my old apartment. My editors assured me they would respect whatever I decided.

I thought about those issues during the next few days, but what I thought about most was whether I wanted people to know. My family, my close friends and a few of my colleagues knew I had been attacked, but that was all. Was I ready to give them — and countless strangers — the whole story? Was I ready to write it down in black and white for them the way it had been written in memory for me?

SPELMAN and its brother school, Morehouse College, had been in an uproar over a freshman student's accusation that four Morehouse men had sexually assaulted her.

I was at my desk when the phone rang. Pamela Crockett, an Alexandria, Va., lawyer and rape activist I had been trying to reach for weeks, was on the other end. Shortly after my attack, I had thrown myself head on into healing. Part of the medicine is keeping in contact with women who work on this issue. She and

From *Emerge: Black America's Newsmagazine*, May 1997, pp. 42-53. © 1997 by Emerge Communications, Inc. Reprinted by permission.

I had met when we both spoke to high school girls about careers. In her opening comments, Pamela had mentioned sexual assault as an important issue, and we both noticed how the girls had responded with a keen interest.

I told Pamela what I was considering. In the past we had talked about the silences and the shame in our communities. How Black women are raped at the same rate as White women but are less likely to report it. How we debate the issue when "heroes" such as Mike Tyson are the accused, but never seem able to find our voices when the victim is our mother, or our daughter, or our sister, our niece, or ourselves. I am still amazed at how many women have a story to tell, either about themselves or someone they know.

I went over my concerns with her about doing a story — not only about Spelman and Morehouse, but about me. Finally, Pamela said simply, "I would do it if I were you."

MAY 19, 1995

IT WAS EXHILARATING being on my own. It hadn't been easy living with my parents for two years, saving up money for an apartment. But I had stuck it out and wound up with a comfortable, one–bedroom apartment in Northeast Washington near Catholic University of America. It was a quiet neighborhood and considered relatively safe.

It was my four–month anniversary of independent living, and I was looking forward to attending my college reunion later that week. After visiting friends that Monday night, I drove home a little before 11:30. As I drove, I prayed for inner peace, hoping to quell the ordinary anxieties that left me feeling down from time to time. I believe now that prayer enabled me to get through what was about to become the worst hour of my life.

"Great, a space across the street from my apartment building," I thought as I drove up. Usually, street parking filled up by 8 or 9 p.m., and I would have to park behind the small, two–story apartment building where I lived. It was always too dark and spooky back there for my taste. Pleased at my good fortune, I parked and walked toward my building, thinking about the exercise video I was going to play and the dishes that needed washing.

I jumped slightly when I saw two brothers. "Funny, I didn't notice anybody walking when I parked," I thought once I had crossed the street. Then I reminded myself that I didn't have any reason to be afraid of two men just because they were Black. I didn't give them a second thought. But as I reached my doorstep, one of them jumped up behind me and said something I didn't understand. I turned around to the barrel of a gun pointing at my head. It took me a second to focus. My eyes bulged as I started to look at who was on the other end of the gun.

"You better not look at me," he spat out.

My heart was pounding hard and fast. I felt weak, as if all the wind had left my body. It struck me then that this is what it felt like to have your life threatened. I handed over my purse.

"You can have anything you want," I squeezed out of my burning, deflated lungs.

They ordered me to open the door, but I couldn't get the key to work. That lock always jammed. My hands were shaking. I was talking out loud. "I know it's this key next to the silver one." After several of my futile tries, one of the men said, "It better open this time."

I stopped struggling with the lock and surrendered to God. This time the key turned. They rushed me up the stairs to my apartment. Once inside, they told me to lie on the floor, then they walked around spouting questions.

"Anybody else live here? Anybody else have a key? You supposed to call anybody when you got home?"

They led me to my bedroom, sat me on my bed and continued asking questions about my belongings, reminding me not to talk so loud. "You better not be lying," one said.

Then I was ordered to lie face down on my full–size bed. They tied my feet to the bottom corners of the bed, and my right arm to the upper right corner. When one asked me for something else to use to tie my left hand, I told him where my belts were. Then they wrapped thick duct tape around my head, covering my eyes and mouth.

"Are they doing this so they can shoot me? Maybe they just want to make sure they have plenty of get-away time." My thoughts raced. What was about to happen hadn't occurred to me. Then, with a knife from my kitchen, one of them spliced up the back of the right leg of my black stretch pants. Then it became clear.

"I'm about to be raped."

I never felt so powerless as at that moment. My underwear was snipped at the side and pulled out from under me. Then I heard the sound of a zipper.

One of the rapists climbed on top of me and barked another order.

"Open it up."

He penetrated vaginally for a few seconds, then anally.

The first guy didn't take as long as the second one. He climbed on top of me and started vaginally, too. Then he jammed his penis into my anus. He also talked a lot.

"We're not crazy or nothing.... Does your boyfriend do this to you?"

The time they pounded at me was probably a matter of minutes, but for me, those minutes seemed like hours. Every second I thought I couldn't take any more of the pain.

"Can I come inside you?" he asked several times. Then, as if he had heard me answer through the duct tape across my mouth, he said simply — and pathetically — "Okay, I'll pull out."

The semen poured over my behind.

I remember wondering what it would feel like if they shot me. Maybe a single bullet in the back of my head. I thought about how terrible it would be if I just didn't show up for work for a few days and people came looking for me. They would find me dead, tied to my bed with no underwear. Then I tried not to think about being shot. I tried not to feel any more of the pain and terror that were consuming me. At some point, I simply let go. I realized that I was powerless and helpless. Who I was, the Lori I had known all my life, receded at that moment. All I wanted was for them to leave. All I wanted was to live.

I waited until the apartment was quiet and I was sure they were gone. Ordinarily a hopeless crier, I wasn't crying at all as I worked to untie myself from the bed. I looked at the clock and noticed only an hour had passed since I had parked my car.

All the electronics from my apartment were gone. So was my car. They took the phone cord, so I summoned up the courage and humility to walk down the stairs and knock on my neighbor's door. When I had to face people, that's when I started to cry.

After calling the police, I called my sister and began the long road to healing.

SPELMAN AND MOREHOUSE

On Nov. 12, I was on USAir Flight 1161 headed south to a place where Black girls are molded into women and sent out to make their mark in the world. I do not know how ready for the world the 17-year-old I met last fall will be when — and if — she graduates from Spelman. If what she says is true, that four Morehouse men raped her and three of them sodomized her, the road to self-realization will be difficult. Thinking about the case reminds me that, in a perverse way, I'm one of the lucky ones. My attackers were armed strangers who forced their way into my home and into my body. No one doubted my story or suggested that the assault was my fault. Statistics show, however, that 60 to 80 percent of rape victims know their attacker. For them, the story is very different.

Except for a brief delay caused by the chaos of the 1996 Summer Olympics, the school year had started off like the others. There was a "freshman week" of activities for all the students in the Atlanta University Center, the six-member college association that includes Spelman and Morehouse. There were special bonding events, such as the annual brother-sister tea for Spelman and Morehouse. Shortly after the semester began, President Cole announced her plans to resign after the academic year. When she took the job in 1987, she promised to stay for 10 years.

She was going out with an incredible record, having exceeded the $81 million capital fund-raising goal by almost $33 million. That, with an endowment of about $143 million, gave Spelman, one of two Black all-women's colleges in the country, one of the richest endowments for a Black college. Who would've guessed that Cole would leave another special mark[?] How many college presidents testify at bond hearings for alleged rape defendants?

When the school year began, the Spelman teenager, who spoke to *Emerge* on condition that her identity not be disclosed, settled into her freshman dorm room with the normal anxieties and excitement of new college students. That summer she had worried about whether she and her roommate would get along, but they hit it off immediately. She was excited about the opportunities college would offer—the new experiences, the new friends. Plus, that September she had celebrated her 17th birthday. She was away from home, away from her sheltered family life and ready to take full advantage of her new independence.

Then late one Friday night, she says, it all changed.

At a hearing on Oct. 30, she told her side of the story. She spoke so softly, court records show, that officials had to repeatedly ask her to speak up. This is her courtroom account:

Somewhere between 9 and 9:30 p.m. on Friday, Sept. 27, the freshman, her roommate and several other friends boarded a shuttle bus to go party at The Casino, a nightclub on Auburn Avenue N.E. Spelman freshmen who live on campus are not allowed to have cars, so piling onto a party-destined bus is virtually a weekend ritual. At The Casino, the young woman said she shared two or three drinks with friends. After a few hours, a male acquaintance — whose name she told the court she does not remember — drove the group to the International House of Pancakes for a late-night meal. That same guy dropped her off at Morehouse's Frank Forbes Hall, where she visited a friend, Lorenzo McFadden, also a freshman. His roommate and another young woman, whom she didn't know, were also there. The four of them played cards in McFadden's third-floor dorm room, then she and the other woman played "Bust- A-Move," a video game. After McFadden fell asleep, the Spelman freshman left, deciding to walk the short distance to her dorm alone.

"I'M ONE of the lucky ones. My attackers were armed strangers who forced their way into my home and into my body. No one doubted my story. . . ."

At the bottom of Forbes' stairwell, she told the court, she bumped into Herman Lamar Banks, a senior and member of Morehouse's basketball team. They had met briefly before at the Robert W. Woodruff Library, which is shared by the six colleges of the Atlanta University Center. At Forbes, Banks was standing with Darren Peter Marshall and Dadon Kimontte Dodd, both sophomore basketball players. She'd never met either of them, she testified. Banks offered to walk her back to Spelman but asked her to wait in his room for a few minutes because he had to get something from another room. It was about 15 minutes before Morehouse's 2 a.m. curfew for Friday and Saturday nights, which requires all visitors to leave the dorms.

Banks never walked her home.

While waiting in his first-floor room in the same hallway where the resident director resides, the young woman testified that she heard a loud banging at the window. Then it shattered. Banks, the Morehouse basketball team's starting point guard, had broken it from the outside, she said. Why he broke it has never been explained.

She was about to leave when the few guys now gathered in the room urged her to wait in another room while they cleaned up the glass. Then she would be walked home. She decided to visit another friend in Forbes Hall, but he was not in. She left him a note before going to wait in Dodd's room.

The room was empty for five to 10 minutes before Dodd came in, she said. His name, he had told her, was Suave. When he sat on the bed, she stood up. She looked through his CDs, selected one and he put it on his disc player. He noticed her looking at his bottle of rum. He offered her some. She told him she couldn't drink it straight. Then they began to hunt for change to buy Cokes. She went to the vending machines in the lobby to get the sodas. She saw Banks and Marshall near the machines.

THE INCIDENT

When she brought the drinks to Dodd's room, he left to find some glasses. He came back with one and told her they'd have to do shots. The young woman said she didn't do shots. She poured the rum and Coke into the glass and took two sips; Dodd drank the rest. In court testimony, she also would say that she had had a couple of hits off a friend's bottle of Boones Farm wine before arriving at Morehouse.

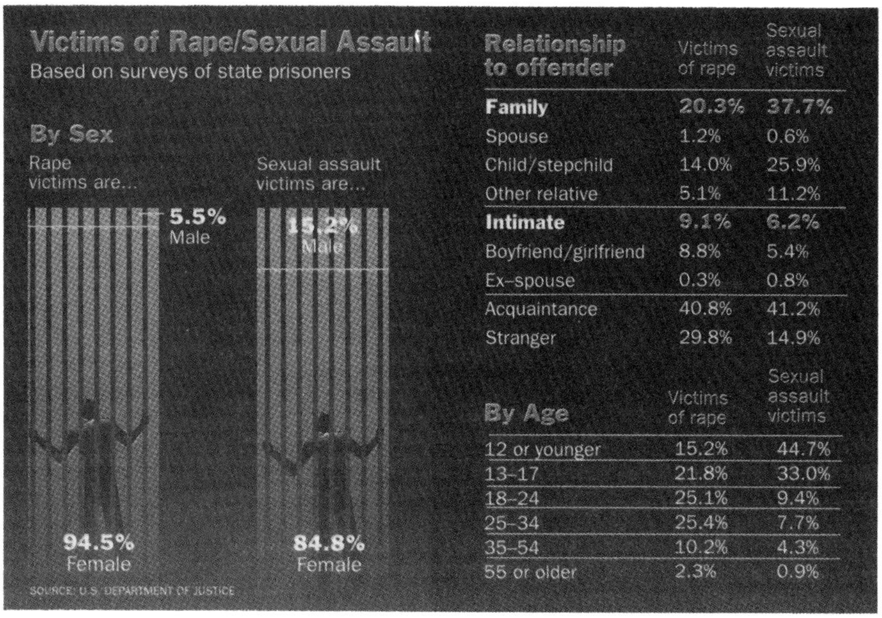

CHART: ROD LITTLE FOR EMERGE

Dodd sat down on the bed again and they began to browse through a photo album, she said. They talked casually about majors. Dodd asked her to sit on the bed. When she did, he asked why she sat so far away. She told him she was leaving soon. By that time, curfew had passed.

Morehouse's curfews are routinely broken. The rules for male visitors on Spelman's campus are strict. Men must be off the grounds by midnight. Guards keep track of male visitors by signing them in and out and by collecting identification. Morehouse is on an honor system, and guards don't track women visitors, a policy officials now say they are re-evaluating.

Dodd slid close to her and began touching her pants, she told the court. He asked what type of material it was. She said she didn't know. He said he thought it was silk. She said she didn't think so. He put his hand in her lap and began to touch her vagina through her pants, she testified. She said she didn't think they should be doing this because they'd just met. He said sometimes people click. She said she didn't feel like they had clicked.

In hearing the testimony, a lawyer asked the Spelman student why, at that point, she didn't leave. She said she still felt safe, that if she asked him to stop he would. Then she added, "Now that I think about things, I look back and say there's so much I could have done but I didn't."

Dodd, she said, reached above his head and turned off the light and began pulling down her pants. She tried to pull them back up, but the 6'6" basketball player eventually got them off, she testified. He stood over her and stuck his penis in her vagina against her will, she testified. She objected and told him that she wanted to go home.

Banks and Marshall entered the room at that point and spoke to each other in whispers, she testified. Then Marshall, also 6'6", stood next to the bed. His pants were off. "This is all for you," she said he told her as he pushed her head toward his penis and stuck it in her mouth. Marshall raped her as Banks put his penis in her mouth, she said.

Morehouse junior Tony Carnell Clark came into the room, the Spelman student said. He stood in the doorway for a moment before telling Banks that his brother was on the phone. The Spelmanite doesn't recall Banks responding. Marshall got off her and Clark then stuck his penis in her vagina, she testified. While Banks was on top of her, Clark stuck his penis in her mouth. Clark also sodomized her, she testified.

She repeatedly said, "I do not want to do this. I want to go home," she told the court. But the young men ignored her.

When they did back off, she was in tears. She grabbed her clothes and ran to the door. Clark stopped her there. "Haven't I seen you before?" he asked her. Disgusted, she shook her head, but he continued. "I remember meeting you at the library, that was the last time I saw you.'" Marshall wouldn't look at her, she said. Dodd focused on a closet. She did not account for Banks.

She ran outside Forbes Hall, but there was a crowd of people there and she couldn't bear to walk past them, so she ran back upstairs to her friend McFadden's room, she testified. She banged on the door, but there was no answer. She called from the pay phone down the hall, but there was still no answer. She banged on the door again. This time his roommate answered. Still crying, she woke McFadden and told him she needed him to walk her home.

"He kept on asking me what was wrong...and I couldn't tell him. I said I just need for you to walk me home," she said. He told her he wasn't going to walk her home until he knew why she was crying. She finally told him.

She also told her roommate, Jackie Holland, daughter of Spelman board chairman Bob Holland, former CEO of ice cream-maker Ben & Jerry's Homemade Inc. It was Holland who called a cab and took her to Grady Memorial Hospital's rape crisis center, where she underwent a rape examination.

The examinations can be physically and emotionally painful. Far worse than any gynecological exam, doctors must scrape inside the body for "evidence." What I remember most about my exam is that it felt like another rape.

Early that Saturday morning, the young woman reported the incident to Spelman's security force. Five days later, on Oct. 2, she filed a report with Atlanta's police department. Banks, Clark, Dodd and Marshall were arrested the next day.

FACE TO FACE

FINDING HER IS EASIER than I thought it would be. I ask around and am eventually directed to her dorm door. I introduce myself to a young woman standing in the door. I tell her who I am looking for and she shakes her head. "I'm just a friend," she says and points to another young woman who is sitting on a bed, talking on the phone. She is a petite, attractive woman. I introduce myself, explain that I am a journalist. I tell her that I am a rape victim, too, but spare her details, saying only that I was attacked at gunpoint in my home. I mention, too, that I am a Spelmanite.

Our situations are so different. She is 17, in her first semester of college. I am already a woman, out of college, working. My story has never been questioned. For her, others' doubts are a given, and their accusatory questions are a fact of life. What was she wearing? What was she doing in the dorm so late? And why was she alone?

Even I must reserve judgment. The four accused men are innocent until proven guilty in a court of law.

Her soft, quiet voice does not fill the tiny room where we sit. The floor is cluttered with magazines, shoes and other items you'd expect to find in a college dorm room. There are lots of pictures of her family and friends on the wall above her bed. She and her mother. Her sister, who is older, out of college and working, like me. Family and friends have been with her in court, and her sister testified at one hearing.

During our brief time together, friends drop in to check on her. She tells me that she rarely goes to class and sees a private therapist. She slowly shakes her head at how much of a spectacle this whole thing has become.

I am not sure if I could have stayed on campus. I never returned to the apartment where I was assaulted. My sister, my boyfriend and other friends moved my things. Police found my car, which the attackers used to get away. I drove it once, from the police station to my parents' home. A short time later, it was traded.

I think, too, about the 15-year-old high school student at New York's Manhattan Center for Math and Science who was forced to perform oral sex on the school's basketball star, Richie Parker, and one of Parker's friends, in January 1994. She was harassed so much that eventually she was forced to transfer. The Spelman freshman has received an anonymous letter implying that she was ruining the lives of four promising Black men.

So why does she stay? "They've already taken so much from me," she says.

The four young men tell a different story. Three say they engaged in consensual sex with the Spelman freshman. The fourth, Marshall, says he had no sexual contact with her at all. They have all pleaded not guilty. Though I have had several conversations with their lawyers, I have not had access to the young men. But within hours of being on campus, I learn that they are well-liked.

On Thursday, Oct. 3, Atlanta police arrested the four on Morehouse's campus, and took them to the Atlanta City Detention Center before eventually moving them to the Fulton County Jail. They would spend nearly a month and a half in jail, their names and faces flashed across television screens, their alleged crimes recounted in print.

The first time I see them it is at a bond hearing. It is Nov. 14, the day before they will be released from jail. They are marched into a crowded courtroom, each wearing a blue prison jumpsuit with "Fulton County Jail" emblazoned in white.

Banks, the shortest of the four at 5'7", is Morehouse's starting point guard. His youthful, light-brown face belies his age. He turned 21 the day before he was freed on bail. Banks grew up in Cambridge, Mass., where his father is a retired police officer. His mother works in the registrar's office of Roxbury Community College. And his sister, Chandra Banks, a 1991 Spelman graduate, is president of the Boston chapter of the National Alumnae Association of Spelman College.

Clark is a Morehouse junior who also grew up in Cambridge, and like Banks, spent his 21st birthday behind bars. He is on academic scholarship and the only defendant not on the basketball team. His father is deceased and his mother teaches preschool.

Dodd, a 20-year-old sophomore, is the youngest and one of the tallest at 6'6". His parents are divorced. His mother, an administrative assistant, now lives in Stone Mountain, Ga., near Atlanta. His father is vice president of a steel company in Detroit. His basketball skills were good enough to win him a scholarship to Morehouse.

Darren Marshall is also a sophomore, but is the oldest of the four at 26. Even with his long, brown face and mustache, he appears younger. A native of Trinidad, he was required to surrender his passport as a condition of his release on bail. A younger brother is also a Morehouse student, and their parents live in New York, but unlike the parents of the other young men, they cannot make the trip to Atlanta.

They are Morehouse men, with family and friends who love them. And, according to a young African-American woman, they are the four men who raped her. For young Black men to successfully navigate the pitfalls and dangers that ensnare so many others, it is particularly painful for their family and friends to believe that their lives may be destroyed. If convicted, they face a minimum sentence of 10 years with no probation or parole, up to life in prison, the maximum for rape in Georgia. At an Oct. 30 court hearing, the sodomy charges, which also carry a minimum 10 years to life, were dropped because the judge believed it would be impossible for the accuser to say which of the students committed it.

"THAT was one of the most emotional courtrooms I've sat in in a long time." People "would run out of the room."

In this drama, their lives and futures have been pitted against the life and future of their accuser.

I have squeezed into a seat in the back of the courtroom. As it was for a hearing nearly a month earlier, on Oct. 16, the room is packed. By all accounts, that October hearing was an emotional, tense and dramatic scene. The Spelman freshman's parents and three of the four defendants' mothers were there. President Cole's testimony that day played a pivotal role in the initial denial of bail.

Spelman senior Cara Grayer, a friend of Clark's, was there.

"That was one of the most emotional courtrooms I've sat in in a long time," says Grayer, whose father is a lawyer. "I was sitting next to Dadon Dodd's mother. . . . They would say 25 years to life. Dadon Dodd's mother would run out of the room. . . . The mother of the girl—[when] they would say [the charge of] 'sodomy', she would . . . run out of the room."

A month later, emotions would be just as high, but there had been a development in the days before that had bolstered the young men's supporters. There had been reports that a security guard had found their accuser in her friend McFadden's dorm room days before the November hearing. She was hiding in a closet, supposedly, with her pants down around her knees.

When I hear this, I, like many, begin to have doubts. I ask her about the accusation when we meet. She does not deny being in McFadden's room. They have grown closer—platonically, she stresses—since the attack. He has become one of the people she talks to and that is what they were doing when she was found in his room. And her pants being down? "He's lying," she says of the security guard's accusation.

At the bond hearing, defense attorneys bring one character witness after another to testify for their clients. Among them were Banks' sister, Dodd's former boss and a Morehouse assistant basketball coach. The young men also take the stand to answer questions about their character. No details of that night are discussed. The most dramatic moment comes when an attorney asks all those present in support of the defendants to stand.

The display of support stuns me. I try to count the people still in their seats, but can't see in front of me because there are so many people standing. I would learn later that the Spelmanite also had been in the courtroom.

The hearing was enough to persuade Judge Gail S. Tusan, a Black woman, to set bail at $30,000 for each of the accused.

In an interview later, Ted Lackland, Tony Clark's lawyer, tells me this case reminds him of the Scottsboro Boys, nine young Black men who in 1931 were falsely accused of raping two White girls. Eight received death sentences and one received life in prison. Their case inspired a successful international campaign for their freedom. "The presumption is that it must have been a rape because that kind of thing is beneath her," he says of this case.

His point leaves me wondering about questions I do not ask. What if the young men accused had been White fraternity boys? What would he have said then? But Black women have always been put in the position of choosing between racial and sexual oppression.

Grayer, like many students on Spelman's campus, is torn. "It's very, very difficult and that's where a lot of students are being put in that position," she says. "They're being asked to choose. ...you either have to stand behind the women or you have to stand behind the men, there's no middle ground. I stand firmly against rape. At the same time, I stand firmly that I hold one of the young men in my heart. And that's what's most disturbing about this case.

"That's what makes it high-profile, when you see the mothers and they're in tears, all of them.... That is a mother's worst nightmare...to send your daughter away to college, and then at the same time to have your young man that you've raised...to know that they've assaulted another woman. I think that that has to be the hardest thing on earth."

Grayer says she has chosen to support her friend, Clark. The circumstances, she says, are questionable anyway, and she does not want to see his future lost.

Hers is a view not foreign to African-American women. I am a Black woman, too, and I understand. I, too, cringe at the thought of one more Black man being turned over to a flawed criminal justice system. I have a brother and a father and other Black men in my life whom I love and respect. My brother was falsely accused and arrested once for mugging an elderly White

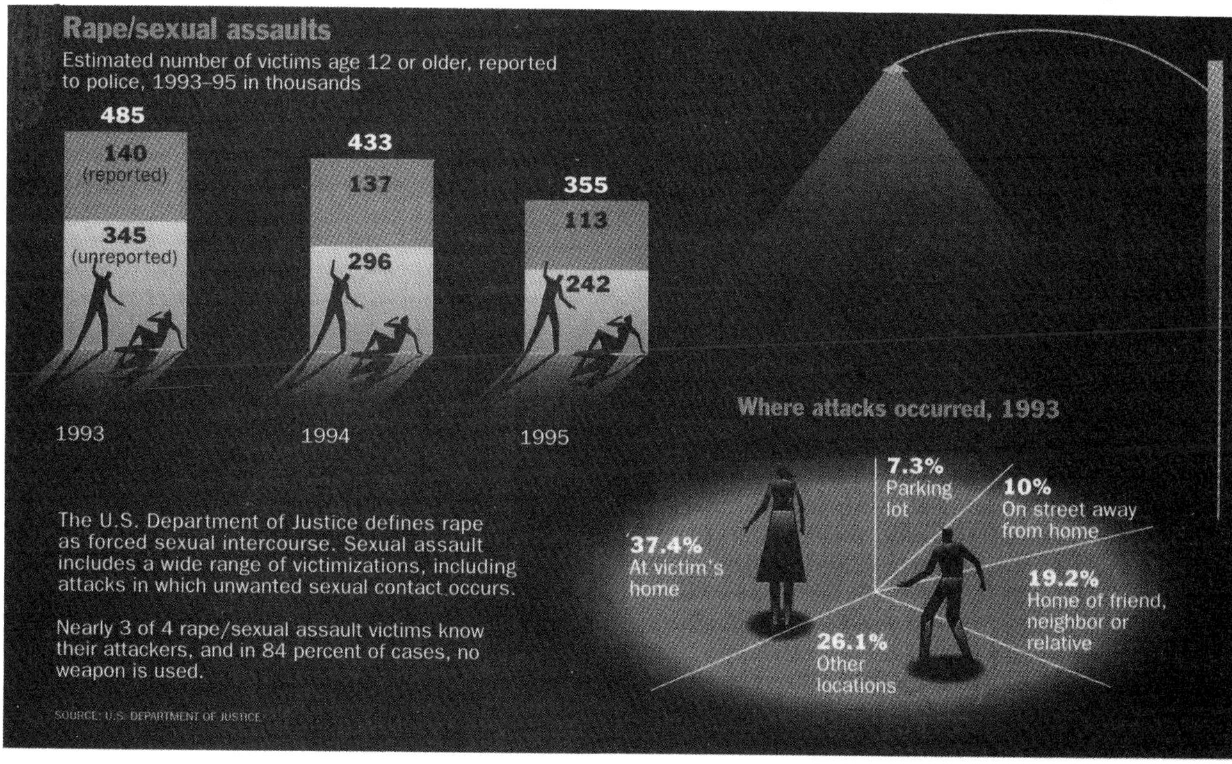

CHART: ROD LITTLE FOR EMERGE

woman when he was in college in Tacoma, Wash. If my father had not had the money to fly across the country and hire a lawyer, who knows how long my brother would have been in jail. The thought of any of my loved ones behind bars — or the thousands of men wrongly jailed — ties me in knots of sadness and anger. But I also know this: One of my greatest fantasies is to castrate the men who raped me.

Evelyn C. White, author of *Chain Chain Change: For Black Women in Abusive Relationships*, says there is a "great sense of racial loyalty that exists among Black women. Black women, because of racism, are very, very aware and understanding and empathetic toward the African-American men who sexually assault us."

Still, questions remain. What if the Spelmanite is lying? It has happened, though I don't understand why someone would put themselves through the emotional or physical horrors of doing such a thing. No matter what, her college years have been ruined. College will not be the wonderful experience it should be. But I am forced to concede that anything is possible.

But what if she is telling the truth? This type of hell I already know the answer to. Rape is a violation that forever changes you. To confront it on a campus or in a courtroom, takes tremendous fortitude. I could not imagine being in a courtroom where a sea of people stand up against me.

A final question comes to me: What if she's telling the truth, and so are the defendants — at least that they believe they are innocent? What if they think that what happened is okay? Nathan McCall writes, in *Makes Me Wanna Holler*, about "running trains" on women — women who may not have fought or resisted, but who were certainly tricked or coerced into a situation that devalued and demeaned them. I listen to students such as Grayer and conclude that that would be the worst of all.

THE CAMPUS

THE SISTER-BROTHER bonds between Spelman and Morehouse have been strained. The case has forced a tight-knit community to examine its attitudes about sexual violence. Some Morehouse students have said they felt betrayed by President Cole's strong support of the Spelman student. They are disappointed, too, in what they consider their own administration's lack of support for their four schoolmates.

"Everybody becomes consumed by it, students, faculty, staff, it's almost like a struggle to try to understand, and people hold on to beliefs," says Vice Provost Eddie Gaffney, a Morehouse graduate who worked at the University of South Carolina for 17 years. "At the University of South Carolina, they'd see [this] as an individual problem. Here, it's a family problem."

For a while it seemed the family was divided into two camps.

Cole set the tone at Spelman. She took the freshman into her home for a few days immediately after the incident. At a town hall meeting, she urged students to support their schoolmate. And when she testified at the hearing where bail for the four accused men was denied, she got the best of a defense lawyer who tried to spar with her. Spelman students followed her lead, attending public meetings and holding discussions on sexual violence. They decorated a board of supportive wishes in the Manley College Student Center. The young woman's friends rallied around her, supporting her decision to remain on campus, getting her assignments from professors, turning them in for her, as she rarely left her dorm.

SHE recalls Spelmanites complaining about an offensive image on a flier advertising a club. But by the next week, they were back partying at the same spot.

There were about 80 women and fewer than a dozen men at a speak-out against sexual violence sponsored by the Women's Research and Resource Center when I was on campus. SGA president Ardenia Johnson talked a lot about personal accountability. She recalled Spelmanites complaining about an offensive image on a flier advertising a club. She said students were ready to burn bras, Snoop Doggy Dogg tapes and anything they could get their hands on that denigrated women. But by the next week, she says, they were back partying at the same spot.

Morehouse's administration wasn't far behind Cole. The school began its own investigation into the matter on Sept. 30. Administrators immediately suspended the four students for the academic year for violation of college rules. It said the suspensions were not related to the criminal charges but the violation of the campus rules regarding conduct.

"For generations, Morehouse has set very high standards of ethics and morality for its students, staff and faculty, standards that must be upheld at all times," said the school's Oct. 7 statement. "The College determined through its investigation that the behavior of the students in this case was not consistent with behavior expected and demanded of Morehouse students.

"The College is deeply concerned and saddened that anyone, especially a student at our sister institution, Spelman College, may have been the victim of violence or abuse. Inappropriate sexual conduct has never been acceptable on the Morehouse campus and will not be tolerated now."

At a school assembly that same day, John H. Hopps, provost of Morehouse College, made similar remarks. Faculty members answered questions about the incident at a forum that night in King Chapel. At least 1,500 students attended the town hall meeting and what faculty and staff heard that night took some by surprise, says Gaffney. "That's when we really found out that a lot of young men had no idea about the sexual politics of present times," he says.

If statistics from the U.S. Centers for Disease Control and Prevention are any indication, such educational efforts are desperately needed on all college campuses, not just African-American ones. From 15 percent to 25 percent of male college students admit to involvement in some level of sexual aggression. Additionally, more than 80 percent of rapes on college campuses are committed by someone the victim knows.

At Morehouse, while there was tough talk about the abuse of women, there was also another side to the discussion. In handouts distributed on college stationery, the administration said it was considering a defense fund for the four accused students. Five lawyers volunteered to teach students about their legal rights.

Beverly Guy-Sheftall, founding director of Spelman's Women's Research and Resource Center, wants to know who will teach young African-American men at Morehouse and around the country about respecting Black women?

"There is an assumption that Black men are being targeted, or that there's actually some conspiracy to destroy Black men," she says. "I think that's the scenario around which these cases get framed and that it's very difficult to separate those notions. "

Lawrence Edward Carter, dean of the Morehouse chapel, didn't help the campus friction much. During regular worship services, a day before the Oct. 7 assembly, Carter suggested that women bring abuse upon themselves because of their attitudes and their dress. Some Spelman students walked out. Later, nine Spelmanites responded in a pointed letter that was printed Oct. 14 in Morehouse's newspaper, *The Maroon Tiger*:

"We found your understanding of the true issues involved in the violent crime of rape to be faulty. As evidence of this, we point to the particularly offensive description of the woman wearing 'a strip of tape,' the woman whose skirt was 'sprayed on,' and that she was 'an accident waiting to happen.' ...You victimized the victim in your remarks, and this was unfair, inappropriate and un-Christian.

"...You suggested that a heinous crime of violence perpetrated against a Spelman woman by Morehouse men should be excused or even justified because the sisters are 'loose,' and the brothers are weak and must be expected to succumb to 'temptation.' Rape is not about lust or attire; it is about power and control."

They demanded an apology. Carter was suspended for an unspecified period. He issued a five-paragraph response/apology, which *The Maroon Tiger* printed the same day, and agreed to attend a joint worship service at Spelman's Sisters Chapel but he did not show up.

Says Hopps: "Let me be very clear. Morehouse College absolutely rejects any such notion. No individual, no man or woman, ever deserves to be abused by virtue of the clothing they choose. We abhor any suggestion to the contrary."

Says Antonio Johnson, Morehouse's student government association president, whose mother was raped when he was a child, "Dean Carter, in my opinion, should be fired. Those statements, I think, were extremely insensitive to women. He knew of the sensitivity of the moment, and that's why I'm so outraged about it."

Some students were disappointed in the Morehouse administration for other reasons.

"I didn't like the positions the college took," says Baimba Norman, a junior from Liberia, who believes Morehouse turned its back on the young men. "I don't think they should have suspended them.... Other people break curfew rules. If it was based on that, on breaking curfew rules, hundreds of people would be suspended because that happens daily."

Another junior, Darnik McAlpin, expressed a common attitude toward the Spelman freshman. "Why was she over here at that time by herself?" asks the Augusta, Ga., native. "Maybe [she] got mad afterwards. . . . There's no justification for doing that, don't get me wrong. . . . But I think she was there, and she had sex with all those guys, and afterwards, maybe she was feeling guilty.

" . . . Like Mike Tyson and Desiree [Washington] . . . one of those things where after they finished with her, instead of letting her stay over or whatever, they're like, 'You better go ahead and get out. . . .' She got mad.

"The law is messed up for the simple fact that a girl can lie. I can have sex with her one night, and then the next day we get in an argument and then she accuses you of rape the night before. . . . My word against hers. I'm already in jail. It's already on my record."

Craig Boyd, who works for Morehouse's sports medicine department and knows all four defendants, says, "Someone

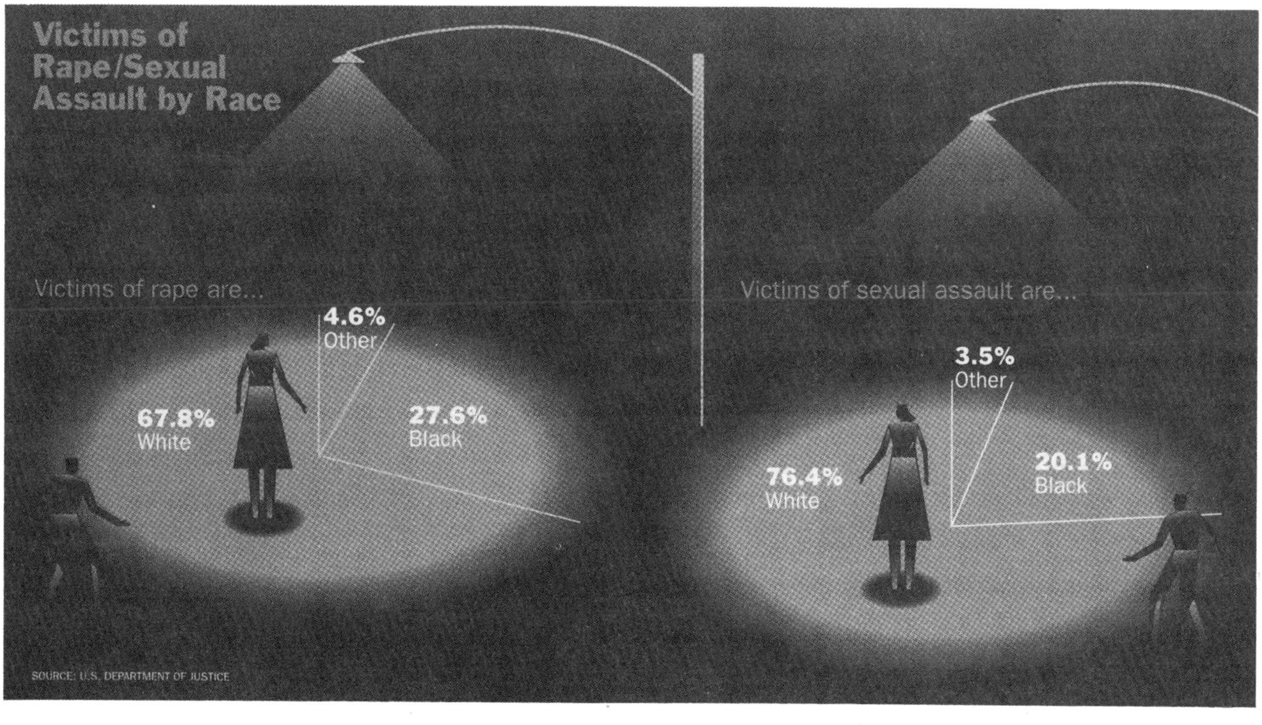

CHART: ROD LITTLE FOR EMERGE

"I DON'T like the positions the college took. I don't think they should have suspended them."

should have said this is wrong," but he does not believe a crime was committed that night.

Kevin Ladaris, a senior and a leader of the campus group Men for the Eradication of Sexism, says he believes so many male students doubt that a rape occurred because they see themselves in similar situations. That is parallel to women blaming the victim, he says, because if the men didn't do anything wrong, then any woman is vulnerable to rape.

Says Rev. Aubra Love, director of the Black Church and Domestic Violence Task Force at the Center for the Prevention of Sexual and Domestic Violence in Seattle, "We have a rape culture which does not accept rape as violence and treats rape as if it has something to do with sex, when in fact, if we could talk plainly, it's like mugging with a body, assault with a penis."

For Kevin Ladaris, of Morehouse, the campus incident has irony. It occurred the same weekend that his organization hosted its forum on violence against women.

At press time, the four men had not been indicted and no court date had been set. "The investigation is still on-going," says Terri Lawson-Adams, a spokesperson for the Fulton County district attorney's office. Atlanta police also are still investigating the charges.

Morehouse officials, meanwhile, have readmitted the four to classes and extracurricular activities. Their original one-year suspensions — for violating college rules and standards of conduct — were appealed and later reduced to one semester.

RECOVERING

THE DAY I LEAVE CAMPUS I am exhausted. I have spent my last hours trying to arrange to speak with the four men. It never works out. I also try to call the accuser, but there is no answer. I walk across the campus and remember that this is where I first learned what it meant to believe in myself and my dreams. For me, like it is for so

Haunted by History

IN ADDITION to the guilt and shame that can accompany sexual assault, Black women often face the additional burdens of race and history, which can encourage them to minimize their own pain and excuse or protect their attacker, say some who have studied the issue. Whether it is the case of Celia, a teenage slave girl who was hanged in Missouri for killing her White rapist, or the film, *Birth of a Nation,* conceived to perpetuate the myth of the Black rapist, African-American women have learned to be silent about sexual assault.

"One of the reasons that historically rape has been more complicated for Black people [is] there is the history . . . of Black men being falsely accused of rape, even though most of that memory is [of being] falsely accused by White women," says Beverly Guy-Sheftall, founding director of Spelman's Women's Research and Resource Center. "So I think that the whole issue of rape is already a contested terrain within the Black community."

Stereotypes of hypersexual African-Americans grew out of the slavery-era ethos. For the first centuries of this nation's existence, it was accepted, even expected for White men to sexually assault Black women slaves, a way for owners to produce more "property" and constantly demonstrate their total ownership of Africans.

One of the most egregious and documented cases was that of Celia, who in 1850, at the age of 14, was bought by Robert Newsom, a 70-year-old farmer. After years of repeated rapes by Newsom, Celia killed him. The court rejected the notion that she had the right to resist. She was charged with first-degree murder and hanged.

Once slavery ended, myths about Black sexuality festered, and the protection of White women's virtue became another rationalization for brutalizing African-American men and women.

In the 1890s, journalist Ida B. Wells reported that about one-fourth of lynching victims were accused of attempted rape or rape. Recorded lynchings from 1882 to 1962 number nearly 5,000, and many more unrecorded murders by White mobs cut short Black lives. Whites also lynched Black men who had attempted to avenge their loved ones who had been raped.

D. W. Griffith's 1915 work, *Birth of a Nation,* went a long way toward immortalizing such ideas. That movie dramatized Civil War and Reconstruction history from a White southerner's perspective, and fictionalized the origin of the Ku Klux Klan. In the film, a lecherous Black man attempts to harm White women. The film concludes with Klan members gallantly riding to the rescue.

Griffith said he wanted "to create a feeling of abhorrence in White people, especially White women, against Colored men."

Considered the technically sophisticated forerunner of today's feature films, the blockbuster grossed more than $18 million and was the first movie screened at the White House. More than anything, however, it reinforced a violent, racist and sexist culture that African-Americans continue to navigate today.

Conversely, Guy-Sheftall says, "Historically, we know that the rape of Black women has been paid absolutely no attention to by the larger society."

That legacy is never far behind, Guy-Sheftall says, arguing that it plays itself out between African-American men and women, both in high-profile media cases and those cases where the rape is never reported.

Says Guy-Sheftall, "In an ironic kind of way, when Black men get accused of rape, the Black woman almost gets put in the same category as White women who accuse Black men of rape, and she becomes the enemy, too."

—*Lori S. Robinson*

many women, it was an academic and social haven. I try to calm my stomach by telling myself if there is a place where lessons will be learned about confronting sexual violence in our communities, it will be here. If we do not, it will continue to eat away at us. The government reports a recent drop in rapes, but the crime remains a serious problem. As it has been true here, as it is true in my own life and the lives of others, rape — or even the allegation of rape — touches more than the accuser and accused. It devastates families, friends, communities.

I do not know how the Spelman student — or even the four from Morehouse — will fare. My own recovery continues and I believe it is a lifelong struggle.

Although I was blessed to never have nightmares, the fears of my waking hours — the fear of disease, of my family being tracked down and hurt by the rapists, of unknowingly bumping into them — left me drained of energy and happiness for months. After all, I never got a good look at the gunman's face, and never saw the other rapist's face. The police told me that the assailants were believed to have raped at least three other women. To my knowledge, they have not been caught.

My biggest obstacles in healing became lingering fears of being harmed again, by the rapists or other men. And I was furious over the disruption in my life, the loss of my treasured independence. I had to change my car, my home, and alter my psyche. My life was turned upside down.

The day after the attack, after I had told my family, I began telling the other people close to me. A girlfriend shocked me with her response, a shrill shriek and then uncontrollable sobbing. It confirmed my concern that even though the rape was not my fault, I now had no choice but to cause pain for those close to me.

When I told my mom, she looked as if she might pass out for a second, then she immediately began to talk about what needed to be done. My boyfriend repeated it back to me. "Did you just say you were robbed and raped?" he said, as if he was hoping he heard wrong. I remember begging for his friendship and support, fully expecting him not to want to deal with a basket case. "This will only bring us closer together," he told me. Nothing could have been more comforting. My family and friends, and the love and tender care of my boyfriend, have helped me survive and to grow stronger in spirit and resolve.

I guess more than anything, what I carry with me as I walk out of this valley in my life is a commitment to help end the silence. A close male member of my family could not bring himself to speak to me about my rape for an entire year. The last time we were both at Spelman was on my graduation day.

I have learned that he cried when told about my rape. I wonder what it would have been like if we had cried — and healed — together.

Where to Find Help

THE RAPE, ABUSE & INCEST NATIONAL NETWORK (RAINN)
24-hour national hot line for instant referrals to local organizations
1-800-656-HOPE

NORTHEAST / NEW YORK
RAPE INTERVENTION PROGRAM
Mount Sinai Medical Center
(212) 241-5461

VICTIM SERVICES
Hot line: (212) 577-7777

NEW JERSEY
SEXUAL ASSAULT AND RAPE ANALYSTS
Newark
(201) 733-7273

MID-ATLANTIC / PENNSYLVANIA
WOMEN ORGANIZED AGAINST RAPE
Philadelphia
Hot line: (215) 985-3333

MARYLAND
SEXUAL ASSAULT & DOMESTIC VIOLENCE CENTER
Baltimore
Hot line: (410) 828-6390

WASHINGTON, D.C.
D.C. RAPE CRISIS CENTER
Hot line: (202) 333-7273

VIRGINIA
SEXUAL ASSAULT OUTREACH PROGRAM
Richmond
Hot line: (804) 643-0888

MIDWEST / OHIO
RAPE CRISIS CENTER
Cleveland
Hot line: (216) 391-3912

ILLINOIS
YWCA WOMEN'S SERVICES
Chicago
(312) 372-4105

MINNESOTA
SEXUAL VIOLENCE CENTER
Minneapolis
(612) 871-5111

WISCONSIN
SEXUAL ASSAULT TREATMENT CENTER
Milwaukee
Hotline: (414) 937-5555

MICHIGAN
DETROIT POLICE RAPE COUNSELING CENTER
(313) 833-1660

MISSOURI
METROPOLITAN ORGANIZATION TO COUNTER SEXUAL ASSAULT
Kansas City
(816) 531-0233

SOUTH / GEORGIA
GRADY RAPE CRISIS CENTER
Atlanta
(404) 616-4861

NORTH CAROLINA
RAPE CRISIS CENTER
Charlotte
Hot line: (704) 375-9900

FLORIDA
SEXUAL ASSAULT CRISIS CENTER (RESPONSE)
Orlando
Hot line: (407) 740-5408

CRISIS CENTER OF HILLSBORO COUNTY, INC.
Tampa
(813) 238-8821

LOUISIANA
YWCA RAPE CRISIS PROGRAM
New Orleans
Hot line: (504) 483-8888

TEXAS
HOUSTON-AREA WOMEN'S CENTER RAPE CRISIS CENTER
Hot line: (713) 528-7273

TENNESSEE
SEXUAL ASSAULT RESOURCE CENTER
Memphis
(901) 272-2020

WEST/ CALIFORNIA
LOS ANGELES COMMISSION ON ASSAULTS AGAINST WOMEN
(310) 392-8381

COLORADO
RAPE ASSISTANCE & AWARENESS PROGRAM
Denver
Hot line: (303) 322-7273

SOURCE: D. C. RAPE CRISIS CENTER

DOMESTIC VIOLENCE Can Be Cured

Tulsa, Okla., has created a task force to establish protection for battered women that could prove to be a model for a nationwide program to combat such abuse.

by Felicia Collins Correia

IMAGINE THIS SCENARIO: You are a woman walking on a street in your community when you are attacked for the *fourth* time this month. You file a report with the police again, although you really don't know why you bother. They know who has been perpetrating these assaults on you, but do little more than talk to him and tell him to refrain from repeating the attacks. The police officers know he will do it again, yet seem apathetic. One cop informs you that, even if they were to arrest him, he would make bond and the crime would be plea-bargained down to community service. They suggest you walk on the other side of the street to avoid him next time.

There are a number of disturbing aspects in this hypothetical situation. For one, it appears that you no longer are safe from violent crime. More alarming is the response of the police force and judiciary. This criminal is free to continue assaulting you without any fear of facing jail time. On top of all of this, you feel powerless.

You may be inclined to dismiss this vignette as something that never could happen in the U.S. Unfortunately for millions of battered American women, the situation is not at all hypothetical. This is their reality:

- Every nine seconds, a woman is abused by her husband or intimate partner. That translates to almost 4,000,000 females each year.
- Women are victims of domestic violence more often than of burglary, muggings, or other physical crimes combined.
- Forty-two percent of murdered women are killed by their intimate male partners.

Injuries received by victims of domestic violence are at least as serious as those suffered in 90% of violent felonies, notes Joan Zorza, editor of the *Domestic Violence Report* of the Civic Research Institute, Kingston, N.J. Yet, in most states, battering still is considered a misdemeanor punishable only by small fines and/or a short time in prison. That presumes, of course, the batterer actually is arrested and charged with the crime.

For all of the latest political posturing about getting "tough on crime," many in the law enforcement and legal communities across the nation do not respond to this type of assault as a crime. Contrary to popular belief, domestic abuse is not a family matter. It is a crime and, as such, a *public* matter that should involve protection for the victims and justice for the batterers. In order to attack the epidemic of family violence effectively, a concerted response from various segments of society is necessary. These include lawmakers, the police, the judiciary, medical providers, educators, employers, and the general public. As public awareness of domestic violence has increased due to growing media coverage, the time is ripe to work toward "systems" changes. It is no small task, but can be done.

The domestic violence movement in the U.S. originated in the mid 1970s as a grassroots crusade led primarily by women's advocates. Part of their agenda involved establishing state coalitions and working collectively to convince politicians and the public that the problem was widespread and serious enough to warrant legal and social attention. These early activists toiled tirelessly at improving the response to domestic abuse by creating legislation and forming domestic violence coalitions. (All 50 states and the District of Columbia now have one.) Their original focus was to encompass legislative, systems, and policy advocacy.

While the problem was being addressed by lawmakers and policymakers, the issue of helping individual victims of abuse remained. This need was recognized formally when the first shelter for battered women opened its doors in 1974 in St. Paul, Minn., to assist individuals in crisis situations and

Ms. Correia is executive director, Domestic Violence Intervention Services, Inc., Tulsa, Okla.

From *USA Today Magazine,* November 1997, pp. 32-34. © 1997 by the Society for the Advancement of Education. Reprinted by permission.

has grown to more than 2,000 shelters in communities across the country. As local domestic violence organizations sprung up, they began providing much-needed treatment and services to individual victims.

After laws to protect women were passed, the state coalitions failed to expand their role to include monitoring local protection systems to ensure that such policies were being enforced. Too many local domestic violence programs did not or could not monitor or implement changes in police, legal, or judiciary responses to domestic violence in their communities. As a result, the focus of domestic violence advocacy shifted from systems to individual clients during the 1980s.

While the strides made in the domestic violence movement have been laudable (shelters, counseling, batterer treatment, the Violence Against Women Act of 1994), there is room for improvement. Politicians who tout the importance of family values must recognize the need for proper legislation regarding violence. How can they promise a return to family values if they can't promise their citizens protection and justice in the face of domestic abuse?

Traditionally, the state coalitions primarily have targeted the "top" of the system—*i.e.*, state and national legislatures—to pass laws that apply to all citizens. While it is crucial to secure these laws, they mean nothing if not enforced in every town and city. Instead of relying on the top-down strategy favored by the state coalitions, local domestic violence groups should employ a bottom-up one, working together with local government, law enforcement, legal, judiciary, medical, and educational organizations to effect changes in their handling of domestic violence. The best way to realize this is to combine systems and individual client advocacy on the local level. Domestic violence agency directors no longer can hope for better community and systems response; they have to pursue it actively. National and state legislation and support are needed to help end family violence. Yet, to witness a real difference in our communities, starting from the ground up is key.

One city's fight

In Tulsa, Okla., cited as an "average city" by *American Demographics* magazine, some progressive steps have been taken. The agency that has effected these changes is Domestic Violence Intervention Services, Inc. Like many other programs across the country, DVIS started as a telephone crisis line in 1975 and began sheltering women and their children in safe homes throughout the city in 1976. Since then, the private, nonprofit agency has expanded its services greatly. In addition to a 24-hour crisis line and a confidential shelter for battered women and their children, DVIS offers outpatient counseling for abusers, victims, and children; court advocacy; a transitional living program; and community education programs.

"... Domestic abuse is not a family matter. It is a crime and, as such, a *public* matter that should involve protection for the victims and justice for the batterers."

These developments alone are notable since few domestic violence agencies across the country offer all of these interventions under one roof. However, its greatest mark of distinction is the agency's commitment to systems change. DVIS could serve as a model for other domestic violence agencies and advocates struggling to bring about significant differences in their communities.

In September, 1992, DVIS staff began tracking the number of women murdered in Tulsa. They only could determine if a murder was related to domestic violence through newspaper accounts, since the law enforcement community did not report domestic violence homicides accurately. By March, 1993, 12 deaths in the Tulsa area were found to have been related to domestic violence. DVIS researched each case to determine the victims' involvement with the various protection systems prior to their deaths.

At the same time, some officers in the police department reportedly were responding negatively to victims of domestic abuse and failing to make arrests even when signs of abuse were visible. Police administrators requested documentation to support these complaints. The outcome was the Police Response Report Form, which would be distributed to all DVIS clients who had interactions with a police officer. All interactions, positive or negative, were noted on these report forms. The chief of police supported the use of the form and assured that internal investigations would be initiated whenever necessary.

What happened next set the stage for the sweeping changes in the systems response to domestic violence. In a span of nine days in the spring of 1993, two Tulsa women were murdered—one by her abusive spouse; the other, a 39-year-old mother of four, hours after being released from a local hospital, where she had been treated for injuries sustained from an earlier attack at the hands of her ex-husband. The first victim, a 35-year-old mother of three, was gunned down in the parking garage of a downtown building, where she worked as a human resources specialist.

In response to these murders, I publicly stated that the system failed these two women and called for the "creation of a review board to investigate domestic-related slayings and to hold the system accountable." Public outcry over the murders was mounting, and a member of the City Council requested that a special task force be appointed to review the system of protection for battered women. Members included the chief of police, the Tulsa County district attorney, the executive director of DVIS, the police commissioner, and a district judge who had worked on the protective order docket in recent years. The four major hurdles this group faced were police sensitivity to the response reports DVIS was maintaining; law enforcement officials not wanting task force members to "point fingers" regarding the recent murders; the D.A.'s contention that his constituents would prefer law enforcement dollars be spent on what they perceived as "more dangerous" crimes; and the belief that nothing could prevent a homicide if the batterer is determined to kill.

After meeting once a week for eight weeks, the task force delivered a report to the City Council that included a recommendation for a permanent city-wide effort to expand the safety net for domestic violence victims. Essentially, it called for a "system overhaul" that would encompass the formation of a domestic violence police unit; a review of the police probable cause policy; recommendation of adopting mandatory arrest of batterers; expansion of DVIS's court advocacy program; the training of all assistant district attorneys by Sarah Buel, a Massachusetts attorney and prosecutor who advocates full prosecution of abusers without victims' testimony; domestic violence training for all city prosecutors and 750 Tulsa police officers within six months; the district attorney, police chief, and DVIS executive director attending a domestic violence conference in San Diego and reviewing that city's system of protection for battered women and prosecution of abusers; and establishing a permanent Family Violence Council to be staffed by the mayor's office and chaired by one of the county commissioners.

The Tulsa Family Violence Council (FVC) was launched in January, 1994, with committees formed to address specifically public education, health and hospitals, data collection, the judiciary, and children who witness abuse. These committees continue to meet on a monthly basis, while a steering committee, made up of committee chairs, outside representatives, and the mayor's staff, meets quarterly. In addition, the entire council of 70 representatives meets semi-annually.

Changes in the police response to domestic violence have been extensive and exemplary. A special unit of eight detectives follows up on all domestic violence cases handled by field officers. The unit's primary goal is to generate arrests and get the batterers into the judicial system at an early stage. These detectives interview the victim and witnesses and collect physical evidence. The responsibility for filing an affidavit to seek an arrest warrant no longer is the victim's; the detectives prepare the affidavits from their investigation. They then can testify in court with the evidence gathered, eliminating the need for the victim's testimony. This is significant because victims often change their minds about testifying against their abusers out of fear of retribution. Tulsa's court system has put into place a domestic violence court with one judge who hears all permanent protective order requests and rules on violations.

Local hospitals have implemented emergency room protocols to screen better for domestic violence injuries. Employers in the local Human Resources Association have been trained on the protective order process and how to assist employees who have been abused and may need time off to appear in court. All businesses listed in the Tulsa Chamber of Commerce Directory received an employer-specific brochure developed by the FVC's Public Education Committee. The court advocacy program has in place a court watch program whereby law students volunteer to monitor protective order hearings as well as divorce and child custody proceedings to ensure that judges consistently are following state law, particularly in regard to domestic violence. In fact, all of the recommendations of the original task force have been implemented, and the FVC is working towards the all-important goal of preventing domestic abuse.

“When asking yourself if battering really does affect each of us, consider this statistic: Children raised in violent homes are 74% more likely to commit assault.”

Some of the positive changes made in Tulsa regarding systems response to domestic violence have been occurring in other communities across the nation. Programs in Duluth, Minn.; San Diego, Calif.; and Denver, Colo., have produced similarly commendable results. Other communities should look to the examples of these programs and cities where law enforcement, the judiciary, and victims' advocates work together cooperatively.

Domestic violence agency directors and other advocates, in gathering the real-life stories from battered women, should be able to identify groups within law enforcement or the judiciary that aren't treating domestic violence as a crime. Once this is done, they should follow the lead of DVIS and join forces with local government leaders, the judiciary, police officials, and others who positively can impact the response to domestic abuse.

Having accomplished this, small domestic violence organizations can begin to implement prevention strategies with help from the state coalitions and the National Family Violence Prevention Fund. Any prevention effort must include increasing public awareness of battering as a problem that affects everyone through continual education and exposure to the issue. DVIS employs a full-time community relations manager whose essential task is to keep domestic violence in the public eye by urging local media coverage.

The Family Violence Prevention Fund is a national organization that is working to change attitudes about violence against women and promote cultural intolerance of abuse worldwide. It has launched a national campaign, “There's No Excuse for Domestic Violence,” with accompanying media advocacy training. The organization's newsletters offer new ideas and facts regarding domestic violence and its prevention. Community-based domestic violence programs need to tap into these and similar resources when working toward systems changes and prevention.

When asking yourself if battering really does affect each of us, consider this statistic: Children raised in violent homes are 74% more likely to commit assault. As First Lady Hillary Clinton said in her address to the Fourth World Conference on Women held in China, “What we are learning around the world is that . . . if women are free from violence, their families will flourish. And when families flourish, communities and nations will flourish. . . .” Treating domestic violence as a crime and its victims with dignity and justice can go a long way toward ensuring a healthier, more productive nation.

The Consequences of Violence against Women

Violence is a vicious cycle that harms women and their families

by Lisa A. Mellman, M.D.
Columbia University

Society is riddled with violence. In 1995 some eight million people were assaulted in the U.S. Homicide was the second leading cause of death among 15- to 24-year-olds and the principal cause of death for 15- to 24-year-old black men. Of the several thousand women murdered each year (4,654 in 1995, according to the Department of Justice), one quarter to one half are killed by their male partners—and many were battered by these men in previous incidents. The homicide rates for children and adolescents have doubled since the early 1960s, and teenage girls are at least 13 times more likely to have been raped or sexually assaulted than teenage boys. The impact of this violence is pervasive, with profound physical, psychological, economic and social consequences for everyone.

Police and doctors are called in for only a small number of cases of domestic violence.

Because violence against women largely takes place at home, it has a particularly insidious character and effect. Women are seven times more likely than men are to experience violence committed by someone close to them, by a lover, spouse or ex-lover. This corruption of trust and intimacy means that primary relationships are disrupted throughout the household and that a vicious cycle is set in motion—one that is at risk of being perpetuated by the next generation.

Violence and neglect beget violence and neglect. All children can become scarred and depressed by abuse that they observe or receive. Although most mistreated children do not become violent adults, one third may become abusive or neglectful parents; one third are at risk of becoming violent. Only by realistically assessing and facing the full scope and consequence of violence against women can health care professionals and political advocates made some headway in combating it. Fortunately, better-designed epidemiological studies are clarifying prevalence and are increasingly documenting the long-term medical and psychological effects of violence on women and their children.

Numbers at Odds

Arguments revolving around statistics have long plagued discussions about how to gauge the prevalence of violence. In part, the problem has arisen from semantics. Survey results differ depending on how exactly terms are defined. For instance, various studies have imprecisely defined terms such as "rape" or "domestic violence." In addition, methodology shapes outcome. Face-to-face interviews, for example, yield higher numbers than do those conducted over the telephone. (The figures given in this article are the best ones available to date, but it is certain that some of them also suffer from these confounding factors.)

Only recently have epidemiologists precisely clarified their terms. Today we know from solid studies that 36 percent of American women—that is, more than 34 million women—report experiencing violent events (including rape and sexual or physical assault) or the homicide of someone they knew well. And between 9 and 12 percent of women report being raped at least once.

The data on violence by intimate partners remain less clear, however, Research using more exact methodology and larger samples is under way, including a large study funded by the Centers for Disease Control and Prevention (CDC) and the National Institute of Justice (NIJ). Results from this study will be available later this year. But for now we have to rely on older estimates: every year between 1.8 and four million women are battered by their partners.

Assessing the medical and psychological aftermath of this violence has been difficult to quantify as well, but for reasons other than terminology. Instead the challenge has been establishing causality between a violent event and a later physical or psychiatric symptom. Women often experience more than just violence: familial dysfunction and neglect usually coexist with physical or sexual abuse, or both. This confluence makes it difficult for physicians to tease apart which factors are contributing to an illness. In addition, abused women may develop more than one psychiatric disorder and may show symptoms long after a traumatic event took place.

These complexities are further compounded by the stigma and shame that abused women feel. According to a report by the Commonwealth Fund, 90 percent of women who described themselves as physically abused by their partner or spouse had never told a doctor. Even when directly asked, women often deny being beaten or assaulted. Some feel embarrassed about their situation and frightened of their batterer; others are understandably terrified about addressing the serious problems of their relationship. To confront the batterer means risking his denial or revenge. To leave means facing the daunting task of securing housing and work—efforts often complicated by the need for child care and the lack of economic or emotional self-sufficiency.

A Nightmare of Body...

Although precise numbers remain elusive for the time being, the medical and psychological effects of domestic violence are nonetheless becoming terribly clear. In 1991 the American Medical Association began a campaign to educate physicians—and the country at large—about domestic violence. Studies have documented that victims of violence and their children make more visits to physicians and have more medical complaints than most people do. Indeed, researchers found that the average number of physician visits increased 31 percent for assaulted women and 56 percent for rape victims in the year after the crime against them. Only in the past few years, however, have physicians begun to be trained to recognize and treat abuse.

Even a cursory look at the injuries women incur explains why the resulting medical costs for domestic violence in the U.S. have been estimated at between $5 billion and $67 billion annually. Women suffer not only transitory injuries such as bruises, cuts, broken bones, concussions and urinary tract infections but also permanent ones: joint damage, hearing or vision loss, chronic pain, irritable bowel syndrome and sexually transmitted disease, including HIV infection.

Pregnant women are especially at risk of complications related to abuse. Studies indicate battered women have almost twice the number of miscarriages as nonbattered women do. Battered women often start prenatal care late in pregnancy and may have a greater number of low-birthweight babies. Because substance abuse is more prevalent among abused women, their fetuses are more likely to suffer drug- and alcohol-related complications.

...and of Mind

The psychiatric consequences of violence are also proving to be wide-ranging and severe. Survivors often describe a pervasive sense of terror and loss of control during and after the assault. Acute stress disorder (ASD) or posttraumatic stress disorder (PTSD) often follows violent events. Both are characterized by flashbacks and nightmares, numbness and avoidance, and heightened alertness—including irritability, vigilance, overresponsiveness to touch or sound, and an increased capacity for being startled.

Domestic violence leaves lasting scars, emotionally and sometimes physically.

Stress disorders are much more prevalent in victims of physical and especially sexual assault than they are in people who have not experienced such violence. In one survey, more than 94 percent of women who had been raped developed ASD within the first month, and 47 percent of these women had PTSD after three months. Extrapolation from several studies suggests that of the estimated 12 million or so American women who have been raped, almost four to five million have suffered PTSD.

Physiological studies demonstrate that the stress response evoked in PTSD is distinct from the normal stress response—and from the response reported in other psychiatric disorders. Individuals with PTSD have low cortisol levels and greater cortisol fluctuation, which indicates that their stress response has been biologically altered. These chemical changes may translate into a more reactive heart rate and a tendency to startle easily.

Violence and abuse are frequently associated with other disorders as well: depression, anxiety, substance abuse and feelings of being disconnected from reality. Women who were repeatedly raped in childhood are three times more likely to develop depression and almost five times more likely to develop anxiety disorders than women who have not suffered in this way. Abused women also suffer from low self-esteem and poor interpersonal skills and feel inherently bad or dirty. They blame themselves for what has happened. These feelings make them unwilling to take care of themselves—and thus unwilling to seek help or to comply with medical care.

Many women who have been victimized are at higher risk of having chronic sexual problems, mutilating themselves, running away from home as teenagers and entering into prostitution. They are more likely to abuse substances; according to one report, 75 percent of women in substance-abuse treatment programs have a history of sexual abuse. The risk of attempted suicide increases dramatically in women who were sexually assaulted before age 16.

The implications for children are immeasurable. Not only is it damaging to grow up with a primary caretaker who is consistently depressed or suffering from PTSD, but as targets of and witnesses to violence, children are deeply harmed. Basic trust, the first developmental stage in psychoanalyst Erik H. Erikson's life-cycle theory, is completely disrupted. Normal expectations—that parents and caretakers are protectors, that daily life is predictable, that your body is your own—may be permanently crushed. When violence is enacted toward a child, it may disrupt normal development, setting the stage for lifelong difficulty.

At least three million children in the U.S. witness parental abuse annually; between 40 and 70 percent of children entering battered women's shelters are abused, mostly by the mother's abuser but sometimes by the mother herself. Children suffer behaviorally and intellectually from seeing violence in abusive environments and from the nomadic life that may ensue. Many develop the same problems that plague abused adults: PTSD, anxiety, depression, suicidal thoughts. Male children are at greater risk of committing a violent offense if they have a history of abuse or neglect; female children who have been sexually abused are twice as likely as nonabused children to be abused in adulthood by their partners.

As more research emerges, the social implications of violence against women are becoming increasingly apparent. The circle of violence set in motion in the home moves out onto the streets and then back into homes, ruining the childhood of another generation and setting the stage for the perpetuation of all forms of violence and abuse. Violence against women is not a discrete phenomenon but one that underlies many aspects of our culture. It is time it was addressed as such.

LISA A. MELLMAN is an associate clinical professor at Columbia University, where she is also the associate director of residency training. Mellman directs the psychotherapy clinic for training and research at the New York State Psychiatric Institute.

The Department of Health and Human Services has a nationwide, 24-hour domestic violence hotline: 800-799-SAFE.

Unit 8

Unit Selections

Key Points to Consider

❖ How does money impact the quality of our health as we age?

❖ How would you define a "good death"?

❖ Which article in this section do you think is the most controversial? Why?

DUSHKINONLINE Links

www.dushkin.com/online/

27. **Lifecycle: Mature**
http://www.womenshealth.org/lifecycle/mature.htm
28. **National Institute on Aging**
http://www.nih.gov/nia/
29. **National Survey of Women's Health**
http://www.cmwf.org/programs/women/whhilite.asp

These sites are annotated on pages 4 and 5.

Special Issues for Older Women

The final section of the book deals with issues of interest to mature women. An interesting phenomenon occurs when one attempts to define the term "older." Somehow, older usually comes to mean older than oneself. It's as if distancing ourselves from the aging process makes it easier to navigate. In asking one of our grandmothers on the occasion of her 90th birthday how it felt to have reached such a milestone, she replied "Oh, are you asking me how it feels to be old?" Tact stripped away, we had to admit that that was what we wanted to know. "I'll let you know when I get there," she replied. With that bit of wisdom, coupled with the humbling knowledge that our students consider 39 to be old, we have used this section to include articles that we hope will be of value to a wide range of ages and interests.

"Midlife Motherhood: Is It Never Too Late?" explores the issue of delayed childbearing from both a biological and a sociological perspective. The question that is posed is: Just because we are able to do something, does that mean we should? "Women & Estrogen: Old Fears, New Hopes" helps to sort out the seeming contradictions in the literature on menopause by providing the reader with the latest information on the risks versus the benefits of estrogen replacement therapy. Also addressing the estrogen debate, "Estrogen to Prevent Alzheimer's?" presents some rather intriguing evidence that suggests yet another benefit of estrogen therapy.

Taking a broader perspective on the aging process, "Can You Afford to Get Old?" explores the link between money and access to health care. While they do not ensure good health, adequate finances certainly do increase a person's health care options.

The final pair of articles in this unit deal with death and the dying process. "A Harder Better Death" familiarizes the reader with the concept of a "good death." Although this may appear to be a contradiction in terms, the author discusses the issues of choice and control over the course of one's own dying process. Similarly, "Taking Care of Mom" describes the odyssey of three "experts" in the field of gerontology as they walk with their parents through both the aging and the dying process.

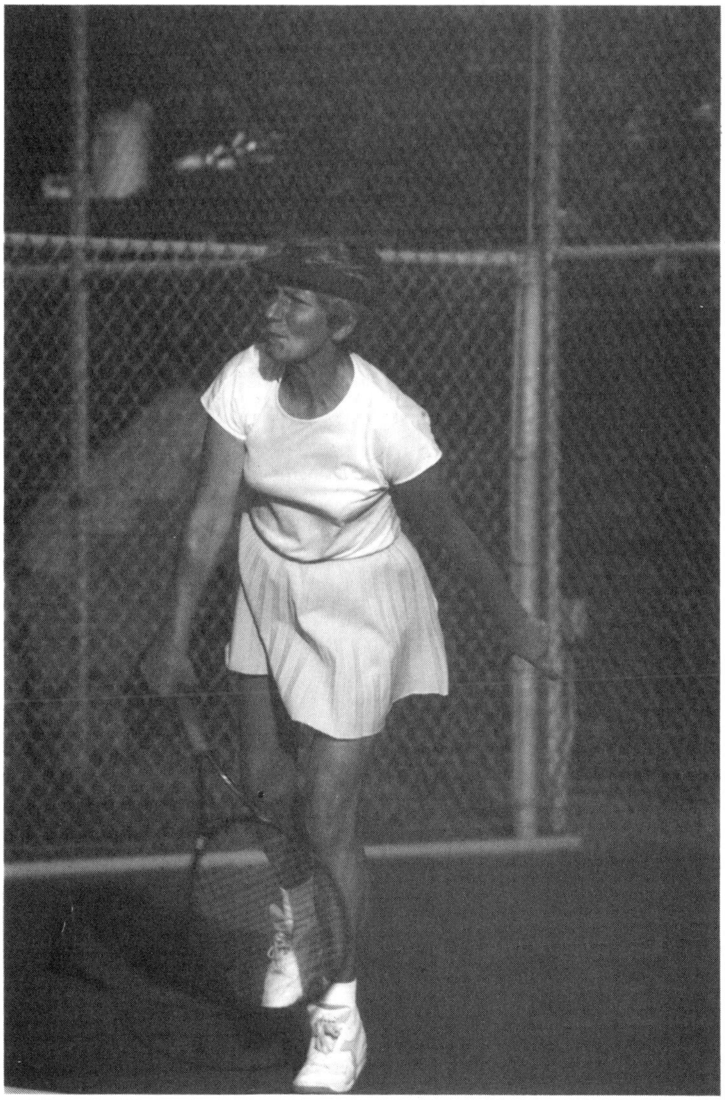

MIDLIFE MOTHERHOOD

IS IT NEVER TOO LATE?

It's time to examine the price—both physical and emotional—that women may pay for turning back their reproductive clocks

BY RITA BARON-FAUST

We've heard a lot lately about the miracle of motherhood for women in their 40s and beyond. (Remember the buzz about the baby born to the 63-year-old woman?) It's amazing that with in vitro fertilization and donor eggs, women can become pregnant at a time in life when an earlier generation might have been cuddling their first grandchildren.

Between 1985 and 1995 the number of births among American women in their 40s more than doubled, from about 29,500 to almost 70,000, according to the National Center on Health Statistics in Hyattsville, MD. Births among women aged 50 and older are also on the rise and are expected to continue climbing.

Yet in all the debate about whether women at midlife should embark on motherhood, the focus has always been on the well-being of the babies. While that discussion continues, *American Health for Women* decided to investigate the other side of the story, the one no one talks about: How do late-in-life pregnancies affect mothers? What impact does carrying a child have on their bodies, their minds and their ability to raise the children they miraculously give birth to?

When Looks Are Deceiving

Baby boomers are a notoriously health-conscious crowd, ever striving to better their bodies and push them as far as they can go. They eat nutritiously, exercise regularly and lately have been taking on perhaps the greatest challenge yet: turning back their biological clocks. And while many women have met with success, researchers are discovering that there's often a price to pay. There are health risks associated with late-life pregnancies, and worse, they're rarely reported on. "Most midlife women coming in for fertility care really don't understand the dangers," says Mark V. Sauer, M.D., director of reproductive endocrinology at Columbia-Presbyterian Medical Center in New York City. "They may be joggers or tennis players and assume that because they're in good shape they won't have problems, and that's not necessarily true."

Late-in-life pregnancy can bring a sense of joy and fulfillment, but it can also create health problems where none existed before, draw out latent conditions and exacerbate existing ones. A woman over 35 is twice as likely to develop high blood pressure during pregnancy as a woman in her 20s, according to a 1996 article in *Obstetrics & Gynecology.* Of course, the odds a midlife woman will have the disorder going into a pregnancy are relatively high: At 45, 42% of white women and 56% of black women have hypertension.

The risk of gestational diabetes also increases with age. Women over 35 have twice as much risk of developing the condition as younger women, according to the March of Dimes Birth Defects Foundation in White Plains, NY. And while diabetes can usually be managed with dietary changes, developing the disease during pregnancy almost doubles one's chances of becoming diabetic later in life.

Then there are the chronic conditions. Having lupus may increase the risk of pregnancy-induced high blood pressure. And the weight gain women experience while carrying a child can provoke further pain and joint damage to those suffering from osteoarthritis, a painful disease in which the cartilage that lines the joints breaks down. Medications for these and other problems often experienced by women in their 40s and older must be carefully chosen and monitored (see box, "Drugs and Pregnancy: What's Safe, What's Not").

Obstetrical complications are more common in post-40 pregnancies, even among healthy women. A study at Mount Sinai Medical Center in New York City found that pregnant women over 40 were two to three times as likely as women under 30 to develop preeclampsia and abruptio placentae. Preeclampsia (also called toxemia) causes high blood pressure after the 20th week of pregnancy and can be fatal for the child and, rarely, the mother. Abruptio placentae, in which the placenta prematurely becomes detached from the uterine wall, can lead to hemorrhage, causing the mother to go into shock and interrupting blood flow to the baby.

In addition, one can't always predict how a midlife woman will tolerate the cardiovascular and hormonal stresses of pregnancy, and that in itself is a risk, says Zev Rosenwaks, M.D., director of the Center for Reproductive Medicine and Infertility at New York Hospital—Cornell Medical Center in New York City. "A woman in her 40s may have a marginal cardiac condition that's not picked up by screening tests but later becomes unmasked due to the physical stresses of pregnancy, " he says.

The Fatigue Factor

Of course, carrying a baby to term is only the beginning. "It's not so much childbearing at 45 or even 50 years of age that's difficult; it's child rearing," says Yvonne S. Thornton, M.D., the Morristown, NJ, author of *Woman to Woman.* Even those who are fortunate enough to get through a pregnancy without any health problems have an enormous challenge in front of them. "Women in their 40s just don't have as much energy as they did in their 20s to care for a newborn and run after a toddler," says Dr. Thornton.

Taking care of a baby means disrupted sleep, which can be particularly taxing for perimenopausal and menopausal women, who already tend to have more sleep problems than younger women, children aside. And the National Commission on Sleep Disorders Research, a committee organized by the National Institutes of Health in 1993, reported that adults who suffer from impaired sleep don't deliver the same quality of child care as those who are better rested.

Also, rates of depression spike during the perimenopausal years. Add the fact that hormonal changes associated with pregnancy and postpartum increase the risk of depression, and the resultis that midlife women often come to pregnancy primed for trouble, explains Deborah Sichel, M.D., director of the Hestia Institute for Women and Families in Wellesley, MA.

Putting the Risks in Perspective

The physical concerns of late-life pregnancies are real, but there's good news too. A recent Harvard Medical School study found that women who have children in their

7 Ways to Safeguard Your Pregnancy

While pregnancies in women over 35 are usually considered riskier than those in younger women, a number of medical advances have been made to help ensure that the outcome is a healthy one for mother and baby, says Denise Guidetti, M.D., a specialist in maternal-fetal medicine at Long Island Jewish Medical Center in New Hyde Park, NY. Not only should older expectant moms follow the basic rules of pregnancy, but they should also speak with their doctors about taking the following tests, according to the American College of Obstetricians and Gynecologists in Washington:

◆ **PRENATAL TESTING** Chorionic villus sampling and amniocentesis can rule out chromosomal abnormalities such as Down's syndrome.

◆ **DIABETES SCREENING** This test should be conducted at 24 to 28 weeks. Women who have preexisting or gestational diabetes should monitor their own blood sugar levels regularly throughout pregnancy with a home test kit.

◆ **BLOOD PRESSURE CHECK** Your doctor should monitor your blood pressure closely throughout your pregnancy. You can also use a home test kit to check yourself.

◆ **PREECLAMPSIA SELF-TEST** In addition to being tested by your doctor, you can use a simple kit to check your urine for excess protein, a symptom of preeclampsia. Be alert to other signs of the condition, which occurs during the third trimester: sudden increase in weight, severe headaches, visual disturbances, vomiting and pain in the upper-right part of the abdomen.

◆ **FETAL GROWTH MONITORING** Sonograms should be performed throughout your pregnancy at the discretion of your doctor to make sure the baby is growing properly.

◆ **FETAL MOVEMENT ASSSESSMENT** Beginning at 30 weeks, do the following on a daily basis: For an hour in the morning and an hour in the evening, lie on your side, and each time the baby moves, note it on a piece of paper. You should count at least four or five movements an hour. Otherwise, see your doctor for additional testing.

◆ **PRETERM LABOR SELF-CHECK** Your physician should be able to tell you how to recognize a contraction, and you can also use a home monitor. Other symptoms of early labor include persistent back pain and pressure in the pelvic area. —*Hilary Macht*

40s live longer than women who give birth at younger ages. The researchers theorize that women who are able to become pregnant later in life have slower biological clocks and therefore age more slowly than other women. While older women are likelier to encounter pregnancy problems than younger women, the actual risk isn't always that high. For example, only about 5% of women over 35 develop gestational diabetes.

The bottom line is, if an older woman is healthy, the odds are still in her favor that the pregnancy won't harm her health. For Richard Berkowitz, M.D., chairman of obstetrics and reproductive science at Mount Sinai Medical Center, this is a deciding factor in advising older women whether or not to become pregnant. "If a woman in her 40s or 50s has no underlying chronic disease," Dr. Berkowitz says, "the risks to her own health when she's pregnant are minimal."

Remember too that women have the power to help ensure a positive pregnancy outcome. That means being in shape and not overweight going into a pregnancy, and caring for yourself properly throughout the entire process (see "7 Ways to Safeguard Your Pregnancy").

DRUGS AND PREGNANCY: WHAT'S SAFE, WHAT'S NOT

As a woman grows older, the likelihood that she'll have a health problem rises, and with it the chance she'll be using medication. The trouble is, some drugs can cause birth defects in a developing fetus. On the other hand, not treating a medical problem can cause serious complications for you and your baby. Fortunately, safer drug substitutes are available for most medical conditions. But be aware that even those aren't always risk free. If you're planning to get pregnant, it's crucial to schedule a preconception visit with your doctor to review your medications and discuss alternatives. Meanwhile, we consulted Anthony Scialli, M.D., director of the Reproductive Toxicology Center in Washington, and outlined some common problems, medications to avoid and safer substitutes. Never start or stop taking a drug without speaking with your doctor.

AILMENT	UNSAFE	SAFER
ARTHRITIS	Methotrexate (Folex, Rheumatrex). It's been shown to cause serious and sometimes fatal birth defects.	Hydroxychloroquine sulfate (Plaquenil) and prednisone (Deltasone). Neither of these drugs has been linked with birth defects, although prednisone has been associated with slightly lower birth weights.
CHRONIC PAIN	Nonsteroidal anti-inflammatories such as aspirin, ibuprofen (Advil, Motrin) and naproxen sodium (Aleve). In the later months of pregnancy, NSAIDS can constrict fetal blood vessels and interfere with lung functioning in a newborn.	Acetaminophen (Tylenol).
DEPRESSION	Antidepressants—both tricyclics and selective serotonin reuptake inhibitors—have not been linked with birth defects. But third-trimester use of these medications has been asociated with neonatal problems such as trouble breathing, eating and maintaining body temperature. In addition, fluoxetine (Prozac), an SSRI, has been found to increase the risk of premature delivery, a potentially serious complication.	If you and your doctor feel you could avoid the use of antidepressants, do so. Consider other options, such as psychotherapy.
DIABETES	Sulfonylureas, a class of oral drugs that includes chlorpropamide (Diabinese). These medications have been shown to produce glucose abnormalities, jaundice and possibly some birth defects in fetuses.	Insulin. It's essential that diabetes is controlled during pregnancy, or you risk harming your own health and having an abnormally large baby, a difficult delivery or a stillbirth.
HYPER-TENSION	Calcium channel blockers and angiotensin-converting enzyme inhibitors. Animal studies have shown that calcium channel blockers can cause limb defects and that, in the later months of pregnancy, ACE inhibitors can impair fetal growth and kidney function.	Thiazide diuretics, methyldopa and labetalol. None of these has been found to cause birth defects, but all have been associated with mild, treatable blood sugar abnormalities in the fetus.

—*Elizabeth Shaw*

"A pregnant 25-year-old woman who hasn't been screened for health problems and is not being followed may be at greater risk than a 45-year-old who has passed the medical screening and whose pregnancy is being carefully monitored," says Richard Paulson, M.D., chief of reproductive endocrinology and infertility at the University of Southern California School of Medicine in Los Angeles.

Certainly for many older women the possibility of problems pales in comparison with the desire for a child and the ability to raise one. "Yes, I'm tired, overworked and constantly barraged by my kids who need me 'right now,' " says Marjorie Peskin, 45, of Newton, MA, the mother of five-year-old twins. "But if had it to do all over again, would I? Absolutely." There are advantages to waiting until later in life, when careers, finances and relationships are usually more stable, says Vivian B. Pender, M.D., a clinical assistant professor of psychiatry at New York Hospital—Cornell Medical Center in New York City. Dr. Pender notes that many older women "have resolved the emotional conflicts of their 20s and 30s and are better prepared for the challenges of parenting."

Martha Henriks, 44, of Toronto, gave birth to her first child when she was 28 and to her second child two years ago. "I can't go back to that high-energy phase of my life, but I'm much more relaxed as a parent now than I was the first time around," she says. "I'm also in a more flexible, higher-level job, so I'm not panicked about getting to work exactly on time."

Older mothers who have waited so long may be more dedicated to the idea of motherhood. "We shouldn't underestimate everything that a mature woman has to give to a child," Dr. Pender stresses. "Older women have a much firmer sense of identity and accomplishment, not to mention a wealth of life experience, all of which are a decided advantage when it comes to raising children."

If you're over 40 and thinking about having a child, talk to your doctor about the pros and cons in order to make the decision that's best and most comfortable for you. Make it your business to learn about all the things you can do before, during and after pregnancy to optimize your physical and psychological health. The goal is to enter this miraculous and transforming experience with open eyes—fully aware of the possible risks, though never forgetting the benefits.

Rita Baron-Faust is an award-winning medical writer in Brooklyn, NY. Her latest book is Mental Wellness for Women.

WOMEN & Estrogen

BY LAURA FLYNN McCARTHY

Old Fears, New Hopes

AT AGE 57, JUDITH LICHTMAN FOUND herself facing a decision that has become an almost universal dilemma for American women: Should she take estrogen replacement therapy (ERT)? She'd sailed through menopause at 46 with only mild symptoms; she was healthy, exercised, ate well and had a sterling family medical history—no breast cancer, heart disease or Alzheimer's in her background and only a little osteoporosis. But when a routine bone scan revealed significant bone loss in her hips and spine, Lichtman, who is president of the National Partnership for Women and Families (formerly the Women's Legal Defense Fund) in Washington, DC, started to consider ERT.

"I read everything I could, spoke to lots of friends and several doctors, including a breast surgeon and a gynecologist," she recalls. "Like many women, I was concerned about the possible link between ERT and breast cancer. But I was also intrigued by evidence that estrogen may help prevent Alzheimer's disease, since memory loss is one of my great fears. Most compelling was ERT's ability to fight osteoporosis."

Last spring, Lichtman began taking Prempro, a combination of Premarin (the top-selling estrogen brand) and progestin (synthetic progesterone). "It wasn't an easy decision," says Lichtman. "Much more research needs to be done, but I had to choose based on the information available today. Still, I don't see it as a one-time decision. As I have ongoing mammograms, bone scans and other exams, and as new studies come out, I'll reevaluate whether to continue or stop. For now, this is the right decision for me."

The Estrogen Explosion

Once seen only as a way to help women negotiate the hot flashes, insomnia and other aggravations of menopause, estrogen is taking on important new medical roles. Today it's one of the most commonly prescribed medications for preventing heart disease and osteoporosis in women. And scientists are trying to develop versions that may be safe and protective for men.

Meanwhile, new studies appear constantly. The latest show ERT may help prevent colon cancer, Alzheimer's and stroke, improve sex, make skin look younger, relieve arthritis and control incontinence (see box "The Estrogen Effects"). But shadowing the benefits are lingering questions about whether taking estrogen increases the risk of breast cancer. (Uterine cancer is also an issue but its threat can be reduced or negated by adding progestin to estrogen.) Still, new "designer estrogens" and other alternatives could make even women who swore they'd never take hormones reconsider their decision. For instance:

✣ Late last year, the FDA approved a new estrogen-like drug, *raloxifene hydrochloride* (brand name, Evista—see box, "Should You Take Raloxifene Instead?"), that appears to strengthen bones and protect the heart without increasing the risk of breast cancer.

From *Remedy*, March/April 1998, pp. 12-20.

Should You Take Raloxifene Instead?

Last year, the FDA approved raloxifene hydrochloride (Evista) to prevent osteoporosis after me-nopause. Many doctors have dubbed it "the first designer estrogen," the leader in a new class of selective estrogen-receptor modulators that target only specific sites—in this case, the bones and heart.

How does raloxifene compare to estrogen? "All of the evidence isn't in but it appears to increase bone density almost as much as estrogen does. It also has some positive effects on cholesterol—reducing total levels and 'bad' LDL," says Dr. Col. "But unlike estrogen, it doesn't increase 'good' HDL." Evista also isn't meant to treat menopausal symptoms. (In fact, it may increase hot flashes.)

There are hints that it may reduce breast cancer's threat.

"As for breast cancer, there's some preliminary evidence that raloxifene may reduce its threat. This is the most promising research; however, much more study is needed to prove it," adds. Col.

So if osteoporosis is a major concern, heart disease is a low one, there's breast cancer in your family and you have no menopausal symptoms, raloxifene may be a good choice for you. But if those medical priorities are reversed—risks of heart disease high, bone thinning and breast cancer low—and if other potential estrogen benefits (such as Alzheimer's protection) are important to you, ERT comes out on top.

Evista may alsobe a good option for women who can't tolerate the menstrual-like symptoms that can occur on estrogen/progestin, and for those willing to be on the cutting edge of drug therapy who take hope from early indications that raloxifene may protect against breast cancer.

Ironically, the exciting "newness" of raloxifene is its greatest drawback. "Targeted estrogens are very interesting drugs but they're so new that we don't know their potential for long-term side effects. That's a concern. By comparison, we have 55 years of research and experience with estrogen, so we've probably seen all the major adverse effects we're going to see," points out Dr. Bush. "Targeted estrogens are promising but they're not the answer yet."

The Soy Factor

Can eating more plan-derived estrogens, such as those in soy, have the same effects as drugs? Perhaps.

◆ Estratab, an estrogen pill derived from soy and yams, has been okayed by the FDA to ease hot flashes and other menopausal symptoms.

◆ Its maker, Solvay Pharmaceuticals, is seeking FDA approval of claims that it can also help prevent osteoporosis.

◆ And last year, a research group of postmenopausal women who ate a very high-soy diet for six months upped bone density by about 2 percent.

Some studies also show that eating even small amounts of soy daily lowers total and bad LDL cholesterol, and raises good HDL. High-soy diets also seem to encourage healthier blood vessels, much as ERT does. "Just a handful of soynuts or a soy milkshake a day can promote these changes," says James Anderson, MD, professor of medicine and clinical nutrition at the University of Kentucky College of Medicine.

Its effects on breast health are also promising. "In animal and population studies, soy protects against breast cancer," says Dr. Anderson. "The studies are so encouraging that soy's being investigated as a way to treat breast cancer."

What Women MDs Do

The biggest single group of ERT users may surprise you: women physicians. A recent survey of more than 1,400 postmenopausal doctors found that on average nearly half of them use hormone replacement therapy—about 60 percent of those in their 40s, 49 percent in their 50s and 36 percent in their 60s.

✥ Other so-called designer or "targeted" estrogens are being used in Europe and may be available soon here. "Within the next five years, there are going to be a lot more choices," says Nananda F. Col, MD, assistant professor of medicine at New England Medical Center/Tufts University School of Medicine and author of *A Woman Doctor's Guide to Hormone Therapy.*

✥ Some studies are testing the best dosage for optimizing benefits while minimizing risks. Others are figuring the smartest length of time to take estrogen.

✥ One firm already has FDA approval to market an estrogen drug derived from soy and yams.

✥ Researchers are examining whether similar benefits can be achieved simply by eating certain foods that are rich in estrogen-like phytochemicals.

Yet many women, like Judith Lichtman, need to make decisions now. And the decision often is based as much on emotions and experiences as on medical history. Any woman who has seen someone suffer through breast cancer may be loathe to take a drug

The Breast-Cancer Connection: How Real Is The Risk?

Just the hint of a breast-cancer link is enough to scare many women off estrogen. Yet while some studies show ERT increases the risk of *getting* breast cancer, others have found that it decreases the risk of *dying from* breast cancer.

Most recently, the ongoing Harvard nurses' study reports that women who take estrogen *for five years or more* are 46 percent more likely to get breast cancer than non-users. But when the American Cancer Society followed more than 422,000 women for nine years, it found that those who used estrogen but then stopped had a 15 percent *decreased* risk of death from breast cancer; those who still used it had *no* increased risk. Several smaller studies have had similar results.

One explanation for some contradictions is that estrogen users tend to be closely monitored, so more breast cancers may be spotted—increasing the cancer rate—but also spotted earlier, decreasing the death rate. Also, higher breast-cancer rates may reflect the fact that estrogen takers, overall, live longer than non-takers, and age ups the risk of breast cancer.

A family history of breast cancer complicates things. Yet even if two or three close relatives have had the disease, ERT may not up the risk as much as most people assume. A woman between 50 and 80 has about a 10 percent chance of getting breast cancer. Add estrogen and the risk goes up to 13 percent. That means 13 out of 100 women will develop the disease—but only three of those cases will be estrogen-related. "And in that same group of 100 women, ERT will spare 30 of them an early death from heart disease," notes the American Cancer Society's Dawn Wills, PhD, MPH.

If your medical history indicates that you are at increased risk of heart disease, the scales tip in favor of estrogen regardless of your breast-cancer risk. "Most women who develop breast cancer die of something else, whereas most women who develop heart disease die from it," points out Dr. Col. (Of course, other medications help fend off heart disease in people at risk, such as cholesterol and blood-pressure drugs, although these carry some risks of their own.)

Still, some doctors feel that the link between ERT and breast cancer may be stronger than current research suggests. They say that several studies on which today's medical advice is based are biased in some critical way. Among these critics is Susan Love, MD, author of *Dr. Susan Love's Hormone Book*, who notes that many of the studies don't consider how long estrogen is used—vital, since breast-cancer risks rise over time.

One possible conclusion from all of this: Women who seem like good candidates for estrogen's heart and bone protection may want to take it—but for a limited period of time, to minimize potential breast-cancer risks. The new Harvard study data suggest that there's a five-year "safety window." "You can use that time to enjoy its benefits," says Dr. Col. "Just remember that you'll lose its heart and bone protection as soon as you stop taking it."

that could increase her own odds of the dread disease. Others worry about the wisdom of putting hormones in their bodies long after nature intended them to be there. And some see ERT as a commitment they're just not prepared to make.

On these pages, the latest, newest findings and how they may apply to you, whether you're starting menopause, long past it or somewhere in between.

Making Your Own Decision

After all the researchers have their say, it comes down to one question: Is ERT right for you? This can be an emotionally-charged medical decision, since so much often depends on feelings as well as facts.

During menopause, of course, the decision may be based mainly on getting short-term relief from hot flashes, insomnia, vaginal discomfort, libido dips and mood swings. "However, while most women only have menopausal symptoms for a year or two and some barely notice them, others have intense problems that can go on for years. Every time they go off estrogen, sweat-soaked hot flashes and other problems return," says Wulf Utian, MD, PhD, executive director, North American Menopause Society.

Start by finding out as much about your family history as possible. For example, if a parent has died of heart disease, that's a concern. But if he or she smoked, overate and under-exercised—and you don't—it may not be such a worry. Similarly, if a grandparent had osteoporosis, that too is a red flag. But if you exercise regularly, don't smoke and eat a calcium-rich diet, you've already reduced your risk. To check, talk to your doctor about having a bone scan.

If your major long-term concern is osteoporosis and you're hesitant to take either estrogen or the new targeted estrogen, raloxifene (Evista), you've now got other options. *Alendronate sodium* (Fosamax) both prevents and improves osteoporosis damage. In studies, it also reduced spine fractures by nearly 50 percent. What's more, it helped prevent repeat fractures in women who had already had bone breaks. These results make Fosamax's bone benefits comparable to estrogen's, but since the drug is quite new, long-term effects aren't certain.

You may also want to ask about *calcitonin*, a hormone recently approved in nasal-spray form (Miacalcin). It inhibits cells that break down bone. Calcium and vitamin D are important to preventing bone loss—doctors recommend 1,500 mg of calcium and 800 mg of vitamin D daily—although they don't help rebuild it.

The Estrogen Effects

Your Life Span

Women who take estrogen during and/or after menopause live longer than those who don't. That's the dramatic finding of three studies.

◆ *At Tufts, researchers combined data from several large studies and found that estrogen users live an average of six months—and sometimes over three years—longer than women who never took the hormone.*

◆ *Researchers at Kaiser Permanente in Oakland, CA, found a 46 percent drop in the death rate from all causes in postmenopausal estrogen users.*

◆ *A large Harvard study of more than 40,000 women also found that ERT reduced death rates—in this case by 37 percent—among estrogen takers vs. those who never took it. The likely reason: better heart and bone health.*

Your Bones

*The latest studies confirm that estrogen not only helps prevent bone loss after menopause but may **increase** its density, giving women more bone to "bank on" later. This is critical since as much as 20 percent of bone mass is lost during the first five to seven years after menopause.*

Other new research shows that bone building occurs whether women begin ERT at menopause or five, 10, even 15 years later. However, bone benefits drop dramatically when estrogen is stopped. But taking estrogen for even five years or so can put off that drop, which may be enough to prevent hip or spine fractures in a woman's lifetime.

Your Weight

Many women won't take estrogen because they believe it causes weight gain. However, several studies show that it doesn't cause women to gain or lose pounds after menopause.

Your Reproductive System

Estrogen eases many effects of menopause on vaginal tissue, including dryness, atrophy and thinning. Unfortunately, it also stimulates the growth of any existing fibroid tumors and, taken alone, ups the risk of uterine cancer. Adding progestin counters this; however, a new study suggests progestin must be taken for at least 10 days a month to get its protective effect. Doctors stress there is no confirmed link between ERT and a higher risk for ovarian cancer.

The Colon, Incontinence And More

A study of more than 2,000 women at the University of Wisconsin found a 46 percent drop in colon cancer among estrogen users. The ongoing Cancer Prevention Study also reports that women who take estrogen have less fatal colon cancer. However, ERT increases the odds of gallstones, though doctors aren't sure why. Finally, an analysis of 23 studies shows that ERT helps control incontinence after menopause, a problem that plagues many women.

Your Skin

Women who take estrogen are a third less likely to have dry skin and extensive wrinkling than those who don't, reports a recent study of 3,875 women. Another smaller study shows that ERT appears to help prevent age-related skin slackness.

Your Heart

Taking estrogen after menopause reduces heart disease. Until recently, the reasons were unclear. Now doctors have some pieces of the puzzle.

◆ ***Improved blood lipids.*** *Estrogen raises HDL ("good" cholesterol) and lowers LDL ("bad" cholesterol).*

◆ ***"Softer" arteries.*** *Estrogen lowers blood pressure by decreasing "hardening of the arteries," making them softer and more pliant. It also fights plaque build-up in blood vessels and makes clumps of it less likely to break off and cause a heart attack. Plus ERT helps keep blood vessels from "clenching" in response to stress, easing angina pain.*

◆ ***Fewer clots.*** *By controlling certain blood-clotting factors, estrogen may cut the risk of stroke or heart attack.*

Your Teeth

Harvard physicians have found that women who take estrogen cut their risk of tooth loss. Why? The hormone strengthens the jaw, as well as other bones, which helps hold teeth in place.

Your Joints

In a study of more than 600 women, ERT reduced the risks of knee osteoarthritis threefold and somewhat decreased the threat to fingers. 1994 research found estrogen cuts osteoarthritis risk by 30 percent.

Your Brain

Exciting new research suggests that estrogen can strengthen verbal memory (such as name recall). It also seems to enhance mood. Most promising, several studies show it may reduce the risk of Alzheimer's and lessen problems in women who already have it. All these findings are still preliminary but large studies are trying to confirm them.

4 Ways To Take Estrogen

In the US, most women choose pills. In other countries, implants and creams are tops. Here is what's available here and some tips on using them.

1. Pills By far the most common and best researched estrogen drug in America is Premarin, a mix of estrogens derived from pregnant mares. (Prempro and Premphase are sister medications that combine estrogen with progesterone or progestin.)

Others include Estrace, Estrovis, Ogen and Ortho-Est. Although not as thoroughly studied as Premarin, all have similar benefits and side effects.

For estrogen/progestin combos, side effects usually mean irregular bleeding for a few months. Five to 10 percent also have breast tenderness, headaches, moodiness and bloating—most of which improve with time. "Sometimes it helps to ease into estrogen by first using a low-dose vaginal cream, just to get the body used to the hormone again. Then switch to pills once every two or three days and work up to daily," says Debra R. Judelson, MD, recent past president, American Medical Women's Association.

2. Estring This new alternative is a soft flexible ring that is inserted into the vagina. It releases a low, steady dose of *estradiol* for 90 days. The ring improves vaginal and sexual comfort, and eases urinary urgency and pain. It doesn't affect overall health because very little estrogen actually gets into the bloodstream. Side effects are rare (possibly vaginal irritation, back pain and headaches).

3. Creams These also primarily relieve dryness and improve sexual comfort. Unless high doses are used, creams have little effect on the heart, bones, breasts, etc. Initially used daily, after a few weeks the dose can usually be tapered down. There are five brands—Estrace, Estriol Cream, Ogen, Ortho Dienestrol and Premarin cream.

4. Patches These coin-sized stick-ons are usually placed on the abdomen or buttocks. So far, studies show that patches are as effective as pills against osteoporosis and nearly so against heart disease.

However, estrogen absorbed through a patch can stimulate the uterine lining, so patch users who haven't had a hysterectomy should also take oral progestin to slash uterine-cancer risks. Some skin irritation is fairly common but usually disappears. Patches need to be replaced once (Climara) or twice (Estraderm or Vivelle) a week.

Patches are good for women with a history of blood clots, or when liver or gallbladder problems are a concern, since less estrogen passes through these organs than with pills.

As for other benefits, most top physicians say it's too early to make estrogen decisions based on any of the exciting new research about Alzheimer's, colon cancer, etc.—but as more data emerges, that could change fast. "The evidence is intriguing, even if it's all still in the promising category," says Dr. Col.

In the meantime, there are a few other factors to consider when making an estrogen decision:

◆ If you've had a hysterectomy, you're not at risk for uterine cancer so you don't need to take progestin with estrogen. This will help to eliminate many of the menstrual-like symptoms caused by taking estrogen/progestin combinations.

◆ Diabetics may need to increase insulin if they take estrogen/progestin, since the duo can upset blood sugar.

◆ Because they're already at increased cancer risk, estrogen may not be right for women who haven't had children or had them after 30; are significantly overweight; or have already had breast or uterine cancer.

◆ ERT can worsen abnormal vaginal bleeding, blood clotting, severe headaches, dizziness or liver disease.

◆ If you drink alcohol, that's an issue. Recent studies show that alcohol increases blood levels of estrogen, which could conceivably increase breast-cancer risks.

Talk with your doctor about any of these and, as always, also discuss any medications you take or have taken (such as birth-control pills) before starting ERT.

The Best Timing

If you do go on ERT, when should you start and how long should you stay on it? Again, answers depend on what you may be prone to. To weigh breast-cancer risks, see "The Breast-Cancer Connection: How Real Is The Risk?" For the best osteoporosis prevention, doctors say take estrogen for at least 10 years—however, some studies show that breast-cancer risks start increasing after five years and rise more after 10. The odds of both heart disease and osteoporosis climb as soon as you go off estrogen, so for the ultimate protection against both of these, ERT may be a lifetime proposition.

"I see estrogen as a year-to-year commitment," says Dr. Utian. "Every year, a woman and her physician should discuss the pros, cons and any new information, then decide together whether to continue or stop."

Although right now most large studies point to positive effects and longer lives, future research may poke some holes in these results. "The 'facts' from just 10 years ago are quite different today," notes breast-cancer surgeon Susan Love, MD. "Knowledge keeps changing."

Some believe it doesn't make sense to treat women with hormones when nothing is "wrong" with them—menopause is a natural, normal part of life. Yet others reply that until about 60 years ago, most women didn't live long enough for the effects of estrogen loss—especially heart disease and brittle bones—to be recognized.

At its best, ERT is a way for women to stay healthy longer. "We weren't designed to live much past 45 and estrogen is helping us to do so," concludes Trudy Bush, PhD, professor of epidemiology and preventive medicine at the University of Maryland in Baltimore.

One message is clear. Whether or not you decide to take estrogen, regular physical exams and screening tests are likely to be more important during and after menopause than at any other time in your life.

Estrogen to Prevent Alzheimer's?

There are plausible reasons why it might work—and tantalizing suggestions that it does

By ROB WATERS

To Howard Fillit, one of the biggest medical stories of the past year or so seems a little like yesterday's news. In journal articles and reports from conferences, he's seen study after study suggesting that estrogen supplements may delay or prevent Alzheimer's disease. Fillit has been trying to convince the research world of that idea since 1984.

A specialist in geriatrics, Fillit ran an Alzheimer's clinic at Rockefeller University Hospital in New York. Treatment there, as elsewhere, amounted to little more than nursing care, but the clinic's practitioners searched diligently for clues to the cause of the baffling disease.

One day Fillit brought a colleague along on his rounds. A patient they saw, Olga,* had been a world traveler and an accomplished artist, but now she lay in bed, staring silently out the window. What day is it? Fillit asked. Where are you? She couldn't answer.

Fillit's colleague, neuroscientist Bruce McEwen, had been studying the effect of hormones on brain activity. In research on rats, he'd seen estrogen boost levels of an enzyme crucial to learning and recall. McEwen wondered aloud: Could Olga's loss of memory and ability to reason stem in part from a lack of estrogen?

Fillit was aware of the hormone's importance to healthy bones in women; the idea that estrogen might also help the brain function properly didn't seem far-fetched. So he set up a study, giving seven women low doses of estrogen for six weeks. For Olga and two others, the hormone made a remarkable difference. "It was as though their brains suddenly became activated," Fillit says. "They were more verbal, their moods were brighter, and their memories improved." Indeed, estrogen made such a difference that the women's families asked Fillit to keep them on it even after the research ended.

Though promising, the study was small. Fillit wasn't able to get funding to take it further, but his ideas began to percolate among researchers.

Today Fillit looks like a prophet. Researchers at Columbia University last August reported that estrogen may cut the risk of Alzheimer's by up to 60 percent; the study was the most rigorous one to date. And in October the largest study so far, of 3,700 California women, came up with similar findings.

The past few years have been the most productive for researchers since Alois Alzheimer first described the disease 90 years ago. Some of the findings—for instance, that a gene called apoE4 triples the odds of developing Alzheimer's—may eventually help doctors predict which patients are likely to suffer from the disorder. But the estrogen research offers the possibility of prevention.

The Columbia study was especially tantalizing, as it minimized a basic problem in Alzheimer's research. Because women who already have the disease might not remember whether they had once taken estrogen (and because reports from worried family members

This name has been changed.

From *Health,* January/February 1997, pp. 40, 42. © 1997 by Time Publishing Ventures, Inc. Reprinted by permission.

MedicalNews

The Pill and Breast Cancer

Doctors have long worried that the daily dose of hormones in birth control pills might raise a woman's risk of breast cancer. A recent study has put their minds at ease: Not only did it fail to find a link, the results suggest that women on the Pill who do get breast cancer are more likely to survive it.

A New Way to Prevent Asthma

Recently approved Accolate is the first asthma treatment breakthrough in more than 20 years. Patients who feel their current medication is failing to prevent attacks may want to ask their doctors about this twice-a-day pill.

Don't Suffer in Silence

The Friends' Health Connection introduces people with similar illnesses, disabilities, or injuries. Members may meet by phone, E-mail, or regular mail. The group also has a network for caregivers. Write to P.O. Box 114, New Brunswick, NJ 08903. Or call 800/48-FRIEND. A $20 donation is requested.

The World's Ten Deadliest Illnesses

1. Pneumonia
2. Diarrhea
3. Tuberculosis
4. Malaria
5. Hepatitis B
6. AIDS
7. Measles
8. Tetanus
9. Whooping cough
10. Roundworm

World Health Organization

Family Docs Overlook Melanoma

In a study at the University of California at San Francisco, primary care doctors missed half the melanomas they saw, while dermatologists missed only 17 percent. If you have a mole with an uneven border or one that's larger than a pencil eraser, see a dermatologist.

might not be reliable either), neurologist Richard Mayeux and his colleagues turned to 1,100 elderly but healthy women, asking them about past or present use of the hormone. Then the researchers settled in for a lengthy follow-up, returning between one and five years later to examine the women.

About 150 of the volunteers had taken estrogen. Of these, only 6 percent developed Alzheimer's, compared to 16 percent of the women who had never taken the supplement. It seemed that women who took estrogen for at least a year gained more protection than those on it for a shorter time, says Mayeux. Other studies also suggest that the longer estrogen is used, the lower the risk.

"It looks like we may be able to prevent maybe two-thirds of Alzheimer's cases in women," says geriatrician Stanley Birge of the Washington University School of Medicine in St. Louis, who wrote a review of recent studies for the *Journal of the American Geriatrics Society.* "And that would be nothing short of miraculous."

Medical researchers know Alzheimer's is largely a woman's disease. One reason is simple: Women live longer, so there are more of them in the over-70 set most vulnerable to the disorder. But many researchers believe there's more to it than that. A number of studies suggest that among people who survive into their seventies, women are up to *three times* more likely to get the disease.

Oddly enough, that jibes with the idea that estrogen may play a crucial role. Both men and women have receptors for estrogen on neurons in the brain, which hints that the hormone has a job to do there. While supply may grow dicey for a woman in the decades after menopause, a man gets his estrogen from a more reliable source: testosterone, which is converted to estrogen in the brain.

How might estrogen protect the brain? Neurons die at a vastly increased rate in people with Alzheimer's. Estrogen seems to raise levels of nerve growth factors, chemicals that help neurons live longer. It also appears to increase the number of connections between neurons, boost levels of an enzyme needed to make the chemical messengers known as neurotransmitters, and improve the flow of blood to the brain.

So researchers can boast exciting findings and plausible reasons why estrogen might work. What they *don't* have is proof. "When I talk to support groups for families of people with Alzheimer's, one of the most frequent questions I get from women is, 'Should I be on estrogen?' " says Alan Lerner, a neurologist at Case Western Reserve University in Cleveland. Lerner is not ready to tell women to take the hormone to combat Alzheimer's—even though he himself has done studies that indicated a protective effect. He points out that there may be other differences between women who choose to take estrogen and those who don't. Women on estrogen tend to be better educated, for instance. Could demanding mental work produce more connections between neurons—essentially creating mental reserves?

To answer such questions, what's needed are large, randomized studies in which some women receive estrogen and others a placebo. One such study is under way; its results, due about 2005, should settle the question of whether estrogen helps preserve healthy brains and, if so, offer a clue as to whether progesterone negates the benefits.

In the meantime Howard Fillit thinks the current findings, however incomplete, will sway many women who are weighing the possible costs and benefits of estrogen replacement therapy. "When they think about their final years," Fillit says, "a far greater fear for 50-year-old women is not whether they're going to break their hip or have a heart attack. It's whether they're going to lose their minds."

Can you Afford to Get Old?

MONEY MAY NOT BUY HEALTH, BUT IT GOES A LONG WAY TOWARD ENSURING LIFELONG MEDICAL CARE

BY MARLYS HARRIS

The first crow's-feet bring with them a disturbing truth: Good habits and healthy living alone won't exempt us from aging. Those of us hitting our 40s and 50s react to this unsettling knowledge by redoubling our efforts to exercise, eat right and behave as virtuously as Barbara Bush. But there's another point that we miss entirely. Our chances of living a long, full life also depend on flagging and treating illness early, and that requires money. Having adequate financial resources is a key element in maintaining physical health. ♦ Anxiety about money has many midlife women slouching toward Medicare, praying that nothing too serious will attack until we reach 65, when the government's health insurance for the elderly kicks in. Even then, though, we won't be free from money worries. Women earn less and therefore retire with less, so we may not have the cash to cover Medicare's many gaps. Add the fact that on average women live about seven years longer than men, and you've got the makings of a real financial—and possible health—crisis.

You may figure that it's too late to get organized. Not so. Just as you boost your odds of living longer at any age by giving up cigarettes or beginning an exercise program, so too can you fortify your finances by taking the first steps right now.

1 Secure Health Insurance

About 13% of midlife women have no health insurance. Until you reach the age when you can be covered by Medicare, you can't afford to go without it. Even a relatively simple operation like an appendectomy can cost $20,000 and push you into bankruptcy if you can't pay the hospital bills.

If your employer provides health insurance, you're set. If not, purchasing a policy should be the most urgent item on your to-do list. Costs vary by state, but a comprehensive indemnity policy—one that covers hospitalization, doctor fees, prescriptions and all medical tests with a $1,000 deductible—for a single, healthy, 50-year-old woman in Connecticut, for example, might run about $150 a month.

An HMO plan for the same woman would cost about $230 a month, slightly more because that fee and a nominal charge at the time of treatment (usually $10 to $20) cover all care, even hospital stays, and all preventive visits, and there's no deductible. You must, however, choose your physician from an HMO list. Then again, many HMO's have added point-of-service provisions that allow you to use doctors outside the plan, reimbursing you for only 70% to 80% of the bill after a $250 to $500 deductible.

If possible, try to avoid buying just a catastrophic health care policy, which covers only hospitalization and certain medical conditions. If you have a serious illness, you could be stuck with frightening bills.

You'll also want to steer clear of so-called dread-disease insurance, which covers costs for diagnosis and treatment of a single disease, such as cancer. These policies can run from $14 to $34 a month and usually pay out as little as 35% of the premiums they take in, according to a study by the U.S. General Accounting Office in Washington. Comprehensive policies pay out 75% or more. It's better to focus on securing high-quality comprehensive health insurance that will cover a variety of costs associated with a wide range of diseases.

But no plan is perfect. According to a 1995 study from the Agency for Health Care Policy and Research in Rockville, MD, about 29 million Americans have health insurance that leaves them with annual out-of-pocket expenses of more than 10% of their incomes. Flexible Spending Accounts (FSA's), offered by many employers,

From *American Health for Women*, July/August 1997, pp. 61-63, 108.

PEOPLE UNDER AGE 60 ARE MUCH LIKELIER TO SUFFER A DISABILITY THAN DIE. THE FINANCIAL EFFECT COULD BE WORSE THAN DEATH. NOT ONLY CAN'T YOU BRING IN ANY MONEY WHEN YOU'RE DISABLED, BUT ALSO YOU'RE STILL SPENDING IT.

can help fill the holes. They allow you to set aside up to $5,000 a year before taxes to pay for medical expenses not covered by insurance. If your plan won't pay for a psychiatrist, for example, but you need to visit one every week, you can use your tax-free FSA funds each year to pay the bill. But you have to use all the money in an FSA by the end of the year or you'll lose it.

2 **Buy Disability and Long-Term Care Insurance** In financial planning, you have to consider the worst-case scenario: an illness or injury so devastating that you can't work for a long time. Disability insurance can protect you. "People under age 60 are much likelier to suffer a disability than die," says Norma Severns, a financial planner in Washington. The financial effect is worse than death, she says. Not only can't you bring in money, but also you're still spending it.

Some employers provide group plans that cover up to 60% of your salary if you're unable to work. Lacking that, you might consider buying your own policy. Your best bet, says Peter Katt, a Mattawan, MI, life insurance adviser, is a plan that covers a shortfall in earnings if you can't continue in your current job but could do something less demanding or work part-time. Policies are expensive, so buy as little as you can safely get away with. Your benefits will be tax-free if you do buy your own policy, so you may not need as much as you think.

For employed people (and their spouses and kids under 16), Social Security will pay a benefit starting six months after you become disabled, based on your total career earnings. (To check your current earnings status, call the Social Security Administration at 800-772-1213 and ask for your free Personal Earnings and Benefit Estimate Statement [Form 7004].) There are holes aplenty in the Social Security safety net, however: the six-month waiting period, a requirement for complete disability and payments that are usually only $200 to $1,400 a month. How can you close those gaps? For starters, every family should have an emergency savings fund equal to six months of expenses. If you don't have such a fund, start paring the budget now to build one.

3 **Prepare for When a Partner Dies or Leaves** Don't think that just because you're married you can breathe easy. Sure, your husband will rush to help if you get sick, but what if something should happen to *him?* Over a million married women in the U.S. rely solely on their husbands for health insurance. Fortunately, the Consolidated Omnibus Budget Reconciliation Act (COBRA) of 1985 allows both widowed and divorced spouses to buy health coverage through their spouse's employer for up to 36 months. After that, you're on your own.

If your husband dies and you have kids under 16, you'll receive up to 75% of his monthly Social Security payments. That and your husband's life insurance (which should be five times his annual salary) should be enough to support children and a nonworking wife indefinitely, particularly if there are savings, other assets and retirement accounts to help. *You* should also have life insurance, to replace earnings that would end with your death.

If you and your husband divorce and you don't work outside the home, do everything you can to preserve your financial security. Many women are able to negotiate a readjustment income for a set number of years to allow them to acquire certain job skills and get on their feet. If you can do this, don't forget to include the cost of your health insurance in your budget estimates. Most employers will continue covering children in health plans after divorce, but not ex-spouses. "If you have to buy your own insurance and you have preexisting

Health Care Sticker Shock

What will it cost you to enjoy a long, healthy *old age? Get a good grip on your wallet: People aged 65 and over racked up bills totaling $7,039 per person in 1995 (by comparison, those under 65 incurred an average of $1,849 in health care expenses). Serious health problems such as those below up the ante even more.*

HEART DISEASE AND STROKE
- One year on Zocor (high cholesterol medication), 10 mg a day: *$591*
- Electrocardiogram: *$30-$135*
- Eight-day hospitalization for a heart attack: *$18,214*
- 10-day hospitalization for a stroke: *$14,175*

OSTEOPOROSIS
- Bone density scan: *$75-$150*
- One year on Fosamax, 5 mg or 10 mg a day: *$544*
- 11-day hospitalization for a broken hip (a common complication of osteoporosis): *$16,871*

BREAST CANCER
- Yearly mammogram: *$70-$175*
- Mastectomy: (breast removal) *$7,415*
- Lumpectomy: (tumor removal) *$7,085*

DIABETES
- Total health care costs for a year, including drugs and doctor visits: *$11,157*
- Six-day hospitalization for diabetes complications: *$6,584*

DEPRESSION
- One year on Prozac, 20 mg a day: *$730*
- Outpatient therapy: *$110 per visit*

—TRINA CHANG

Figures are representative of typical or average charges as provided by various doctors, health care organizations, pharmaceutical companies and government data. Hospitalization figures are based on a sample of community hospitals and include room, board and treatment but exclude physician payments. Drug costs are based on wholesale prices.

BY THE YEAR 2010, ALMOST HALF OF AMERICAN WOMEN WILL BE AT LEAST 50 . . . WOMEN ARE ONLY HALF AS LIKELY AS MEN TO RECEIVE A PENSION FROM A FORMER EMPLOYER.

conditions, you could wind up paying an extraordinarily high amount annually or not get insurance at all," says Gail Koff, president of Jacoby & Meyers, a national law firm.

You'll also be entitled to a cut of the assets: everything you and your ex accumulated during your marriage, including your husband's employee retirement plans, such as his 401(K) and pension. Many states consider these assets marital property and will award a wife her due, if she asks. You're also entitled to half the amount your husband saved during the years you were married, plus interest and dividends. It may not sound like much, but add on 15 to 20 years of interest or earnings in the stock market and you might be looking at real money when it's time to retire—when chronic health problems with their accompanying costs start creeping up on you.

4 **Maximize Your Savings** Because women usually live longer and earn less than men, they need to save more of what they do earn, says Stanford University economics professor Douglas Bernheim, Ph.D. If you haven't developed the savings habit yet, start now to ensure that you'll have the money you need to live comfortably. Using retirement plans offered by your employer is the least painful way to save, because the money is deducted from your paycheck and stashed in an investment account before you ever get your hands on it. The 401(K), the most common plan, allows you to invest up to 15% of your pay or a maximum of $9,500 each year. You don't have to pay taxes on the money when you invest, and the earnings grow tax free. Generally you can't withdraw the money until age 59½ without paying a stiff 10% penalty (plus taxes).

If your employer doesn't offer a retirement plan, establish an Individual Retirement Account (IRA), where you can contribute up to 15% of your pay, to a maximum of $2,000 a year, tax free. If you're a non-earning homemaker, you can establish an IRA in your own name, and this year, for the first time, you can make the same maximum contribution as a wage earner. (Previously you could set aside only $250 a year.)

The tax-free buildup of your money in either an IRA or an employer-sponsored plan makes it worthwhile to tie up the money. A 50-year-old woman in the 28% tax bracket who stashes away $2,000 a year in a money-market fund or savings account earning 8% would have $48,331 at age 65. If she put it in a tax-protected plan, her money would grow to $54,233. The self-employed can get the same plans designed for them—either the Keogh or a Simplified Employee Pension plan.

5 **Forgo Nursing Home Insurance** Eventual residence in a nursing home is a possibility no woman should ignore. Medicaid, the government's health program for the poor, will pay nursing home expenses, but only if you've spent practically all your assets. Nursing home or long-term care insurance, heavily promoted by salesmen to people as young as 40, supposedly fills this gap. At this age, however, it's not a very good deal.

Premiums generally rise with age, but even if you buy young to lock in a low annual premium, as many salesmen suggest, the insurance company can raise rates if its costs go up—and you can bet they will. By the time you're 70 and living alone on a fixed income, that once reasonable premium could be too huge to pay. But if you stop paying, you could lose everything you've invested over the years unless you buy a policy that returns a portion of your premiums.

Is there any other way to fend off the nursing home threat? Yes: Save more money for your future. The funds will be there for you if you need care.

You've probably already taken some steps to fortify your finances. Even so, doing the rest can look overwhelming. Chances are you won't need to do everything, but even taking the smallest steps now will help prepare you for a long, healthy life.

Marlys Harris is a writer in Westport, CT, who specializes in finance.

ASSISTED SUICIDE: DO WE REALLY KNOW WHAT WE WANT?

A Harder Better Death

My father and I would have helped my mother end her life if she'd asked. Instead she wanted to die naturally, at home. As difficult as that became, **hospice made it the right choice.**

BY PETER FISH

I UNDERSTOOD THINGS WERE NOT GOING TO BE ALL RIGHT the moment the plane landed. It was a small commuter airport in Southern California. We'd made our descent over lemon orchards and a bright bend of the Pacific, touched down, taxied to a stop in front of the terminal. I saw my father leaning against a chain-link fence. For the first time in my life I was watching him cry. § WE WERE A FAMILY WHO JOGGED, watched our cholesterol, and scheduled annual checkups. Dying took us by surprise. A few weeks before, my mother had complained of a pain in her ribs. She was a three-times-a-week golfer, a yoga enthusiast, an ocean swimmer, a woman who at 72 looked easily ten years younger. She assumed she had merely pulled a muscle. But the pain refused to disappear. She scheduled an appointment with the family doctor. "I can't see what could be wrong with someone as healthy as you," he said. § BUT THE DOCTOR ORDERED AN MRI, and then a CAT scan and a biopsy. What they revealed was the reason my father stood among strangers crying. An aggressive adenocarcinoma of unknown origin—perhaps breast, perhaps lung, we never found out—had metastasized throughout my mother's ribs and spine. § "I THINK YOUR MOTHER is going to have a lot of trouble with this

From *Health,* November/December 1997, pp. 108-114. © 1997 by Time Publishing Ventures, Inc. Reprinted by permission.

cancer," said the oncologist when we got to the hospital.

A lot of trouble. That wasn't the half of it.

Sitting in a quilted nightgown in her hospital bed, my mother was tanned, cheerful, and stunned. A few weeks earlier she and my father had been planning summer cruises. Now they were planning the remaining months of her life.

I asked her how she felt. "Mad," she said. That was it. We would always have a hard time discussing her illness. Optimism was such a family creed we lacked the vocabulary for crisis. But my mother did make it clear that she did not want to remain in the hospital. She wanted to go home.

Until that moment *hospice* was a word I associated with made-for-TV movies in which guest stars died uplifting deaths in garden settings. Now, we were told, hospice could help us care for my mother at home. Suddenly, and for the next few months, hospice became the center of our lives.

Our house acquired the grim energy of a military headquarters. We accumulated bedpans, walkers, safety railings. We installed a buzzer my mother could press when she required pain medication; its alarm sawed the air like the horn on a navy submarine. Chilling in the refrigerator was an array of narcotics I had not realized private citizens could legally possess. We had a new bed: a heavy electric device designed to lift my mother's frail body on a cushion of air, with coils and baffles that hissed as malevolently as Darth Vader. Most important, we had the hospice staff—doctor, nurses, social worker—making sure my father and I could handle the bed and bedpans, the narcotics and buzzers, the reality of my mother's dying.

March, April, May. The cancer was, as the oncologist promised, aggressive. Each month, each week, each day was a diminishment. My mother was confined to downstairs, then to her bedroom and bathroom, then to her bed. My father brushed her hair and massaged her legs and feet. The hair turned brittle and fell out; she lost all feeling in her legs. I read to her. We examined family photo albums. Shots from the fifties and sixties: my parents glamorous at the Coconut Grove, laughing with golf buddies during some Sweethearts' Tournament. In later snapshots I was present: cradled by my mother at Bryce Canyon in Utah, capped and gowned beside her at college graduation.

Sometimes as my mother and I flipped through these Kodak moments of a life now drawing to a close, I would reassure myself: At least we are home. Home was nothing fancy, just a Southern California beach house, the kind of place where you stowed your surfboard in the carport and then tracked sand into the living room, and when you opened any window you heard the sound of the sea. But my mother loved it here. How well we were doing, I told myself, that she could remain.

Or I thought we were doing well, until one night I was driving up the Pacific Coast Highway. It had been a lousy week. My mother was paralyzed now, and drifting in and out of consciousness. My father and I had argued. It was suddenly clear that despite everyone's hard work and good intentions she was going to die, and sooner than we had thought possible. Each half mile I stopped the car and threw up at the side of the road. By the time I reached Mugu Rock, a plug of granite jammed into the Pacific, I was propped against the car thinking, She can't go on, I can't go on, none of us can go on. For the first time in my life I considered the act usually referred to as euthanasia. No details entered my mind, just the simple fact: My father and I could end this.

I expected a thunderclap. I possessed—still possess—a strong if untutored religious faith and a clear sense that ending someone's life was sin. Yet there I stood thinking any sin would be preferable to continuing this nightmare.

The moment passed. I did nothing. The ending came on its own, soon enough. My mother grew weaker, aging with the withering that cancer brings. She drifted away. It was as terrible and powerful a thing to witness as seeing someone pulled from you by the tide. She died on Father's Day. I had bought my father a card and a bottle of cognac that we were drinking when we heard her breathing stop.

This was a death whose particulars were orchestrated by a hospice program. For two decades the hospice movement has been aiding families like mine. Hospice offers the hope that death need not be painful, impersonal, or entangled in technology. It offers the hope that death, while inevitable, need not be unendurable.

"What do Americans say they most want to avoid?" asks Ira Byock, a Missoula, Montana, physician who is president of the American Academy of Hospice and Palliative Medicine. "They don't want to die in pain. They don't want to die isolated and abandoned. They don't want to be a burden—particularly a financial burden—on their families." Hospice, Byock and his allies maintain, can ease all of these fears.

Given our current frustration with the American way of death, hospice should be enjoying a moment in the sun. Instead the movement finds itself out in the cold—not under direct attack so much as threatened with irrelevance. As I did, a lot of Americans are standing by a dark highway and saying, This can't go on. They're wondering if the best death isn't the quickest death. And unless they have a change of heart, the hope that hospice holds out may simply be . . . beside the point.

RIGHT NOW IT APPEARS the country is intent on living out that Woody Allen joke: "It's not that I'm afraid to die. I just don't want to be there when it happens." Organizations such as the Hemlock Society and Compassion in Dying lobby for physician-assisted suicide with the kind of can-do grassroots enthusiasm we expect from the Sierra Club or Mothers Against Drunk Driving. In Oregon they passed the Death With Dignity Act, legalizing physician-assisted suicide. They have pushed their arguments up to the U.S. Supreme Court. In the meantime pathologist Jack Kevorkian has helped more than two dozen people end their lives, some by injection, others by inhaling carbon monoxide in the back of his van. One poll showed that 90 percent of Americans believe they should have some control over the place and even the time of their deaths.

To be sure, many physicians and ethicists count the current debate on the right to die as long overdue. At least we are finally acknowledging that American medicine, so good at so many things, does a poor job of helping people who are dying.

"We're doing terribly badly," says geriatrician Joanne Lynn, director of George Washington University's Center to Improve

Until that moment *hospice* was a word I associated with made-for-TV **MOVIES IN WHICH GUEST STARS DIED UPLIFTING DEATHS IN GARDEN SETTINGS.**

Care of the Dying. In a recent study on the last days of the hospitalized terminally ill, Lynn and fellow researchers tracked 2,500 patients. They found that four out of ten suffered from severe pain and eight out of ten from severe fatigue. Of dying in America, Lynn says, "It is reasonable to be afraid."

"I have a terrible time with Jack Kevorkian," says Connie Holden, executive director of Hospice of Boulder County in Colorado and one of the nation's most articulate advocates of improving end-of-life care. "I find his methods repugnant. But he turned the light on a topic that needed to have attention paid to it." Likewise, the suicide-minded Hemlock Society may seem morbid and extreme. But, Holden says, "They are just regular folks who have had a bad experience in dying."

Avoiding a bad experience in dying. That is what hospice is all about.

One way of understanding hospice is that it is the only medical institution designed solely for the dying. When a patient is given a terminal diagnosis of six months or less and agrees to hospice care, he or she abandons aggressive treatment of the disease. Generally patients will not receive chemotherapy or blood transfusions nor be connected to respirators or feeding tubes. Typically, they will not be cared for in a hospital or nursing home but in their own homes.

In giving up a hospital's aura of stainless steel crisis, patients and their families put their faith in the ministrations of the hospice team—physicians, nurses, nurse's aides, and social workers, all trained in end-of-life care. The team makes sure that symptoms are managed, pain is controlled, and family members are not shattering under the pressure of illness. Medicare and private insurance plans normally cover the visits.

My father and I knew nothing of hospice before we scanned the local program's tasteful pastel brochures. We knew nothing about anything. To imagine how ill-suited we were to tending a terminally ill patient full-time, you would have to imagine Abbott and Costello starring in "ER."

But we managed. We got better at it. A few times a week (more often as my mother neared death) someone from hospice would visit to check that my mother was reasonably comfortable, to monitor the cancer, to see whether my father and I were beginning to crack. Our favorite was the social worker: a dark-haired, athletic woman not unlike my mother in her youth. She radiated the kind of good health you think will rub off on you, and she did not seem bothered that when my father and I spoke with her we often began to cry.

Nurses and nurse's aides were more problematic. We were hard on them. One nurse arrived a half hour late. We demanded a replacement. Another was brusque. We replaced her, too. Later I understood that we'd been focusing our anger at the cancer on these people. But eventually we found the perfect nurse, who bustled pleasantly and told my mother how pretty she looked. She knew what her patient needed to hear.

Our biggest fear was that my mother would experience intolerable pain. But my mother did not suffer horribly. That, say hospice experts, is usually the case. "Pain management has gotten much better," says Laurel Herbst of the San Diego Hospice. "We have a much clearer understanding of the physiology of pain. Ninety-five percent of patients stay awake, alert, and pain-free." Prescription painkillers including morphine can lessen physical discomfort; steroids can lift, a bit, the dying patient's profound fatigue. If pain increases as death approaches, morphine may be given in higher and higher doses, easing the slide into unconsciousness.

It was in those last days that hospice was of particular help to me. I had not seen anyone die before; in the most rudimentary sense I did not know what to make of the process, did not know what to do. Use swabs to moisten her mouth, the nurse told me. Hold her hand. That breathing you hear is called Cheyne-Stokes; it tells you life is drawing to a close. Her senses are dimming, but hearing will linger. Tell her you love her.

For hospice advocates, deaths like my mother's are examples of the succor hospice can provide. And at best, they say, hospice can do more than that, making death not just an ending but a kind of culmination. When Byock first began encountering dying patients and their families, he didn't believe this was possible. "But every once in a while a person would tell me, 'This has been the most wonderful time of my life,'" he says. "It took several of those incidents before it finally dawned on me that the universe was trying to teach me something."

Byock's new book, *Dying Well,* tells the stories of a dozen of his hospice patients. Byock doesn't ignore the messy terrifying aspects of death—the IVs, the incontinence, the pain. But he shows how they can be managed and sometimes transcended. A brassy hard-living woman reconciles with her estranged sister. Stricken with an inoperable brain tumor, a middle-aged man lets go of his deep-seated anger and expresses love for his wife and children.

"If you control symptoms," Byock insists, "if you provide basic support to people and families, you see enormous growth at the end of life. Erikson, Maslow, Piaget all said human development is a lifelong process. We in hospice have shown they are right. Some of us know that end-of-life care doesn't have to be that bad. There are robust alternatives to suicide even at the very end of life."

WHEN IT'S TIME for HOSPICE

THE DECISION TO ENTER A HOSPICE PROGRAM is never easy. Doctors, patients, and family members must all admit a life is ending, stop trying to cure the disease, and shift their goal to helping the patient die at home surrounded by the people and things he or she most loves. If you find yourself facing the death of someone close to you, here's what you might want to know.

WHEN HOSPICE SHOULD START As difficult as it is, families ought to turn to hospice months rather than days or weeks before death seems imminent, experts advise. This gives caregivers time to adjust to the stresses of their role, and increases the likelihood of a rewarding close to the loved one's life. Medicare and most other insurers will pay for hospice as long as a physician certifies that the patient appears to have less than six months to live.

WHERE HOSPICE TAKES PLACE Nearly always in the patient's home, with the bulk of care provided by family and friends. Residential hospices are rare, and much of their cost isn't covered by Medicare.

WHAT HOME HOSPICE PROVIDES A variety of assistance to caregivers: training in attending to a dying patient; a nurse available by phone 24 hours a day; several weekly visits by professionals who might include a doctor, a nurse, health aides, or a social worker; medication for pain and symptom control; supplies; durable medical equipment; chaplain services; and bereavement counseling.

HOW TO CHOOSE A PROGRAM Ask if it is certified by Medicare, which ensures that physicians, nurses, social workers, health aides, volunteers, and chaplains are on staff. To select among certified hospices, ask the patient's doctor, nurse, hospital social worker, or discharge planner for advice. Also, pay attention to your impressions. "The first contact with a hospice program is important," says Connie Borden of Hospice by the Bay in San Francisco. "Does someone come out to the home and take the time to listen to your concerns and answer your questions?"

WHEN IT'S COVERED Medicare and many private plans will pay for the program. "Even if hospice *isn't* covered, be persistent," says Borden. "Talk with the insurer's case manager. There may be a pot of money for care."

FOR MORE INFORMATION Call or write the National Hospice Organization, 1901 N. Moore St., Suite 901, Arlington, VA 22209; 800/658-8898. Find the NHO's home page at www.nho.org. *A Consumer Guide to Hospice Care,* a 32-page booklet published by the National Consumers League, includes a helpful checklist for evaluating programs. Send a check or money order for $4 to 1701 K St. NW, Suite 1200, Washington, DC 20006; or call 202/835-3323.

—P.F. and Anne Johnson

IF HOSPICE PROMISES COMFORT, dignity, and even growth at the end of life, why don't more Americans embrace it? The nation's 3,000 hospice programs currently tend 15 percent of America's dying—about 390,000 deaths a year compared to the 1.3 million who die in hospitals. Experts like Joanne Lynn believe that hospice programs could well serve twice that number. Indeed, Lynn feels that if hospice developed less intense and less expensive variations, it might be appropriate for *anyone* dying of a chronic illness—about 70 percent of the dying. Meanwhile, polls reveal that most Americans are aware of hospice and support—in theory—its goal of dying at home. So what's holding us back? What's standing between us and the good death we say we want?

The biggest obstacle is one that's existed since the first American program opened in 1974: Many doctors are reluctant to refer patients to hospice, seeing the proposal as a painful admission of defeat. Doctors often suggest more treatment rather than face a patient and his or her family with the news that there's no hope. This tendency is changing as more doctors see hospice's advantages. But even now, says Jennifer Morales of the National Hospice Organization, "We have to get away from the notion that death is a failure for a physician."

Reluctance isn't limited to physicians. Many patients and family members also balk at stopping treatment. Doctors say families frequently hesitate to sign the consent forms required to place someone in hospice, a step that would concede death was on the way. Says Holden, "There is always a certain discomfort patients and families have."

Current Medicare rules are another stumbling block. Medicare will reimburse the costs of hospice care only if a doctor certifies that the patient has less than six months to live. That requirement works fairly well for patients with late-stage cancer, a disease whose course is relatively predictable, and in fact about a third of cancer deaths occur in hospice. But hospice is now stretching to care for patients with emphysema, AIDS, congestive heart failure, and neurological disorders like Parkinson's disease. All of these illnesses progress in less predictable ways, making it difficult for doctors to determine when a patient might die. This year Holden polled local physicians about the biggest problem they experienced in referring patients to hospice. More than 80 percent said it was judging whether a patient had just six months to live.

It hasn't helped that the Department of Health and Human Service's Office of Inspector General is currently auditing hospice programs to see if they have violated Medicare rules. The office charges that some hospices have gotten Medicare to pay for patients' care even when it was clear the patients would not die within six months. The National Hospice Organization counters that most of these cases involve simple differences of medical opinion. Given the timing, hospice administrators find the investigations dispiriting. "It's having a significant chilling effect on extending hospice care," says Byock. Adds Holden, "We've been accused of being cancer focused. But about the time we open up to other illnesses, we get our hands slapped. Right now would be a scary time to start a hospice program."

Combine reluctant doctors and families with hospice directors watching their backs, and the result is that Americans are spending more time in the grips of hospital machinery than makes sense either financially or emotionally. A recent study of 6,500 hospice patients by Nicholas Christakis of the University of Chicago highlighted the scope of the problem. He found that the patients who'd had the longest hospital stays—at least a month—died on average after just a month of hospice. One in seven patients died within seven *days* of moving home. Christakis's overall conclusion was that even among people who do eventually enter hospice, the majority are receiving hospital care long after it has stopped benefiting them. "People are clamoring for better care for the dying," he says. "And hospice offers that. People need to ask for it earlier."

To allow more dying patients to take advantage of hospice, advocates would like legislation to loosen Medicare's six-month limit. Just as much, they'd like a deeper understanding—among physicians and the public both—of the advantages of hospice.

And this is why the debate over assisted suicide troubles most hospice professionals. For who can pay attention to hospice when Jack Kevorkian dominates the headlines and talk shows? The controversy may have helped Americans recognize the ways in which medicine fails the dying, but it has also distracted us from the real challenge of providing decent end-of-life care. "In a sense," says Byock, "the attempt to legalize assisted suicide is an extension of our cultural denial about dying."

The hospice establishment has taken a strong stand against assisted suicide. In the cases before the Supreme Court, the National Hospice Organization filed a brief opposing its legalization. After passage of Oregon's Death With Dignity Act, one prominent hospice announced that its staff would not attend patients who wanted to die with a doctor's help.

This antipathy can partly be explained by hospice's roots. Most of the earliest hospices were affiliated with churches, and even today many hospice workers share a moral aversion toward the taking of life. Others look abroad with alarm. They note that the Netherlands, a nation where physician-assisted suicide has been decriminalized, has a weak hospice program, and they worry that legalizing suicide for the dying might similarly weaken hospice in the United States. Psychiatrist Herbert Hendin, author of *Seduced by Death,* a report on the Dutch experience, sums up the concern: "When assisted suicide is legalized, assisted suicide becomes the easier option, and hospice is a casualty."

Most hospice physicians and nurses maintain that when a patient asks for help committing suicide, the problem is likely not with the patient but with the nature of care being given. "It's a red flag," says Holden. "In the great majority of times it is a cry for better symptom management and more emotional support. And if, in fact, you address those needs, the person's desire for suicide goes away."

In other cases, caregiver burnout is responsible. "Have I ever wanted to help someone kill themselves?" Byock asks. "You bet. And anyone in this profession who says they haven't is lying. But it always turned out it wasn't about the patient. It's when *I've* felt overwhelmed, when *I've* felt helpless."

And yet, within the hospice movement there are people who think that assisted suicide and hospice are not mutually exclusive. One is New York internist Timothy Quill, a champion of hospice care who nonetheless argues that for a small percentage of the terminally ill, physician-assisted suicide should be an option. Holden is another. She was one of a group of hospice professionals who filed a brief in the Supreme Court cases arguing in favor of legalization; she believes that even given the best possible care, some patients simply cannot endure their agony. "There are a small number of people who, as they perceive it, are suffering so much they don't wish to tolerate it any longer." When that happens, expediting death may tempt not just the caregivers but the patient, too. "Patients begin hoarding pills, usually sleeping medication," Holden says. "Doctors sometimes prescribe them knowing that's what's going on. It's unreported, it's unregulated, and the fact that suicide is illegal forces everyone to act in secrecy.

"I think hospices sometimes tend to wear rose-colored glasses," says Holden. "I have had deaths in my family that were quite beautiful and gratifying. My father died in a hospice unit, and he had a very peaceful death. I was able to be at his bedside with my two daughters. And we had no desire to hasten it. But for some people, dying is very difficult and quite dreadful."

> If hospice promises comfort and growth at the end of life, why don't we embrace it? **WHAT'S STANDING BETWEEN US AND THE GOOD DEATH WE WANT?**

DIFFICULT AND DREADFUL. That describes my mother's last weeks. Even with the best of assistance, amateur caregivers make mistakes. When the mistakes involve a terminal illness, they can be grievous. Misreading the physician's instructions, my father and I gave my mother far too much morphine. The overdose caused her to hallucinate; we thought we might be killing her. She was

This was not a learning experience. It was no grand reconciliation. **IT WAS JUST THAT FOR ONE EVENING WE COULD ENJOY OUR OLD LIFE TOGETHER.**

rushed back into the hospital for a day and then rushed home with accompanying ambulance sirens in both directions.

Other crises were beyond anyone's control. The electric bed had not been engineered to withstand power failures. When our neighborhood went dark one evening, the bed's air-cushioned mattress deflated, dropping my mother's frail ribs and spine onto a spiky nest of coils and pipes. She screamed while my father screamed into the telephone, demanding that the electric company turn on the power *right now.* It did not.

These were the moments I dwelled on while I stood beside the Pacific Coast Highway, thinking this couldn't go on any longer. These are the moments I relive when I realize that I don't take the strong stand against assisted suicide I once did.

Serious illness is a journey to a foreign country. You don't speak the language, the inhabitants are strangers, you cannot know how you will behave until you arrive. St. Thomas Aquinas condemned suicide because it violates God's authority over life. I believed that. And one of my favorite writers, Flannery O'Connor—herself the victim of a slow death at a young age—wrote, "Sickness before death is a very appropriate thing and I think those who don't have it miss one of God's mercies." I believed that, too. Now I believe that there is suffering that is ennobling but also suffering that strips the humanity from a person, that is so unendurable you would be wise not to predict your reaction to it until you confront it.

But inner strength, too, is unpredictable. Often during the past few years of heated debate over assisted suicide, I have listened to people plead that they could not possibly endure the final illness of someone they love—or endure their own final illness. And I find myself thinking, Don't sell yourself short. Don't be so sure. It will be bad. But perhaps not as bad as your worst fears. I have reached an age where people I know—parents of friends, aging relatives—are receiving terminal diagnoses with some regularity. I find that once I hear the grim news, the second or third sentence out of my mouth is "You'll want to find a hospice program."

For after I stopped by the side of the road and thought I couldn't go on, we went on. That could not have happened without hospice. We struggled through a few more very bad days. But later that week we had a good day. It was May in Southern California, with mustard blazing yellow on the hills and the ocean half in mist and half in sunlight. My mother felt better. The hospice nurse had made her comfortable. The nurse's aide had set her hair.

We made a small celebration of this good day. My father barbecued steaks and tossed a caesar salad. I hit every florist in town trying to find a dozen yellow roses, my mother's favorite. My mother didn't eat more than a bite of steak and salad, but she said they looked delicious. She liked the roses. We opened the windows, and you could hear the ocean and smell a breeze that carried the start of summer on its shoulders.

This day was not a learning experience for us. It was no grand reconciliation. It did not offer us any moment of particular insight. It was just that the three of us were home, and for one warm May evening we could enjoy a brief piece of our old life together. It had been for all of us a happy life. The kind of life you would want to hold on to for as long as you could.

Peter Fish is a senior writer at Sunset *magazine.*

How three of America's leading elder experts protect *their* parents' health

taking care of mom

BY LISA COLLIER COOL

What would you do if your mother or father became seriously ill or incapacitated? Though you'd probably prefer not to think about it, you should, says the National Family Caregivers Association in Kensington, MD. Over 5 million baby boomers are struggling with the worry of caring for an ailing parent, and that number will continue to grow.

To learn the best ways to cope with the most challenging situations you're likely to face as your parents age, we consulted three geriatric specialists who confronted these problems in their own lives.

BE THE BEST ADVOCATE POSSIBLE

"That my mother regained as much functioning as she did is testimony to what can be done with proper support."

—ANITA WOODS, PH.D.

Doctors held out little hope that Maxine Woods would survive after she suffered a terrible fall in her Vancouver, Canada, home in 1984 at the age of 68. The accident left her with a fractured skull, broken ribs, a collapsed lung and other internal injuries.

"From my professional experience I knew that many physicians think elderly people can't recover from severe injuries, and that's just not true," says Woods's daughter, Anita Woods, Ph.D., an assistant professor of medicine at Baylor College of Medicine and a faculty associate at the Huffington Center on Aging, both in Houston. "Older patients often have more physical and psychological strength than doctors realize."

So when her mother was admitted to the hospital, Dr. Woods, one of three children, took her own advice. "I told the doctors I wanted aggressive medical intervention for my mother," she says. "Most of her injuries were reversible, and I knew that she was a strong person who could recover."

GETTING GOOD HOSPITAL CARE

Anita Woods, PhD., recommends the following:

1. Look for a teaching hospital with a *geriatrics program.* For referrals to geriatricians in your parents' area, call the American Geriatrics Society at 800-247-4779.
2. Arrange to have a trusted *family doctor or geriatrician* be a consultant in your parent's care. It's important to get a second opinion, particularly from someone who knows her medical history.
3. Designate a *family advocate.* It's confusing for doctors to get conflicting instructions from different family members or to field the same inquiries from a series of people.
4. *Educate yourself* about your parent's illness and treatment. Ask your parent's doctor and the hospital staff for relevant materials (books, brochures, videos) and for good sources of additional information.
5. Ask to speak with a *hospital social worker* to take advantage of any guidance or support she can give.

From *American Health for Women,* July/August 1998, pp. 89-92. © 1998 by Lisa Collier Cool. Reprinted by permission.

ASSISTED LIVING: WHAT REALLY COUNTS

Neal E. Cutler, Ph.D., says answering these questions will help your parents identify their priorities and find a group residence where they can feel at home.

- Would you live in a *smaller space* in order to stay in the same neighborhood?
- *How far away* would you be willing to move to get a bigger place at the same cost?
- Are you willing to *change your doctors and your church or temple?*
- Would you prefer to be with people of your *religion or ethnic group* or to have a more diverse group of neighbors?
- How important is it to find a place that permits *pets?*
- Would you pay extra to have your *meals brought to you,* or would you prefer to eat with the other residents?
- What *housekeeping services* do you require?
- Would you like to be on the *first floor or a higher floor* with a better view?

When her mother was finally well enough to begin rehabilitation, Dr. Woods pushed the physical therapists not to be satisfied with a slight improvement. "That my mother regained as much functioning as she did is testimony to what can be done with proper support," she says. (For more on how to get top notch care see "Getting Good Hospital Care").

Until two years ago, Neal E. Cutler, Ph.D., a gerontology professor at Widener University in Chester, PA, and the director of survey research at the National Council on the Aging in Washington, never worried much about the 3,000 miles that separated him from his then 83-year-old mother, Mary B. Smiley, a widow living alone in Los Angeles. At the time, Smiley was healthy and self-sufficient. But she began having leg and back problems that made it difficult for her to climb the stairs to her apartment.

"I felt guilty about being across the country when my mother needed help," remembers Dr. Cutler, an only child, "but since I couldn't uproot my family and move to California, I thought it was time for her to think about an assisted living situation"—in other words, a group residence that provides meals, housekeeping and other aid for relatively independent, elderly people.

FINDING THE BEST FACILITY FOR YOUR PARENT

"It's not just the physical attributes of a place, but how the whole environment fits a person's preferences."

—NEAL E. CUTLER, PH.D.

When Dr. Cutler began to research residences for his mother, however, all he found were checklists to help rate facilities. "They focused on factors like how clean the place looked and how friendly the staff was," Dr. Cutler remembers. "I felt there was a lot more to it."

Over the next six months, Dr. Cutler and his mother had a series of heart-to-heart phone conversations. "Initially she wanted to stay in the same neighborhood, but as we talked further, she realized that most of her friends there were dying or becoming incapacitated," Dr. Cutler says. "Ultimately my mother decided that other things were more important to her—for example, living in a place with people from different ethnic groups."

These talks inspired Dr. Cutler to get a research grant to study what other senior citizens considered most important in choosing a new home (see "Assisted Living: What Really Counts"). "The general feeling was that it's not just the physical attributes of a place, but how the whole environment fits a person's preferences and values," he says.

The next challenge was actually finding a place for his mother. Dr. Cutler followed the advice he's given in journal articles: He hired a geriatric care manager. This professional, usually a social worker, nurse or family therapist, has extensive knowledge of local resources for the elderly.

"The care manager acted as my eyes and ears in making the first cut of dozens of assisted living places," says Dr. Cutler. "She also picked up my mother at her apartment, drove her to the places, showed her around and took her home. After they got the list down to two or three, I flew out and helped make the final selection." (To locate a case manager in your parent's area, order a directory for $15 from the National Association of Professional Geriatric Care Managers, 1604 North Country Club Rd., Tucson, AZ, 85716; 520-881-8008.)

Even though she has cared for hundreds of elderly patients, geriatrician Fran E. Kaiser, M.D., an adjunct professor of medicine and geriatrics at St. Louis University School of Medicine and a geriatrician on *American Health for Women*'s advisory board, acknowledges that she never went through all the necessary "what-ifs" about her mother's aging. "On some level, you always think your parents will live forever," she says.

Until three years ago, Dr. Kaiser's optimism seemed justified. Even though her mother, Bronia Kaiser, then 81, lived almost 900 miles away in New York City, she was still in good shape and running her jewelry business. But after a series of small strokes, Kaiser's memory became cloudy, and she was soon diagnosed with vascular dementia, a condition that causes progressive mental and physical deterioration.

MANAGING AT-HOME CARE

"My sister said, 'You're the geriatrician; can't you fix this?' "

—FRAN E. KAISER, M.D.

"My sister said, 'You're the geriatrician; can't you fix this?' " Dr. Kaiser remembers. "I felt tremendous frustration that I couldn't turn this disease around and terrible guilt that most of the burden of care would fall on my sister because she lived nearby." At first, Dr. Kaiser's mother could participate in making plans and told her daughters that as a Holocaust survivor, she viewed nursing homes as being almost like concentration camps. Dr. Kaiser and her sister promised to do everything they could to keep her at home.

Honoring that commitment has been more difficult than Dr. Kaiser ever imagined.

ANNUAL EDITIONS: WOMEN'S HEALTH 99/00

NO POSTAGE NECESSARY IF MAILED IN THE UNITED STATES

BUSINESS REPLY MAIL
FIRST-CLASS MAIL PERMIT NO. 84 GUILFORD CT

POSTAGE WILL BE PAID BY ADDRESSEE

Dushkin/McGraw-Hill
Sluice Dock
Guilford, CT 06437-9989

ABOUT YOU

Name Date

Are you a teacher? ☐ A student? ☐
Your school's name

Department

Address City State Zip

School telephone #

YOUR COMMENTS ARE IMPORTANT TO US !

Please fill in the following information:
For which course did you use this book?

Did you use a text with this *ANNUAL EDITION*? ☐ yes ☐ no
What was the title of the text?

What are your general reactions to the *Annual Editions* concept?

Have you read any particular articles recently that you think should be included in the next edition?

Are there any articles you feel should be replaced in the next edition? Why?

Are there any World Wide Web sites you feel should be included in the next edition? Please annotate.

May we contact you for editorial input? ☐ yes ☐ no
May we quote your comments? ☐ yes ☐ no